D0848474

Syringomyelia and the Chiari Malformations

AANS Publications Committee
John A. Anson, MD,
Edward C. Benzel, MD,
Issam A. Awad, MD, Editors

Neurosurgical Topics

The American Association of
Neurological Surgeons

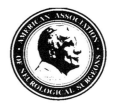

Library of Congress Catalog
ISBN: 1-879284-42-1

Neurosurgical Topics ISBN: 0-9624246-6-8

Copyright 1997 by The American Association of Neurological Surgeons

Printed in U.S.A.

The American Association of Neurological Surgeons
22 South Washington Street
Park Ridge, Illinois 60068-4287

All rights reserved. None of the contents of this publication may be reproduced in a retrieval system or transmitted in any form or by any means (electronic, mechanical, photocopying, recording, or otherwise) without prior written permission of the publisher.

This publication is published under the auspices of the Publications Committee of the American Association of Neurological Surgeons (AANS). However, this should not be construed as indicating endorsement or approval of the views presented by the AANS, or by its committees, commissions, affiliates, or staff.

Daniel L. Barrow, MD, Chairman
AANS Publications Committee

Gay Palazzo, AANS Staff Editor

AANS1.75M1096

Neurosurgical Topics SERIES

FORTHCOMING BOOKS

Subarachnoid Hemorrhage: Pathophysiology and Treatment
Edited by Joshua B. Bederson, MD

Neural Tube Defects, Volumes I and II
Edited by J. Gordon McComb, MD, and Joan L. Venes, MD

Patients and the Law
Edited by Howard H. Kaufman, MD, and Jeff Lewin, JD

Contents

LIST OF CONTRIBUTORS

Issam A. Awad, MD, MSC, FACS
Professor of Surgery (Neurosurgery)
Section of Neurosurgery
Yale University School of Medicine
New Haven, Connecticut

John A. Anson, MD
Assistant Professor, Division of Neurosurgery
University of New Mexico
Albuquerque, New Mexico

Nevan G. Baldwin, MD
Assistant Professor, Division of Neurosurgery
University of New Mexico
Albuquerque, New Mexico

Ulrich Batzdorf, MD
Division of Neurosurgery
University of California, Los Angeles
UCLA Medical Center
Los Angeles, California

Edward C. Benzel, MD
Professor and Chief
Division of Neurosurgery
University of New Mexico
Albuquerque, New Mexico

Richard Brownlee, MD
Department of Clinical Neurosciences
Division of Neurosurgery
University of Calgary
Foothills Hospital and
    Alberta Children's Hospital
Calgary, Alberta, Canada

Alain C. J. de Lotbinière, MD, CM,
    FRCS(C), FACS
Section of Neurosurgery
Yale University School of Medicine
New Haven, Connecticut

Richard G. Ellenbogen, MD
Chief and Program Director
Neurosurgery Service
Walter Reed Army Medical Center
Washington, DC

Graham Flint
Consultant Neurosurgeon
Syringomyelia Clinic Neuroscience Centre
University Hospital
Birmingham, England

Mark G. Hamilton, MDCM, FRCS(C)
Department of Clinical Neurosciences
Division of Neurosurgery
University of Calgary
Foothills Hospital and
    Alberta Children's Hospital
Calgary, Alberta, Canada

Andrea L. Halliday, MD
Assistant Professor, Division of Neurosurgery
University of New Mexico
Albuquerque, New Mexico

R. Patrick Jacob, MD
Assistant Professor
Department of Neurological Surgery
University of Florida
Chief of Neurosurgery
Veterans Administration Medical Center
Gainesville, Florida

Matthew B. Kern, MD
Assistant Professor, Division of Neurosurgery
University of New Mexico
Albuquerque, New Mexico

David G. Malone, MD
Assistant Professor, Division of Neurosurgery
University of New Mexico
Albuquerque, New Mexico

Paul McCormick, MD
The Neurological Institute
New York, New York

David G. McLone, MD, PHD
Professor of Surgery (Neurosurgery)
Northwestern University Medical School
Divison Head, Pediatric Neurosurgery
Children's Memorial Hospital
Chicago, Illinois

Arnold H. Menezes, MD
Department of Surgery
Division of Neurosurgery
University of Iowa Hospitals and Clinics
Iowa City, Iowa

Nazih Moufarrij, MD
Assistant Professor
Division of Neurosurgery
American University of Beirut
Beirut, Lebanon

S. Terrance Myles, MD, FRCS(C)
Department of Clinical Neurosciences
Division of Neurosurgery
University of Calgary
Foothills Hospital and
    Alberta Children's Hospital
Calgary, Alberta, Canada

John G. Piper, MD
Department of Surgery
Division of Neurosurgery
University of Iowa Hospitals and Clinics
Iowa City, Iowa

Albert L. Rhoton, Jr., MD
Department of Neurosurgery
College of Medicine
University of Florida
Gainesville, Florida

Paul M. Ruggieri, MD
Section of Neuroradiology
The Cleveland Clinic Foundation
Cleveland, Ohio

Mari Schenk, MD
Section of Neuroradiology
The Cleveland Clinic Foundation
Cleveland, Ohio

Bernard Williams, MD, CHM, FRCS
    (deceased)
Syringomyelia Clinic
Midland Centre for
    Neurosurgery and Neurology
West Midlands, England

Seth M. Zeidman, MD
Neurosurgery Service
Walter Reed Army Medical Center
Washington, DC

AANS Publications Committee

Daniel L. Barrow, MD, Chairman
Michael L.J. Apuzzo, MD
Edward C. Benzel, MD
John A. Jane, MD (ex officio)
Howard H. Kaufman, MD

Christopher M. Loftus, MD
Robert J. Maciunas, MD
J. Gordon McComb, MD
Warren R. Selman, MD
Setti S. Rengachary, MD

The American Association of Neurological Surgeons is accredited by the Accreditation Council for Continuing Medical Education (CME) to sponsor continuing medical education for physicians.

The American Association of Neurological Surgeons designates the continuing medical education activity as 15 credit hours in Category I of the Physician's Recognition Award of the American Medical Association.

Dedication

Bernard Williams
(1932 - 1995)

Six feet three inches tall, with keenly observant eyes, Bernard Williams presented an imposing figure in one-to-one contact. A conversation with him soon revealed his sharp intellect and, although his ideas may sometimes have seemed a little unconventional, it was evident that here was a man with a great enthusiasm for life and a particular ardour for medicine. What also became apparent was his open-minded approach to any problem and his complete honesty. He was free thinking and uninhibited and this was one of the secrets of his professional success. He possessed many talents including considerable technical skill as a surgeon. He also had an extraordinary memory and seldom forgot people he met, be they colleagues or patients. He was an extremely caring human being and always willing to listen to patients and their concerns. He was supportive of his staff. He welcomed medical students with enthusiasm and tried to show them the fascination of medicine.

Bernard spent the greater part of his professional career in Birmingham, England but achieved international recognition for his work, particularly in the field of syringomyelia and disorders of cerebrospinal fluid circulation. He wrote extensively on this as well as other topics and regularly gave lectures in his own witty and entertaining style. He read extensively beyond medicine and had a particular interest in the English language. He was prone to introduce neologisms into his conversation and introduced new terms in his areas of clinical interest, for example "hindbrain hernia" as a descriptive term to replace the eponymous "Arnold-Chiari" malformation.

He was in his early 60s but remained young at heart with youthful ideas and habits. On a bright summer morning in July 1995 he mounted his 750-cc motorbike to travel from Birmingham to London. Within half a mile he fell victim to the impetuous haste of morning rush hour traffic. He died three weeks later without regaining consciousness. Tragically premature, the manner of his death was somehow in keeping with his charismatic lifestyle. The world of neurosurgery has lost one of its most enthusiastic members but, through his writings, he has taught us a great deal and has significantly advanced our understanding of syringomyelia, to the benefit of a great many patients worldwide. Those who knew him well learnt the virtue of being honest. Bernard was a genuine man of immense talent and without malice, who was nevertheless self critical, ready to acknowledge and learn from his mistake, and always striving to improve himself.

Graham Flint
Consultant Neurosurgeon
Syringomyelia Clinic Neuroscience Centre
University Hospital
Birmingham, England

Publications by Bernard Williams
On the Subject of Syringomyelia

The distending force in the production of "communicating syringomyelia." **Lancet 2:**189-193, 1969

Current concepts of syringomyelia. **Br J Hosp Med:** 331-342, 1970

The distending force in the production of communicating syringomyelia. **Lancet 2:**41-42, 1970 (Letter)

Communicating syringomyelia presenting immediately after trauma. A case description and some theoretical concepts. **Acta Neurochir 24:**97-106, 1971 (with E Turner)

Further thoughts on the valvular action of the Arnold-Chiari malformation. **Dev Med Child Neurol (Suppl) 25:**105-112, 1971

Sciatica caused by sacral-nerve-root-cysts. **Lancet 1:** 137, 1971 (Letter)

Combined cisternal and lumbar pressure recordings in the sitting position using differential manometry. **J Neurol Neurosurg Psychiatry 35:**142-143, 1972

Is aqueduct stenosis a result of hydrocephalus? **Brain 96:**399-412, 1973

Syringomyelia and its surgical treatment. **Nurs Times 69:**662-665, 1973

Syringomyelia produced by intramedullary fluid injection in dogs. **J Neurol Neurosurg Psychiatry 36:** 467-477, 1973 (with RO Weller)

The valvular action of the Arnold Chiari malformation, in: **Intracranial Pressure. The Proceedings of the First International Conference on Intracranial Pressure.** Berlin: Springer-Verlag, 1973, pp 338-342

A demonstration analogue for ventricular and intraspinal dynamics (DAVID). **J Neurol Sci 23:** 445-461, 1974

Why do central arachnoid pouches expand? **J Neurol Neurosurg Psychiatry 37:**1085-1092, 1974 (with AN Guthkelch)

Cerebral biopsy and assessment of brain damage in hydrocephalus. **Arch Dis Child 50:**763-768, 1975 (with RO Weller)

Cerebrospinal fluid pressure differentials in hydrocephalus in association with spina bifida cystica, in: **Proceedings of the VIIth International Congress of Neuropathology.** Amsterdam: Excerpta Medica, 1975, pp 633-639

Cerebrospinal fluid pressure-gradients in spina bifida cystica, with special reference to the Arnold-Chiari malformation and aqueductal stenosis. **Dev Med Child Neurol 17 (Suppl 35):**138-150, 1975

Expansion of central arachnoid pouches. **Childs Brain 1:**364-367, 1975 (with AN Guthkelch)

Theoretical aspects of the attenuation of pressure pulses within cerebrospinal-fluid pathways. **Med Biol Eng 13:**861-869, 1975 (with P Lockey and G Poots)

Cerebrospinal fluid pressure changes in response to coughing. **Brain 99:**331-346, 1976

Cerebrospinal fluid pressure changes in response to coughing. **J Physiol (Lond) 256:**103P-104P, 1976

CSF pressure recordings in spina bifida. **J Neurol Neurosurg Psychiatry 39:**916-917, 1976

Aqueduct stenosis. A case review and discussion. **J Neurol Neurosurg Psychiatry 40:**521-532, 1977 (with JJ McMillan)

Cervical vertebrae measurements in syringomyelia. **Clin Radiol 28:**395-400, 1977 (with J Lee)

Difficult labour as a cause of communicating syringomyelia. **Lancet 2:**51-53, 1977

Foramen magnum impaction in a case of acro-osteolysis. **Br J Surg 64:**70-73, 1977

On the pathogenesis of the Chiari malformation. **Z Kinderchir 22:**533-534, 1977

Three cases of communicating syringomyelia secondary to midbrain glioma. **J Neurol Neurosurg Psychiatry 40:**80-88, 1977 (with WR Timperley)

A critical appraisal of posterior fossa surgery for communicating syringomyelia. **Brain 101:**223-250, 1978

Craniovertebral malformations. European Association of Neurological Societies - European Course in Neurosurgery. Barcelona, Spain, September, 1979

Errors in velocity measurement by the Pitot principle in fluids with slowly propagated pressure waves. **J Biomed Eng 1:**50-54, 1979 (with JR Jackson)

Orthopaedic features in the presentation of syringomyelia. **J Bone Joint Surg (Br) 61:**314-323, 1979

Subarachnoid pouches of the posterior fossa with syringomyelia. **Acta Neurochir 47:**187-217, 1979

Cough headache due to craniospinal pressure dissociation. **Arch Neurol 37:**226-230, 1980

Experimental communicating syringomyelia in dogs after cisternal kaolin injection. Part 1. Morphology. **J Neurol Sci 48**:93-107, 1980 (with J Bentley)

Experimental communicating syringomyelia in dogs after cisternal kaolin injection. Part 2. Pressure studies. **J Neurol Sci 48**:109-122, 1980

Investigations on the pathogenesis of syringomyelia. **Adv Neurosurg 8**:277-283, 1980

The measurement of cerebrospinal fluid flow. **Phys Med Biol 24**:1196-1208, 1980 (with DR Prytherch and MJA Smith)

On the pathogenesis of syringomyelia: a review. **J R Soc Med 73**:798-806, 1980

Radiographic studies of the ventricles in syringomyelia. **Neuroradiology 20**:5-16, 1980 (with RJ West)

A case of high-pressure intracerebral pouch. **J Neurol Neurosurg Psychiatry 44**:918-923, 1981 (with AN Al-din)

Chronic herniation of the hindbrain. **Ann R Coll Surg (Engl) 63**:9-17, 1981

Simultaneous cerebral and spinal fluid pressure recordings. I. Technique, physiology, and normal results. **Acta Neurochir 58**:167-185, 1981

Simultaneous cerebral and spinal fluid pressure recordings. 2. Cerebrospinal dissociation with lesions at the foramen magnum. **Acta Neurochir 59**:123-142, 1981

Syringomyelia as a sequel to traumatic paraplegia. **Paraplegia 19**:67-80, 1981 (with AF Terry and HWF Jones)

Aqueduct stenosis, in Cavanagh, Smith (eds): **Advances in Neuropathology.** 1982, Ch II

Birth injury: a possible contributory factor in aetiology of primary basilar impression. **J Neurol Neurosurg Psychiatry 45**:879-883, 1982 (with RD Battersby)

Spinal extradural arachnoid pouches. Report of two cases. **J Neurosurg 57**:849-852, 1982 (with C McCrum)

A critical appraisal of "terminal tentriculostomy" for the treatment of syringomyelia. **J Neurosurg 58**:188-197, 1983 (with G Fahy)

A suprasellar subarachnoid pouch; aetiological considerations. **J Neurol Neurosurg Psychiatry 47**:1066-1074, 1984 (with O Binitic and CP Case)

Progress in syringomyelia. **Neurol Res 8**:130-145, 1986

Surgery of arachnoid pouches. **Z Kinderchir 41 (Suppl 1)**:18-21, 1986

Syringomyelia. **Spinal Injuries Association Newsletter 35**:22-23, 1986

Syringo-pleural shunting for syringomyelia. **J Neurol Neurosurg Psychiatry 49**:1332, 1986 (Abstract) (with N Page)

Hindbrain hernia headache. **Lancet 1**:731-734, 1987 (with S Nightingale)

Surgical treatment for syringomyelia. **Nurs Times 83**:34-37, 1987

Surgical treatment of syringomyelia with syringo-pleural shunting. **Br J Neurosurg 1**:63-80, 1987 (with N Page)

Syringomyelia in paraplegics. **Paraplegia News 41**: 26-27, 1987

Syringomyelia. **Rehabilitation Gaz 28**:2-4, 1987

Arachnoid cysts of the middle fossa and subdural haematoma. **J Neurol Neurosurg Psychiatry 51**:467, 1988 (Letter)

Syringomyelia. **Auditorium No 5 Vol 15**, 1988 (Taped series produced by Winthrop)

Headache due to hindbrain herniation, in Rose FC (ed): **New Advances in Headache Research.** Smith-Gordon, 1989, Chapter 4, pp 25-30

LP shunting in cases of Chiari malformation. **J Neurosurg 71**:950-951, 1989 (Letter)

Post-traumatic syringomyelia: an update. **Paraplegia 28**:296-313, 1990

Post-traumatic syringomyelia. **Br J Neurosurg 4**: 356-357, 1990 (Letter)

Surgical management of syringomyelia, in Torrens MJ, Dixon RA (eds): **Operative Spinal Surgery.** Edinburgh: Churchill Livingstone, 1991, pp 281-299

Syringomyelia as a complication of paraplegia. **Spinal Injuries Association Newsletter 56**:25-27, 1990

Syringomyelia. **Neurosurg Clin North Am 1**:653-685, 1990

Hindbrain migration after decompression for hindbrain hernia: a quantitative assessment using MRI. **Br J Neurosurg 5**:141-152, 1991 (with MJ Duddy)

Malformations, in Swash, Oxbury (eds): **Clinical Neurology.** London: Churchill Livingstone, 1991

Pathogenesis of syringomyelia, in Batzdorf U (ed): **Syringomyelia: Current Concepts in Diagnosis and Treatment.** Baltimore, Md: Williams & Wilkins, 1991, pp 59-90

Surgical features in post traumatic and post arachnoidic syringomyelia, in Brock M, Banerji AK, Sambasiram M (eds): **Modern Neurosurgery 2. Spinal Neurosurgery.** World Federation of Neurosurgical Societies. Trivandrum, 1991, pp 377-384

Syringomyelia in paraplegia. **Rehabilitation Gaz 31**(1): 1-6, 1991

What is syringobulbia? **J Neurol Neurosurg Psychiatry** 54:664, 1991 (Abstract)

The Chiari deformity. Link - Association for Spina Bifida and Hydrocephalus, 1992, Vol 139

Pathogenesis of post-traumatic syringomyelia. **Br J Neurosurg** 6:517-520, 1992 (Editorial)

Post-traumatic syringomyelia (cystic myelopathy), in Vinken PJ, Bruyn GW, Klawans HL (eds): **Handbook of Neurology. Vol 61: Spinal Cord Trauma.** Amsterdam: Elsevier, 1992, pp 375-398

Syringomyelia, in Findlay G, Owen R (eds): **Surgery of the Spine: a Combined Orthopaedic and Neurosurgical Approach.** Oxford: Blackwell Scientific, 1992, pp 891-908

Syringomyelia, in Teasdale GM, Miller JD (eds): **Current Neurosurgery.** London: Churchill Livingstone, 1992, pp 221-253

Ball-valve and cyst formation. **J Neurosurg** 79:476, 1993 (Letter)

Pathogenesis of syringomyelia. **Acta Neurochir** 123:159-165, 1993

Post traumatic syringomyelia, in Floman Y, Farcy JP, Argenson C (eds): **Thoraco-Lumbar Spine Fractures.** New York, NY: Raven Press, 1993, pp 429-448

Pyomyelia: an intramedullary spinal abscess complicating lumbar lipoma with spina bifida. **Br J Neurosurg** 7:419-422, 1993 (with C Hardwidge and J Palsingh)

Sensory loss in syringomyelia: not necessarily dissociated. **J R Soc Med** 86:519-520, 1993 (with WP Honan)

Surgery for hindbrain related syringomyelia. **Adv Tech Stand Neurosurg** 20:107-164, 1993

Surgical treatment of syringobulbia. **Neurosurg Clin North Am** 4:553-571, 1993

Syringobulbia: a surgical appraisal. **J Neurol Neurosurg Psychiatry** 55:1132-1141, 1993 (with D Morgan)

Syringobulbia: a surgical review. **Acta Neurochir** 123:190-194, 1993

Thecoperitoneal shunt for syringomyelia: report of three cases. **Neurosurgery** 33:327-328, 1993 (Letter)

A blast against grafts—on the closing and grafting of the posterior fossa dura. **Br J Neurosurg** 8:275-278, 1994

Hindbrain herniation and syringomyelia, in Hadley M (ed): **Perspectives in Neurological Surgery.** St Louis, Mo: Quality Medical Publishing, 1994

Overview: session on hindbrain herniation, in Samii M (ed): **Skull Base Surgery.** Basel: Karger, 1994, pp 1114-1117

Pathogenesis of post-traumatic syringomyelia. **Br J Neurosurg** 8:114-115, 1994 (Letter)

Severe exacerbation of post traumatic syringomyelia after lithotripsy. Case report. **Paraplegia** 32:694-696, 1994 (with ND Lorenzo and A Maleci)

Spina bifida and syringomyelia. Link - Association for Spina Bifida and Hydrocephalus, July 1994, Vol 152, pp 18-21

Valvular factors in hydrocephalus. **Childs Nerv Syst** 10:36-42, 1994

The cystic spinal cord. **J Neurol Neurosurg Psychiatry** 58:649-654, 1995 (Editorial)

Outcome of post-traumatic syringomyelia. **J Neurol Neurosurg Psychiatry** 58:124, 1995 (Abstract) (with S Sgouros)

Severe exacerbation of post-traumatic syringomyelia after lithotripsy. **Br J Urol** 75:806-807, 1995 (with D Lorenzo and A Maleci)

A critical appraisal of drainage for syringomyelia. **J Neurosurg** 82:1-10, 1995 (with S Sgouros)

Surgical management of non-hindbrain-related post-traumatic syringomyelia, in Schmidek H, Sweet WH (eds): **Operative Neurosurgical Techniques.** 3rd ed. Philadelphia, Pa: WB Saunders, 1995, pp 2119-2140

Management and outcome of posttraumatic syringomyelia. **J Neurosurg** 85:197-205, 1996

Management schemes for syringomyelia: surgical indications and nonsurgical management in Anson, JA, Benzel EC, Awad IA (eds): **Syringomyelia and the Chiari Malformations.** Park Ridge, Ill: American Association of Neurosurgeons, 1997, pp 125-143

IN PRESS

El-Shafei and Sophy valve shunting. **J Neurol Neurosurg Psychiatry**

Hydrocephalus, in Swash M, Wildin J (eds): **Outcome in Neurological and Neurosurgical Disorders.** Cambridge: Cambridge University Press

Meningeal fibrosis after listeria meningitis. **Br J Neurosurg**

Syringomyelia and syringobulbia, in Guthkelch AN, Misulis K (eds): **Scientific Foundations of Neurology.** Oxford: Blackwell Scientific

Syringomyelia and syringobulbia, in Long D (ed): **Neurosurgical Quarterly.** New York, NY: Raven Press

Syringomyelia, in Swash M, Wildin J (eds): **Outcome in Neurological and Neurosurgical Disorders.** Cambridge: Cambridge University Press

CHAPTER 1

HISTORICAL CONSIDERATIONS

ALAIN C. J. DE LOTBINIÈRE, MD, CM, FRCS(C), FACS

Comme beaucoup d'affections du névraxe, la syringomyélie doit être considérée comme une modalité anatomo-pathologique qui peut être amenée par des facteurs multiples.
Au point de vue pathologique, il n'y a pas une syringomyélie, il y a des syringomyélies.

— Georges Guillain, 1902

Although Charles Prosper Ollivier d'Angers (1796-1845) (Figure 1) is credited with coining the term "syringomyelia" in 1827,[111] others before him described cavities in the spinal cord. Charles Estienne (1503-1564), alternatively known by his Latin name Carolus Stephanus, was a contemporary of Andreas Vesalius. Two years following the publication of Vesalius' *Fabrica* in 1543, Estienne's *De dissectione partium corporis humani*[154] appeared in Latin and was followed in 1546 by a French edition[46] (Figure 2). Estienne's work had been printed up to the middle of the third book by 1539, four years before the publication of Vesalius' *Fabrica*; however, the printing was interrupted as a result of a trial, proving that the book had been compiled entirely independently of Vesalius' work. As Rath[126] has pointed out, Estienne's place in the history of anatomy has been neglected despite a number of anatomical discoveries which can be found in his work, not the least of which is the first description of the central canal in the spinal cord. Subsequently, pathological descriptions of cavitations in the cord were noted by Brunner[25] in 1688 and Morgagni[104] in 1761, the latter author remarking on the frequent association of spina bifida and cystic dilatations of the spinal cord.

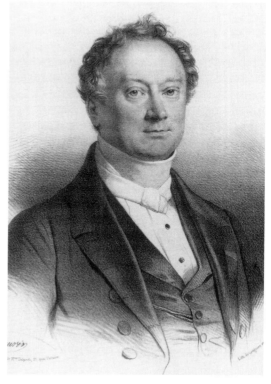

Figure 1: Charles Prosper Ollivier d'Angers. Lithograph by N. B. Maurin. (Illustration kindly provided by the Wellcome Institute Library, London)

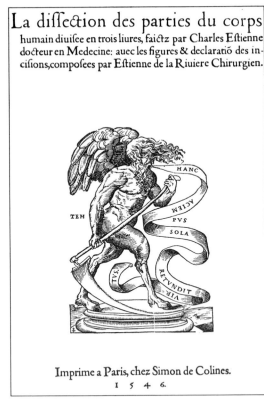

Figure 2: Title page of *La dissection des parties du corps humain divisée en trois livres* (1546). (Illustration kindly provided by the Countway Library, Harvard University)

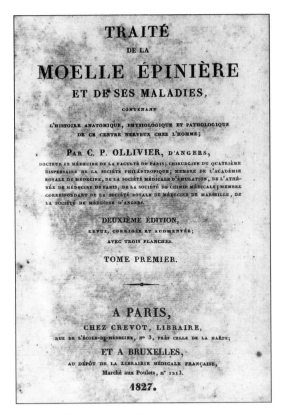

Figure 3: Title page of Ollivier's second monograph, *Traité de la Moelle Épinière et de ses Maladies* (1827). (Illustration kindly provided by the Wellcome Institute, London)

The first description of a clinical presentation of syringomyelia (albeit not with the classic segmental dissociated sensory impairment) accompanied by subsequent pathological examination of the spinal cord is ascribed to Antoine Portal (1742-1832), who in 1803 published his *Cours d'Anatomie Médicale*.[123] In it he described a servant of the duc de Crouy who noted the onset of numbness affecting both lower extremities followed by an ascending paralysis. At autopsy a cavity within the cervical spinal cord was noted extending to the level of the third thoracic vertebral body "dans lequel on eût pu introduire une grosse plume à écrire." Subsequently, Portal was appointed by Louis XVIII to become *le Premier Médecin de sa Majesté* and is remembered as having been the founder of the Académie Royale de Médecine in 1820, after having obtained the king's approval.[54]

As pointed out by Ballantine et al,[9] the term "syringomyelia" first appears in the second edition of Ollivier's monograph, *Traité de la Moelle Epinière et de ses Maladies*, published in 1827[111] (Figure 3). In his earlier monograph of 1824, *De la Moelle Epinière et de ses Maladies*,[110] Ollivier noted the presence of cavities in the spinal cord in stillborns with meningoceles (hydrorachis) and spina bifida. In two cases of anencephaly which he dissected, Ollivier observed that the fourth ventricle communicated with a cavity ending inferiorly in a "cul-de-sac." A critical review of this text and subsequent writings clearly reveals that Ollivier restricted the definition of "syringomyelia" to a pathological dilatation of the central canal, as the subheading in the second chapter of the third edition[112] states: "syringomyélie, ou cavité centrale dans la moelle épinière." He denied that it existed "dans l'état naturel" and surmised that it resulted from a developmental arrest of the spinal cord, noting that it could be observed in normal fetuses during the early intrauterine period. In support of his argument, he cited other authors who had observed that communication between the central canal and the fourth ventricle persisted until the sixth month of intrauterine life and on occasion until term delivery. That the symptomatic condition could develop postnatally was nevertheless recognized, Ollivier cited the case reported by Rullier in 1823[132] in which a progressive paralysis of both hands was described beginning 10 years prior to the subject's death at the age of 44, accompanied by wasting of the muscles of the hands and a progressive kyphoscoliosis. At autopsy, a cystic cavity filled with clear fluid was observed extending from the upper cervical to the upper thoracic spine, approximately six to seven inches in length, giving the appearance of "une hydropsie de la moelle." The significance of the findings for François Magendie, whose comments follow the autopsy description, was in the observation that sensation was preserved in the arms despite a complete paralysis of both upper extremities and that movement and sensation in the lower extremities were intact.

In 1856, the first volume of Stilling's monumental work, *Neue Untersuchungen über den Bau des Rückenmarks,*[155] appeared and clearly demonstrated the persistence of the central canal into adulthood. Henceforth, authors began to abandon the term "syringomyelia," replacing it with the term "hydromyelia" to describe abnormal dilatations of the central canal. In 1869, Charcot and Joffroy[30] suggested that some of the cases previously referred to as hydromyelia might in fact result from a "melting down" of pathological tissue developed in the midst of the central portions of the spinal cord. The following year, Hallopeau[68] proposed that the pathological lesion leading to cavitary formation was a chronic periependymal myelitis, noting that the cavitations were separated from the central canal and that they were associated with a diffuse "sclerosis." Based on this and similar studies, Simon[149] in turn proposed that the term "syringomyelia" be reserved for the latter entity and that "hydromyelia" be restricted to dilatations of the central canal. Controversy

regarding the pathogenesis and appropriate terminology to describe the condition persisted throughout the 19th century. Joffroy and Achard[77] proposed that both terms be rejected in favor of "myélite cavitaire," after they reviewed autopsy material suggesting a chronic inflammatory process surrounding the cavities in the spinal cord. Schultze,[142] who is credited by Charcot as giving the first clinical description in 1882 of the classic dissociated sensory impairment synonymous with the syndrome, went further to conclude that the process was due to an abnormal development of ependymal cells with subsequent breakdown of proliferating glial cells, suggesting a neoplastic pathogenesis of the syndrome. By the turn of the century, attempts to reconcile these opposing theories resulted in the proposal by Philippe and Oberthür[120] that syringomyelia be classified into a "true" syringomyelia, to be restricted to the cavitary and pachymeningitic forms, and "pseudo-syringomyelia," the latter to include hydromyelia, hematomyelia, vascular cavities, and post-traumatic cavities.

Lack of agreement among authors as to what constituted "true syringomyelia," together with the recognition that cavities could arise from a multiplicity of causes, led to the proposal by Ballantine et al[9] that the distinction between hydromyelia and syringomyelia be discarded in favor of "syringohydromyelia" and, more recently, by Hoffman et al[73] that "hydrosyringomyelia" be used. Further confusion was added when Williams[172] proposed the term "communicating syringomyelia" to distinguish it from other causes of syringomyelia in which cystic dilatations existed without any connection to the fourth ventricle, as only a minority of syringeal cavities can be shown to have a radiologically demonstrable communication with the fourth ventricle in the presence of a hindbrain anomaly. For practical purposes, it would seem reasonable to return to the etymological definition of syringomyelia, which, according to the Oxford English Dictionary,[150] is derived from the Greek συριγξ (syrinx) meaning pipe, tube, channel, or fistula and μυελος (myelus) meaning marrow, and is alternatively defined as "dilatation of the central canal of the spinal cord" or "formation of abnormal tubular cavities in its substance." This definition is consistent with the observation that syringomyelia represents a disorder which is multifactorial in origin, has a variety of clinical presentations, and a diversity of associated pathological changes.[100]

An examination of the multiplicity of theories regarding the pathogenesis of syringomyelia prior to the formulation of the hydrodynamic hypothesis of Gardner reveals that the majority can be grouped into two broad categories: theories propounding the congenital origin of the lesion and theories suggesting an acquired origin, the latter including neoplastic or inflammatory origins and theories stressing a degeneration or disintegration of the central gray matter. Many of these theories overlap each other in attempting to explain the variable manifestations and associated conditions of the disorder that is now referred to as "syringomyelia," regardless of its etiology.

THEORIES OF A CONGENITAL ORIGIN

As noted earlier, Ollivier championed the theory that syringomyelia resulted from a developmental arrest of the spinal cord. Leyden[87] in 1876 postulated that the formation of the syrinx was due to incomplete fusion of the primitive fold. The congenital theory was largely championed in the German literature by authors such as Gerlach,[61] Schlesinger,[140] Bielchowsky and Unger,[21] and Hennenberg and Koch.[72] According to this embryological conception, the incomplete fusion of the two folds of the primitive medullary groove results in a derangement of the germinal cell layer, which gives rise to both the ependyma and the glia. This process may result in dilatation of the central canal or malformation of the median dorsal raphé. "Excessive proliferation" of the glia results in formation of secondary cavitations. Cells of mesodermal origin, some of which line the cavities, proliferate forming increased amounts of connective tissue and blood vessels in the spinal cord, occasionally drawing in dermal elements and producing teratomas.[94] In support of the congenital origin of the cavities, Schlesinger[140] in 1902 pointed to several factors which added together to form what was felt to be convincing evidence: the association between spina bifida and syrin-

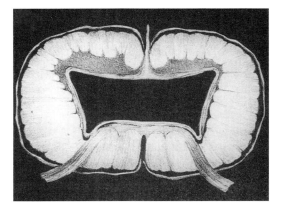

Figure 4: "Illustrating Dr. Gull's case of enlargement of the ventricle of the cord in the cervical region." (Reprinted from reference 66)

gomyelia, the occasional familial occurrence of syringomyelia, the presence of ependymal cells lining the cavities, communication between the cavities and the central canal, and the frequent coexistence of hydromyelia and hydrocephalus.

In the English literature, the congenital theory received support in the report of Gull dated 1862. In it he described a case entitled: *Progressive atrophy of the muscles of the hands: enlargement of the ventricle of the cord in the cervical region, with atrophy of the gray matter: (hydromyelus).*[66] The patient presented with a 13-month history of an inability to extend the fourth and fifth digits of the right hand accompanied by numbness and a sensation of coldness. Three weeks prior to his admission to the hospital "the three inner fingers of the left hand became weak and flexed in the same way, but without any numbness." The patient contracted typhus while in the hospital and died a month following his admission. At autopsy, a large cavity was discovered extending from the fifth cervical level down into the upper thoracic segments; this was illustrated by an accompanying plate (Figure 4). Complete destruction of the central gray matter was observed apart from a small amount of residual tissue noted in the anterior horns. Gull speculated that the atrophy was the result of "distention of the ventricle of the cord, by an accumulation of fluid in it." He compared the process to a chronic hydrocephalus and therefore termed the condition "hydromyelus," predating the hydrodynamic theory of Gardner

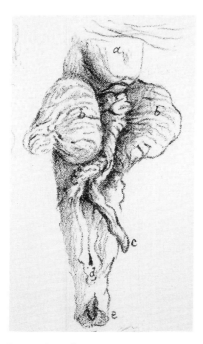

Figure 5: Drawing of Cleland's Case 1. The inferior portion of the vermis (c) has been lifted off the fourth ventricle, revealing the underlying obex (d) extending inferiorly into the cervical canal. The superior recess of the syringeal cavity (e) is illustrated, no apparent communication being visible between it and the floor of the fourth ventricle. Note also the hypoplastic cerebellar hemispheres (b) and "beaking" of the tectal plate (a). (Reprinted from reference 34)

by almost 100 years. Unfortunately, the autopsy was limited to the spinal cord, so no comment regarding the hindbrain could be made.

The association between hindbrain anomalies and hydromyelia was clearly recognized by John Cleland (1835-1925), who in 1883 published a paper entitled "Contribution to the study of spina bifida, encephalocele, and anencephalus" in the *Journal of Anatomy and Physiology*.[34] In it he described a case of hydrocephalus associated with spina bifida in which he observed dilatation of the central canal, elongation of the fourth ventricle, and an absence of communication between the two. The accompanying illustration clearly demonstrates a downward displacement of the cerebellar vermis and medulla oblongata in addition to a deformity of the tectal plate (Figure 5). Cleland speculated that "distention of the canal, after closure, caused its dilatation above, and led to its rupture below"

into the open spina bifida. Further on he hypothesized that the developmental abnormalities which he had described were the consequences of "overstimulation in early embryonic life," concluding that primary dysgenesis of the brain stem was responsible for the malformation. As Carmel and Markesbery[29] have stated, it is unfortunate that Cleland's work did not achieve wider dissemination given the importance of his observations. Two years prior to the seminal publication of Cleland, Langhans[82] reported a case of cerebellar heterotopia associated with a syrinx in addition to three other cases of tumors of the posterior fossa. It remained for Hans Chiari (1851-1916), Professor of Morbid Anatomy at Charles University in Prague, to describe the anomalies which now bear his name.

In 1891, there appeared a publication bearing the title, *Über Veränderungen des Kleinhirns in Folge von Hydrocephalie des Grosshirns*[32] (Concerning changes in the cerebellum due to hydrocephalus of the cerebrum). In this original account, Chiari described three types of hindbrain anomaly of increasing severity associated with hydrocephalus, illustrating each of these types with a single case. Five years later, Chiari published an expanded report entitled *Über Veränderungen des Kleinhirns, des Pons und der Medulla Oblongata in Folge von Congenitaler Hydrocephalie des Grosshirns*[31] (Concerning changes in the cerebellum, pons, and medulla due to congenital hydrocephalus of the cerebrum). It initially appeared as a monograph in 1895 (Figure 6), before it was published in 1896 in the *Denkschriften der Kaiserlichen Akademie der Wissenschaften* in Vienna.[31] In his second publication, Chiari described the three types of hindbrain anomaly, adding a fourth type, cerebellar hypoplasia without protrusion through the foramen magnum, which was unrelated to the three previously described malformations and has therefore been abandoned. A total of 24 cases were reported, with extensive illustrations accompanying the text. In three of 14 cases illustrating the Type I malformation (Figure 7), dilatations of the central canal were observed, whereas in the Type II malformation (Figure 8) the majority (five out of seven cases) demonstrated this finding. The accompanying illustrations clearly demonstrate the salient features of the Type II malformation (Figure 8) together

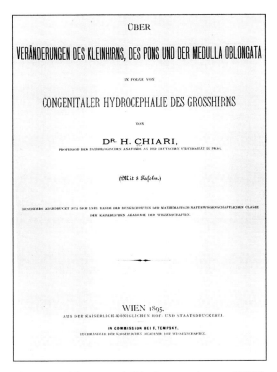

Figure 6: Title page of Chiari's second paper (1895).

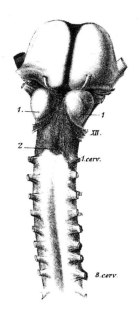

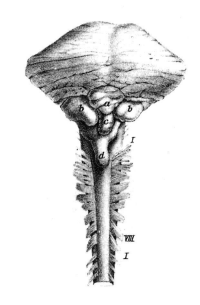

Figure 7: Illustration of Chiari I malformation demonstrating the downward course of the 12th cranial nerves and horizontal course of the upper cervical nerve rootlets. (Reprinted from reference 31)

Figure 8: Illustration of Chiari II malformation demonstrating the inferior displacement of the vermis (c) and the fourth ventricle (d) into the upper cervical canal, together with the upward course of the upper cervical nerve rootlets. (Reprinted from reference 31)

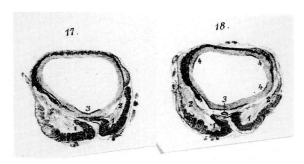

Figure 9: Adjacent segments of the thoracic spinal cord illustrating the lining of the ventral surface of the syringeal cavity by ependymal cells (3) on the left, whereas on the right, the ependymal cells line the central canal (3). (Reprinted from reference 31)

with cross sections of the spinal cord which show a communication between the central canal and the cystic cavity in the immediately adjacent segment (Figure 9). Chiari acknowledged Cleland's contribution at the end of the monograph; however, Cleland's name was omitted by subsequent authors and the name of Arnold was added to Chiari's name by Schwalbe and Gredig[144] in a publication in 1907 to become the eponymous Arnold-Chiari malformation, despite Arnold's meager contribution to the study of the malformation.[135]

That the significance of the association between hindbrain anomalies and syringomyelia was largely ignored by subsequent authors is underscored by the fact that over the following 40 years, discussions regarding the pathogenesis of the condition barely mention the name of Chiari. For example, in a publication dated 1920, Hassin[70] regarded syringomyelia as a developmental anomaly of the glia which he termed an "abiotrophy," comparing it to developmental deficiencies of the neurons in progressive muscular atrophy. He proposed that "deficient" glia break down, disintegrating to become walled off by connective tissue which, in turn, proliferates. The hyperplastic thickening of the vessels accompanying the connective tissue was thought to be "absolutely pathognomonic of syringomyelia," giving it the stamp of a distinct anatomopathological entity. Only those spinal cavities that exhibited the characteristic changes of the glia and accompanying connective tissue were to be referred to as syringomyelia. This restrictive

view was further championed by Tamaki and Lubin,[158] who stated that syringomyelia was a specific developmental anomaly "caused by imperfect formation of the central canal by primitive medullary epithelium." They argued that the resultant cell rests later underwent gliosis, cavitation being the end result of "poorly nourished gliotic tissues."

It was not until Russell and Donald[133] examined the relationship between the Arnold-Chiari malformation and hydrocephalus, in a series of 10 cases of meningomyelocele and in a single case of meningocele, that attention was once again brought to the developmental anomalies of the hindbrain. They proposed that it was the hindbrain anomaly itself which might be the cause of the hydrocephalus and suggested that decompression of the spinal cord at the foramen magnum might facilitate the circulation of fluid in the leptomeningeal spaces. Lichtenstein[88] noted that compression of the neuraxis from a variety of developmental defects at the level of the foramen magnum could result in degeneration of the central portion of the cervical spinal cord, with the production of a "syringomyelic-like state." He speculated that the formation of cavities could be due either to a combination of vascular ischemia and venous stasis resulting in liquefaction necrosis, or to "an obstruction of the outlet of the fourth ventricle secondary to the Arnold-Chiari malformation, stating "the accumulating cerebrospinal fluid dilates the central canal and, in some instances, is associated with perforation of the ependymal lining and the spread of the fluid into the posterior columns." This mechanistic explanation of the pathogenesis of syringomyelia was to become the basis of the hydrodynamic theory of Gardner.

THEORIES OF AN ACQUIRED ORIGIN

The observation that syringomyelia was not infrequently associated with tumors of the spinal cord was reported well over 100 years ago in the literature. Tamaki and Lubin[158] noted that Simon[149] was the first to comment on the association in 1875 and Langhans[82] reported an additional four cases in 1881. Detailed descriptions of cases were subsequently reported in the German literature by Baümler,[17] Schultze,[141] Dimitroff,[39] Schlesinger,[138] and Oppenheim.[114] In the English literature, Harris[69] and Bullard[27] each noted the coexistence of cavities in the spinal cord and medullary tumors. As noted above, Schultze had initially proposed that syringomyelia was secondary to the degeneration of an abnormal proliferation of ependymal cells, coining the term "gliosis" to describe the condition. He theorized that it represented an earlier stage of glioma formation, comparing the two as "a hill to a mountain." Jonesco-Sisesti,[78] in an extensive monograph, came to the conclusion that syringomyelia and intrinsic spinal cord tumors were at opposite ends of an unbroken series, and that intermediate forms could be recognized. This view was championed by Mackay and Favill,[94] who reported the autopsy findings of a case of "ependymoblastoma" and coexistent syringomyelia. According to their view, the syringomyelia and the ependymoblastoma were "only slightly different manifestations of the same proliferative process." Similar views regarding the common origin of intrinsic spinal cord tumors and syringomyelic cavities were expressed by authors such as Lichtenstein and Zeitlin,[89] Wyburn-Mason,[182] and Poser,[124] further blurring the distinction between congenital and acquired processes. Based on pathological examination of tissue removed at autopsy, Feigin et al[48] proposed that edema was the major factor in the formation of cavities, whether or not the syrinx was associated with a spinal cord tumor. Despite the fact that

these theories are no longer tenable, the truth remains that the boundary between what constitutes intramedullary "gliosis" and what can be said to be a low-grade intramedullary "glioma" is not often a sharp one.

Initially proposed by Hallopeau,[68] the infectious theory of the origin of syringomyelia was elaborated by Joffroy and Achard[77] in 1887. They speculated that a chronic inflammatory periependymal myelitis preceded the development of the syringomyelic cavity, noting in autopsy specimens an excessively profuse vascularization of the spinal cord in the presence of venous stasis and arterial thrombosis; necrobiosis of the central gray matter ensued, followed by the formation of cavities. Support for this theory was subsequently obtained in the experimental work of Camus and Roussy.[28] Using an emulsion of fatty acids, sodium nucleinate, and talc, Camus and Roussy performed a series of injections into the cervical subarachnoid space of 11 dogs, producing an acute cervical meningitis. After the animals had succumbed (the majority within a few days of the injections), cavities associated with perivascular inflammatory cells and adjacent areas of necrosis were observed within the spinal cords of several animals. Camus and Roussy were struck by the analogy between these experimental findings and the condition previously described in human pathology by Charcot and Joffroy[30] and designated as "pachyméningite cervicale hypertrophique." They theorized that the same phenomena preceded the formation of cavities in the human following a chronic cervical meningitis, which they surmised was possibly syphilitic in origin. Further support for the infectious origin of syringomyelia was obtained from the experimental work of Levaditi and coworkers,[85] who noted the presence of an extensive syringomyelic cavity in the spinal cord of a fox whose brain was inoculated with a neurotropic virus. Achard, whose comments follow the paper, felt that these experiments provided irrefutable evidence that syringomyelia could be caused by viral infections of the nervous system.

The role of ischemia in producing cavities in the spinal cord was subsequently emphasized by multiple authors. Tauber and Langworthy[160] noted the presence of cavities in the spinal cords of cats after a ligature had been passed around the ventral portion of the spinal cord, occluding the anterior spinal artery. They surmised that impairment of the blood supply to the cord was at the origin of the formation of cavities, preceded by necrosis and glial scarring. Netsky,[106] in a bold and provocative theory based on clinicopathological material, suggested that congenital intramedullary vascular anomalies were responsible for the development of syringomyelia, which occurred as a result of occlusion of the blood supply of the central portion of the spinal cord, leading to infarction and cavitation. In support of his theory, Netsky pointed to the frequent association of intramedullary vascular malformations and syringomyelia, the presence of anomalous vessels found in and around "true" syringes, and the frequently observed gliosis and proliferative connective tissue, which he surmised was best explained as originating from an increased number of blood vessels. Further support for the role of ischemia in producing spinal cord cavitations came from the work of McLaurin and coworkers[98] who performed a series of elegant experiments by injecting a suspension of kaolin into the cisternal subarachnoid space of 13 dogs. Neurological deficits were observed in the days and weeks following the injections, consisting of unsteadiness of gait, diminution of pain perception and, at later stages, spasticity of the limbs. After the animals were killed or had died from other causes, autopsy revealed the presence of hydrocephalus in every dog, accompanied by a variable degree of cavity formation in their spinal cords. McLaurin et al postulated that the cavitations were secondary to ischemia resulting from compression of vessels in the meninges by a fibrosing arachnoiditis, although the presence of some degree of hydrocephalus may have contributed to vascular insufficiency at the foramen magnum. They were quick to point out that the degree of hydrocephalus correlated poorly with the severity of spinal cord damage and that pressure at the foramen magnum was therefore not likely to be the principal agent. Subsequent studies[40,181] confirmed the findings of McLaurin and coworkers; however, the role of the kaolin-induced granulomata in producing vascular impairment has been questioned by other investigators,[67,175] and a more recent experimental study[183] revealed a close correlation between the degree of cervical

vascular insufficiency and tonsillar herniation resulting from gross hydrocephalus.

Despite the controversy regarding the relative importance of ischemia as an initiating factor in the formation of cavities in the spinal cord, the association of spinal arachnoiditis and syringomyelia in the clinical setting has continued to receive attention in the literature since the initial report of Charcot and Joffroy. Extensive pachymeningitis secondary to subarachnoid hemorrhage, the use of intrathecal contrast agents, and infections secondary to tuberculosis, syphilis, or other pathogens, may be associated with the development of cavitation in the spinal cord. Alternatively, syringomyelia has been reported in association with focal spinal arachnoiditis.[165] Prior to the advent of postmyelographic computed tomography (CT) scanning and magnetic resonance imaging (MRI), the ability to detect syringes in the setting of arachnoiditis was extremely limited. Barnett[11] reviewed the reports in the literature prior to 1973 and found that only seven cases of syringomyelia could be conclusively related to spinal arachnoiditis, adding an additional seven cases of his own; in the latter series, only one patient demonstrated myelographic signs of syringomyelia, despite the fact that all had evidence of spinal arachnoiditis on myelography. In the majority of cases, syringes were discovered at the time of surgical exploration. It would therefore seem probable that the majority of cases of progressive myelopathy, occurring years after spinal arachnoiditis (whatever the cause), may have been due to the development of syringes, rather than an "ascending neuritis" of unknown etiology.

The role of trauma in initiating the formation of cavities was first described by Bastian[15] in 1867 and by Strümpell[156] in 1880. However, the experience of gunshot wounds to the spinal cord during World War I received a more extensive report in 1915 by Holmes,[74] who provided detailed clinical descriptions and micrographs of autopsy material documenting the formation of cavities above and below the area of injury. Holmes observed that the cavities had a predilection for the dorsal funiculi, noting the absence of ependymal lining and that they extended several segments beyond the lesion. Nevertheless, the presence of necrotic material in the cavities raised questions as to whether or not they might have been the result of hemorrhage at the time of the initial injury, following which resorption of blood products took place.

As has been pointed out by others,[131] the paucity of reports prior to the 1950s on the late deterioration of retained neurological function following spinal cord trauma can be largely attributed to the short life span of paraplegic and quadriplegic patients. The development of a progressive myelopathy following traumatic paraplegia may take many years to manifest, Vernon et al[162] noting a range from two months to 23 years. In a retrospective series, Barnett and coworkers[13] noted the presence of clinical features suggestive of syrinx formation in 1.8% of 319 patients. However, the development of syringes as a delayed complication of traumatic spinal cord injuries, is being noted with increasing frequency[22,145,152] and may be more common with lesions in active young paraplegics due to a combination of tethering of the spinal cord at the site of injury and the increased compensatory movements of the cervical spine.[115] Rossier and coworkers[129] found the incidence of posttraumatic cervical syringomyelia to be higher in patients with cervical spine fractures. In a more recent study by Schurch et al,[143] a group of 449 patients were followed prospectively with yearly MRIs; 20 (4.4%) developed symptoms of posttraumatic syringomyelia, occurring as early as two months and as late as 30 years after injury.

The pathogenesis of posttraumatic syringomyelia has provoked a lively debate and is by no means fully understood. Although Gardner and McMurry[60] claimed that all cases of syringomyelia were due to a patent communication between the fourth ventricle and the central canal, the majority do not demonstrate a connection with the fourth ventricle and have no evidence of a posterior fossa abnormality.[178] Hemorrhage into the spinal cord at the site of the injury is usually followed by localized arachnoid adhesions. This in turn results in delayed ischemia, tethering of the spinal cord, and impairment of the flow of cerebrospinal fluid (CSF) within the spinal subarachnoid space.[12] Extension of the syringeal cyst subsequently occurs with repetitive flexion and extension due to the relative immobility of the spinal cord, with abrupt deterioration occurring at times following Valsalva maneuvers. Rupture of the syrinx into the subarachnoid space has been noted occasionally to arrest the progression of neurological deficits.[99]

THE HYDRODYNAMIC AND SUBSEQUENT THEORIES

The explanation of the pathogenesis of syringomyelia initially proposed by Lichtenstein was adopted by Gardner and Goodall[59] after they had reviewed the first 17 adult cases of the Chiari I malformation treated by suboccipital decompression at the Cleveland Clinic. As Gardner[56] subsequently pointed out, the concept evolved serendipitously because of an inadequacy in the radiological equipment at the hospital in the 1930s. Expecting to find a tumor at the level of the foramen magnum, a congenital hernia of the hindbrain was occasionally discovered, below which there appeared a dilated cystic spinal cord. "As a result of such experiences the light gradually dawned that this was symptomatic syringobulbia with asymptomatic syringomyelia." Gardner and Goodall viewed the malformation as "merely a foraminal herniation of intracranial structures produced by an obstructive hydrocephalus" and termed the condition "congenital obstructive hydroencephalomyelia with foraminal hernia." Gardner and Angel[57] subsequently postulated that the obstructive hydrocephalus was due to a failure of the fourth ventricular foramina to open during embryonic life. Based on Weed's[166] experiments with living pig embryos, their explanation was centered around the theory that either a premature development of the choroid plexus or a delayed attenuation of the rhombic roof results in a pathological state of embryonic noncommunicating hydrocephalus. Herniation of the hindbrain structures through the foramen magnum follows, giving rise to the Chiari malformation (its severity being determined by the degree of herniation into the upper cervical canal). Subsequent to the development of the malformation, the rhombic roof becomes permeable to the egress of CSF, resulting in a compensated hydrocephalus with restoration of a normal ventricular size. Hence, even though the intracranial pressure is rarely elevated in patients with the

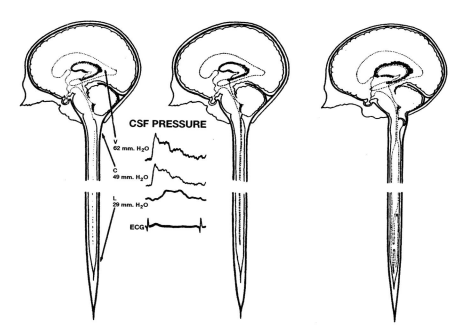

Figure 10: *Left:* Normal adult relationships with progressive dampening of the CSF fluid pulse wave as it reaches the lumbar thecal sac. *Center:* Normal embryonic relationships with the fourth ventricle foramina closed by semipermeable membranes. *Right:* Syringomyelia with hindbrain hernia. CSF passes into the central canal forming a diverticulum below. (Reprinted from reference 58, with permission)

Chiari malformation, the "water-hammer" effect of the CSF pulsations (described by Bering[19]) is directly transmitted to a patent central canal, resulting in dilatation and rupture of the ependymal lining, in turn leading to cord cavitation (Figure 10). In support of this "hydrodynamic" mechanism, which is based on the hypothesis that the syrinx maintains its communication with the fourth ventricle, three observations were noted: 1) indigo carmine injected into the lateral ventricles could be recovered from the syrinx; 2) fluid aspirated from the syrinx at the time of operation was identical in composition to CSF; and, 3) chronic adhesive arachnoiditis in the experimental animal led to "communicating" hydrocephalus and multiple cavitations in the spinal cord.

Williams[172] challenged Gardner's hypothesis, pointing out that the enormous dilatation of cord cavities in the presence of only "modest" hydrocephalus would argue against the arterial pressure wave as being the prime distending force of the syrinx. Furthermore, in many cases the foramina of Luschka were patent and not covered by a permeable membrane. Williams proposed that venous distention produced by activities such as coughing, sneezing, and voiding in patients with defective intracranial drainage resulted in a state of disequilibrium, following which the intracranial pressure was elevated with respect to the spinal intrathecal pressure forcing CSF through a patent central canal into the syrinx (Figure 11). He suggested that all patients with communicating syringomyelia had had at one point in time a brief episode of hydrocephalus producing the initial dilatation of the central canal, corresponding to the "compensated" enlargement of the ventricles, and that blockage of the outlet of the foramen magnum was the factor responsible for the subsequent distending force within the syrinx via a patent communication with the fourth ventricle.

Williams subsequently modified his views,[171] noting that it was not the venous engorgement of the head, but the rebound downward movement of the CSF caused by the pressure gradient between the intracranial and intraspinal com-

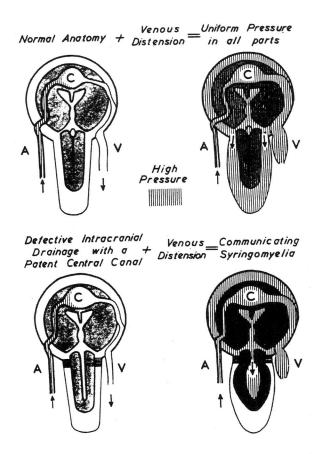

Figure 11: Schematic description of effect of venous distention with normal anatomy *(upper)* and with defective intracranial drainage and patent central canal *(lower).* (Reprinted from reference 171, with permission)

partments following a Valsalva maneuver which resulted in dilatation of the syrinx. Williams referred to this cranial-spinal pressure dissociation as "suck" and was able to measure the differential by recording pressures simultaneously from both the ventricle and the spinal subarachnoid space when asking patients to cough or blow into a mouthpiece. He noted that in patients with hindbrain hernia, pressure differences of over 100 mm Hg could be recorded between the head and the spine.[173] To explain progression of the syrinx cavity in the absence of communication with the fourth ventricle, Williams proposed that surges in pressure of intrasyrinx fluid could occur, a mechanism which he referred to as "slosh" (Figure 12).

Acute exacerbations in symptoms resulting from abrupt changes in the size of cord cysts had been previously noted by Bertrand,[20] who underscored the importance of dynamic factors governing the evolution of syringomyelic cavities. He noted that coughing or straining produced strong pressure gradients between the poorly communicating fluid spaces on either side of the arachnoidal block at the craniocervical junction, occasionally resulting in forceful dissection of the cyst fluid upward into the gray matter of the medulla, producing syringobulbia. Positive contrast ventriculography was found to be a useful tool to demonstrate patency of the central canal and anomalies of outflow from the fourth ventricle, particularly where conventional oil myelography followed by gas myelography and pneumoencephalography had failed to

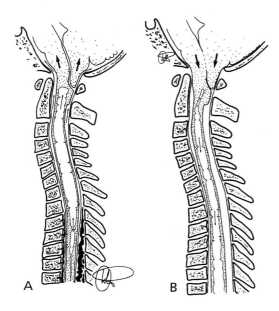

Figure 12: Mechanism of "slosh" illustrated. **A)** Upward movement of CSF during a Valsalva maneuver. **B)** Rebound phenomenon with further impaction of tonsils. (Reprinted from reference 174, with permission)

show the abnormalities at the foramen magnum. Du Boulay and coworkers[42] also stressed the importance of sudden changes in the spinal venous pressure produced by coughing and straining in extending the syringomyelic cavity once the cyst had formed. Based on animal experimentation and on observations of patients with hindbrain anomalies, they hypothesized that the basal cisternal pulse occurring with each heartbeat produced an increase in the peak height of the pressure wave around the brain stem, which in turn resulted in a downward pulsatile systolic thrust of the cerebellar tonsils into the cervical canal. Under certain conditions, such an increased pressure wave could result in reflux of CSF from the cisterna magna into the fourth ventricle and displacement of the fluid into the central canal. Acting as a ball-valve, the cone of cerebellar ectopic tissue would not only accentuate the rise of pressure in the posterior fossa, but might also "milk" fluid along the slit-like central canal to form an underlying syrinx further caudally. Aboulker,[3] in a comprehensive monograph summarizing the

pathogenesis of syringomyelia and its surgical treatment, emphasized the combined role of obstruction to the flow of CSF and venous stasis of the epidural venous plexus. He theorized that the latter might give rise to a state of CSF hypertension within the spinal canal in the face of a blockage to the outflow of CSF at the level of the foramen magnum. Hence, CSF would be forced into the spinal cord, possibly via the dorsal rootlets, giving rise to edema, subsequent breakdown of the gray matter, and formation of cavities within its substance.[2]

In an attempt to reconcile elements of the hydrodynamic theory of Gardner with the cranial-spinal pressure dissociation hypothesis of Williams, a new theory was proposed by Oldfield and coworkers[109] to explain the pathophysiology of syringomyelia associated with the Chiari I malformation. Based on dynamic MRI, they observed abrupt downward movement of spinal CSF and intrasyrinx fluid in the upper portion of the spinal canal during systole and upward movement during diastole, but minimal movement across the foramen magnum. Intraoperative ultrasound studies further demonstrated abrupt downward movement of the cerebellar tonsils during systole, synchronous with sudden constriction of the spinal cord and syrinx. Based on these studies, they proposed that the "piston-like" effect of the movement of the impacted tonsils during systole imparts an accentuated systolic pressure wave to the spinal subarachnoid CSF, abruptly constricting the surface of the cord and underlying syrinx. CSF is thereby forced into the spinal cord expanding the underlying syrinx (presumably via enlarged Virchow-Robin spaces, as was surmised by Ball and Dayan[8] in 1972). Further abrupt increases in intrathecal pressure produced by coughing or severe straining could act in a similar fashion on the cord surface, thereby explaining the occasional acute progression of neurological deficits seen in these patients. Oldfield et al emphasized that their proposed mechanism for the progression of syringomyelia required no communication with the fourth ventricle, unlike the hydrodynamic theory which postulated that acute systolic *expansion* of the syrinx took place with each heartbeat. It also gave a satisfactory explanation for the clinical improvement or stabilization that occurs in the majority of patients after surgical decompression of the craniocervical junction alone, without further incising the arachnoid or plugging the obex. Due to the relative paucity of cases studied, further observations will be required to lend support to this compelling theory.

A review of the theories of pathogenesis leads to the inescapable conclusion that syringomyelia is not a distinct disease entity in itself, with a well-defined anatomic substrate, but instead, a pathological condition common to a variety of disorders, all of which produce cavitation within the substance of the spinal cord. It is not surprising, therefore, that no theory of pathogenesis can hope to embrace all aspects of this condition. Each theory undoubtedly has its place and "raison d'être" in the multifaceted spectrum which characterizes the varied manifestations of this disorder. Many theories have been abandoned, and many have undergone extensive modifications to account for new and, seemingly, contradictory data. It is to be anticipated that new theories will arise in the future, challenging our understanding of this complex and fascinating disorder.

TREATMENT OF SYRINGOMYELIA

Radiation Therapy

By the turn of the century, the prevalent theory regarding the pathogenesis of syringomyelia suggested that it represented a disorder of abnormal proliferation of neuroglia with subsequent breakdown of proliferative tissue and destruction of surrounding neural elements, which eventually resulted in the formation of cavities in the spinal cord. It seemed logical, therefore, that radiation therapy might halt the progression of symptoms by inhibiting the formation of "gliomatous tissue," thereby allowing cells not irreversibly damaged to undergo repair and regeneration.[83] It was not long after Roentgen's discovery of x-rays in 1895[63] that the therapeutic use of its properties was directed at conditions such as syringomyelia, multiple sclerosis, and tabes dorsalis. By 1905, Raymond[127] was able to report the case of a 16-year-old seamstress with syringomyelia treated with x-rays, who experienced a marked improvement in both motor and sensory symptoms. Wilson[179] recalled the use of radiation therapy for syringomyelia by Byrom Bramwell as far back as 1902 when he was his house physician, although this case was never reported. Enthusiasm for its use subsequently spread to many clinics in France, Italy, and Germany. By 1912, Sahatchieff[134] was able to summarize the results of 30 published cases, adding a further six of his own: improvement was noted in 80%. Delherm and Morel-Kahn[37] published a statistical summary of cases covering the period up to 1930, estimating that there were 150 cases published to date; to these they added 16 of their own from the Hôpital de la Pitié. Approximately 72% of the published cases showed marked improvement, some of whom were believed to have been "cured," whereas improvement was noted in about 60% of their own. Variability from center to center in the total dose and number of treatments was noted by the authors, who recommended using "penetrating, but not deep, radiotherapy" at frequent intervals for an extended period of time. By using these techniques, they were able to give doses up to 24,000 rad and more, apparently without causing radiation dermatitis! In 1932, Markow et al[95] reviewed the experience at Minsk, adding a further 32 cases of their own to the literature. In 47% there was both objective and subjective improvement with decrease in pain, reduction of hyperhydrosis and cyanosis of the extremities, restitution of sensitivity to touch, and reappearance of tendon reflexes in the arms and decrease of spasticity in the legs. A brief clinical standstill of the disease was noted in 37%. Two years earlier, Czerny and Heinismann[36] reported their results from Kiev, noting improvement in 75% of patients who had been followed for a minimum of two years. Soon afterward, Giese and Ossinskaja[62] reported their series of 128 cases, of which 55 showed evidence of bulbar symptoms. Remarkably, they stated that these last patients "did particularly well under treatment," with 50% showing improvement in their condition and 30% an arrest of the disease.

In contrast to the large number of reports on the use of radiotherapy for syringomyelia in the French, German, and Italian literature, the English and American literature is marked by a paucity of publications. In 1935, O'Brien[107] reported the results of 30 cases treated at the Boston City Hospital: 61% were noted to have experienced "definite improvement." Haworth[71] reported six cases in 1934, noting improvement in some and, in others, progression of the neurological deficits, despite subjective relief of their pain. This is perhaps why neurologists in the United States and England remained skeptical of the use of radiotherapy; in 1934, Grinker[65] stated that the treatment was questionable, although he acknowledged that there was frequently relief of central pain in a progressing lesion. Frazier and Rowe[53] stated that they had never seen "more than very transitory results" from the use of irradiation. Tauber and Langworthy[160] felt that x-ray therapy had no logical basis for non-neoplastic conditions associated with syringomyelia. Netsky[106] noted the lack of controlled studies, stating that "sham radiation might have as much subjective value as genuine radiation." He questioned the rationale for x-ray therapy, especially in light of the knowledge that radiation myelitis could occur years later. Logue,[91] on the other hand, was quick to point out that *any* improvement in a patient's subjective condition was a worthwhile goal even though there might not be improvement in the overall neurological condition.

The value of radiation therapy in the treatment of syringomyelia is, nevertheless, questionable in this day and age, with the exception of cases of syringomyelia secondary to inoperable or incompletely removed spinal cord tumors. Boman and Iivanainen[23] reviewed the group of patients who were followed at the University of Helsinki from 1920 to 1965. Of the 22 patients who underwent radiation therapy, no differences in the progression of the disease could be appreciated when compared with the untreated group. In over one-half of all patients, treated or untreated, stabilization of the neurological condition was noted lasting 10 years or more.

A somewhat unusual alternative to the treatment of syringomyelia by radiation therapy was presented in the report of Borysowicz[24] in 1967, describing the use of systemic nitrogen mustard in a group of 50 patients treated between 1956 and 1961. Based on the assumption that syringomyelia was a neoplastic condition characterized by "an excessive proliferation of neuroglia," a course of treatment consisting of 0.02 mg of nitrogen mustard per kilogram body weight was administered every second day for a total of five injections. The course was repeated every 6-8 weeks until an arrest of the disease progression was obtained and improvement maintained. Most patients received between two to five courses of treatment. All patients were reassessed in 1962. Remarkably, improvement in sensory abnormalities was reported by 78% of patients, motor strength improving in 47%. In those patients who experienced pain, 81% noted improvement. Borysowicz acknowledged that follow-up in many was relatively brief and that there was a "lack of pathological confirmation." Unfortunately, no information was given as to how the diagnosis of syringomyelia was made, although this paper leads one to believe that it was on the basis of symptoms and signs alone. Furthermore, measures of outcome were "often based on the subjective statements of the patients," making any definitive conclusions of the efficacy of this treatment tenuous to say the least. To date, no further reports on the use of chemotherapy in syringomyelia have appeared in the literature.

Surgical Therapy

As has been pointed out by Batzdorf,[16] the surgical treatment of patients with syringomyelia and the Chiari malformation has evolved mainly from the prevalent theory of genesis of the syringeal cavity. Hence, the initial efforts were directed at the cystic cavity itself and not the malformation at the level of the cranioverterbral junction. This can be explained in part by the lack of radiological tools to diagnose the malformation prior to the introduction of contrast myelography using iodized oil (Lipiodol) by Sicard and Forestier[147] in 1921. Abbe and Coley[1] were the first to report a successful surgical approach to a syringeal cavity in 1892, four years after Horsley performed the first successful removal of a spinal tumor.[64] Abbe and Coley exposed the spinal cord after performing a thoracic laminectomy, expecting to find evidence of a tumor or transverse myelitis. At operation, a swollen cord was discovered, expanded twice its normal size by a "lemon"-shaped cystic cavity. The cyst was aspirated through the posterior columns, which resulted in collapse of the cord.

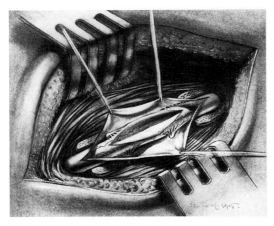

Figure 13: Drawing showing the appearance of the cord after a hydromyelic cavity has been incised. (Reproduced from Ellsberg CA: *The Diagnosis and Treatment of Surgical Diseases of the Spinal Cord and Its Membranes.* Philadelphia, Pa: WB Saunders, 1916, p 288)

Temporary improvement in the spasticity in the lower extremities was noted postoperatively; however, six months later the patient showed increasing signs of spasticity and subsequently succumbed after developing cystitis.

In 1916, Elsberg[45] reported that he had incised the cord "on several patients" near the posterior median septum, following which there was "marked improvement" which lasted for a number of years (Figure 13). Wilson[179] reported that Horsley incised the syringomyelic cord of one of Gowers' patients in 1907 at The National Hospital, during the time in which he was the house physician, although this case was never published. Poussepp,[125] apparently unaware of any prior reports in the medical literature, described in 1926 two cases in which he performed myelotomies for syringomyelia; substantial improvement in both motor and sensory function resulted, although follow-up was limited to a few months in each case. By 1931, Peiper[118] was able to publish the first review in the literature of patients treated by open surgery, documenting a total of 44 cases. The following year, Schaeffer[136] wrote an extensive review, tabulating the results from 18 different papers in which 50 cases were reported with follow-up ranging from two weeks to two years. Not surprisingly, the results of surgical inter-

vention were reported as "improved" or "much improved" in the majority of cases.

In 1936, Frazier and Rowe[53] were able to report two of their own cases with "long-term" follow-up of two years in the one and 14 months in the other. They argued that the sustained benefits of myelotomy, when combined with stenting, gave a superior result, noting that both patients who underwent myelotomy alone required a second procedure due to a relapse. At reoperation "not a trace of the first incision was found in either patient." They concluded that incisions into the syringeal cavities subsequently closed secondary to arachnoid adhesions or gliosis and suggested that "a foreign non-absorbable material" should be used to maintain drainage of the cavity, even though it might prove "irritating" to the tissues. Frazier[52] recommended the use of gutta percha, whereas Sharpe recommended the use of silk thread. Peiper,[118] proposed excision of a window of cord tissue, Mixter[103] advocated suturing the lining membrane of the cavity to the surrounding arachnoid, and Mucenieks[105] and Oppel[113] both advised using dura mater. Subsequently, others have recommended the use of silk sutures,[93] tantalum wire,[79] and Silastic wicks.[128] Two years later, Adelstein[5] was able to review the postoperative results of 87 cases collected from the world literature; 120 cases having been reported to date: 66 were noted to improve, 10 stabilized, and 11 were noted to worsen. Follow-up ranged from one month to seven years, the majority of reports noting improvement lasting "over 6 months." Later, the introduction of biocompatible tubing allowed for the placement of shunts from the syrinx to the subarachnoid space,[81,116,130,159] or from the syrinx to the peritoneal[10,84,121,122] or pleural cavities,[177,180] and, more recently, from the syrinx to the posterior fossa cisterns.[101] Although encouraging short-term results were reported by a number of centers using these techniques, Sgouros and Williams[146] recently reviewed their considerable experience with the use of drains, with long-term follow-up ranging from 12 months to 20 years. Only one-half of the patients remained clinically stable after 10 years; the remainder required reoperations or experienced deterioration as a result of the intervention. Sgouros and Williams concluded that permanent drains had questionable value given the fact that they frequently became blocked and might be the cause of late deterioration by inducing or provoking gliosis inside the spinal cord.

The injection of contrast agents into the cystic cavity of syringomyelic patients for both diagnostic and therapeutic purposes was initially reported by Sicard et al[148] in 1926. They injected 2 cc of Lipiodol into the cavity of a syrinx exposed at the time of surgery after aspirating 10 cc of fluid, following which clinical improvement was noted in the patient. The following year, Jirásek[76] described his technique of endomyelography to outline the syringeal cavity prior to surgical exploration in four patients. In 1928, Vitek[163] reported his percutaneous technique with favorable results, subsequently describing a modification of the technique to empty the cyst by outlining its inferior pole.[164] In his opinion, the therapeutic aspect of the percutaneous aspiration of fluid contained in the syringomyelic cavity was a purely palliative procedure, which needed to be followed by x-ray therapy. Westberg[169] subsequently perfected the technique of cervicothoracic percutaneous puncture, and Ellertsson[44] reported that percutaneous puncture produced gratifying results in patients who had distended cords, with objective improvement in two-thirds of the patients. Pantopaque was used by Schlesinger et al[137] for percutaneous puncture, leading at times to a dramatic relief of the clinical picture, although repeat punctures were often required to "stabilize a deteriorating syndrome." The use of sclerosing agents to obliterate the cavity has been contemplated by some; however, Williams[170] cautioned against their use before the development of an adequate animal model, stating that "in the present state of knowledge a surgeon would be bold to attempt such measures."

Although the name of Gardner is frequently associated with the development of a direct approach to the abnormality at the level of the hindbrain, it is important to note that others before him had attempted to relieve the compression at the foramen magnum. In 1945, Russell and Donald[133] suggested that in cases of spina bifida and myelomeningocele the hydrocephalus frequently found to accompany the Arnold-Chiari malformation might be caused by the anomaly itself. In that case, they argued,

decompression of the spinal cord at the foramen magnum would be desirable "to facilitate the circulation of fluid in the leptomeningeal spaces." They stated that such an operation had not yet been undertaken; however, in a footnote to the paper they noted that C. J. van Houweninge Graftdijk[161] had written a monograph in 1932 entitled *Over Hydrocephalus*, which had only recently come to their attention while the paper was in press. In it the author described his attempts to relieve the obstruction at the craniovertebral junction by resecting the tongue of redundant tissue (presumably the tonsils) or by resecting the bone over the posterior surface of the malformation and incising the underlying dura. Unfortunately, his patients "died either from the effects of the operation or from postoperative complications."

In 1938, Penfield and Coburn[119] described the case of a 29-year-old woman with a past history of repair of a thoracic meningocele at the age of three, who presented with a two-year history of hearing loss, decreased vision affecting the right eye, occasional double vision on looking to either side, and weakness of the right side of the face. Bilateral acoustic nerve tumors were suspected; however, a Type II Chiari malformation was discovered during an operation with the tonsils, which were excised for histological study, extending down to the arch of C3. Postoperatively, the patient never regained consciousness and died two months later. Penfield and Coburn suggested that in future operations the tonsils be left intact, the arachnoid opened, and the posterior margin of the foramen magnum removed along with the arches of C1 and C2. They postulated that the malformation at the level of the hindbrain was caused by a cicatricial contraction at the site of the myelomeningocele acting on the cord, which exerted a traction on the brain stem and cerebellum; this, in turn, resulted in an obstruction to the outflow of CSF from the fourth ventricle, producing an "internal" hydrocephalus. Hence, the recommendation of exposing the myelomeningocele to free the spinal cord from its surrounding attachments was emphasized as a necessary step in dealing with the malformation in its entirety.

The same year, McConnell and Parker[97] reported the results of treatment of five patients with the Chiari I malformations, two of whom had successful outcomes. Subsequent reports by D'Errico,[38] List,[90] Ogryzlo,[108] Adams et al,[4] Bucy and Lichtenstein,[26] Steele,[153] and Chorobski and Stepien[33] described attempts to surgically approach the hindbrain malformation with varying degrees of success. By 1950, Gardner and Goodall[59] were able to collect a total of 17 adult patients with the Chiari I malformations who had undergone operations directed at the craniovertebral junction; to these they added a further 17 cases of their own which had been accumulated over the past 10 years. In 13 instances a cystic cervical spinal cord was encountered, which on puncture yielded a clear, colorless fluid whose protein content was identical to CSF. In each case, an attempt was made to reopen the foramen of Magendie to facilitate communication between the fourth ventricle and the subarachnoid space; the dura was left open. Thirteen patients improved, three were made worse, and one died.

On the basis of the formulation of the hydrodynamic theory of syringomyelia, Gardner began to plug the obex in 1957 in an attempt to seal off the hypothetical communication between the syrinx and the fourth ventricle, although no opening of the syrinx onto the floor of the fourth ventricle could be identified at the time of the surgical exposure. Gardner believed that the operative results were improved in patients in whom the obex was plugged, although no proof of such an assertion was provided. By 1965, twenty-five years after his initial publication, Gardner[56] was able to report on 74 cases of syringomyelia associated with a congenital deformity of the hindbrain. Plugging of the obex was performed using a bit of muscle or wisp of cotton in 33 of the patients. Improvement in some of the symptoms was noted immediately following the operation in 52 patients, no change was noted in 11, worsening of the preoperative symptoms in six, and five patients died from postoperative complications. Gardner's demonstration that the correction of the hindbrain anomaly alone often led to a significant clinical improvement in patients with syringomyelia and the Chiari malformation resulted in the widespread adoption of his surgical technique, despite the fact that no proof could be offered that plugging the obex actually improved the outcome.

This uncritical and enthusiastic adoption of a surgical procedure of questionable value was underscored by Williams,[170] who in 1978 retrospectively analyzed the morbidity and mortality rates of the collected cases of posterior fossa surgery in the literature. Complications included sudden respiratory arrest; exacerbation of hydrocephalus; aggravation of cerebellar, brain stem, and spinal cord neurological signs; postural hypotension; descent of the cerebellum; nuchal and occipital headache; and progression of the condition despite seemingly successful decompression of the craniovertebral junction. In addition, a mortality rate of 12.5% was documented in Williams' own series. Williams argued that the correction of the cranialspinal pressure dissociation should be the primary objective, noting that the patients who underwent decompression alone had just as good results as those who had their hypothetical communications blocked.

This view was echoed by Logue and Edwards[92] in 1981, who reviewed their series of patients treated surgically for syringomyelia: 35 patients underwent Gardner's operation (foramen magnum decompression with plugging of the obex), whereas 33 underwent decompression alone. An analysis of the outcome revealed that there was essentially no difference between the two groups, although the incidence of complications was higher in the former. If the arachnoid was left intact, it was noted that the incidence of complications in the latter group was practically nil (discounting a wound infection). With the notable exception of a few, others have confirmed these findings on retrospectively reviewing their own personal series.[86,96] Hoffman et al[73] found that their results were improved following plugging of the obex, although the very small number of patients who underwent posterior decompression alone makes any comparison somewhat tenuous. The fact that their retrospective analysis was confined to the surgical management of syringomyelia in childhood (a large percentage having Chiari II malformations) may explain in part the radically different conclusions. Dyste et al[43] also believed that "superior results" were obtained when posterior fossa decompression was combined with obex obliteration, fourth ventricle shunting, and a dural graft. However, close inspection of their report reveals that only six patients underwent posterior fossa decompression and dural grafting alone, whereas 33 patients underwent the more extensive procedure. In their skilled hands "there were no major operative complications or deaths." Peerless and Durward[117] also reported that in their series of 34 patients who underwent foramen magnum decompression procedures, better results were noted in patients who had plugging of the obex combined with a fourth ventricle to subarachnoid drain when compared to foramen magnum decompression alone, although follow-up was limited in the eight patients who underwent the former procedure. Sensibly, they cautioned against enthusiastic endorsement of this potentially hazardous microsurgical procedure "until tested by the fullness of time."

Due to the morbidity associated with craniovertebral junction decompression procedures mentioned above, together with the realization that many patients with seemingly "successful" responses to surgery might relapse years later, other less risky approaches to decompress the syringomyelic cavity were attempted. In 1977, Gardner et al[58] published a report on terminal ventriculostomy for syringomyelia. Of the 12 patients reported, seven had undergone a prior craniovertebral junction decompression (five having had an initial good result). The remaining five patients underwent terminal ventriculostomy as an alternative to the more invasive Gardner procedure. Good results were reported in all but two patients, with follow-up ranging from 12 to 30 months. One patient suffered postoperative complications contributing to a poor result. For reasons not elaborated upon, it was recommended that "terminal ventriculostomy deserves a further trial as a substitute for craniovertebral decompression in the treatment of syringomyelia."

Soon after this report was published, other surgeons,[151] encouraged by these seemingly impressive results, began utilizing the procedure primarily in patients whose symptoms progressed despite undergoing posterior fossa decompression. Williams and Fahy[176] reviewed the combined results of terminal ventriculostomy from several centers totaling 31 cases, including 12 of their own. The majority had undergone prior surgical interventions, mainly in the form

of craniovertebral junction decompression procedures. Contrary to Gardner's optimistic report, sustained improvement was noted in only a few patients; although many patients claimed improvement in their preoperative symptoms, the condition in a majority of these proceeded to deteriorate. More than one-third of the patients were not improved, even subjectively, after surgery. Williams and Fahy concluded that although terminal ventriculostomy might have a place in the management of syringomyelia, their review of the accumulated experience from several neurosurgical centers did not substantiate Gardner's claim that it could be considered as a viable alternative to hindbrain hernia decompression. They argued that probably less than one-third of patients with syringomyelia had a functional communication between the syringomyelic cavity and the filum terminale and that only a minority of syringomyelic cavities extended the length of the cord, the majority becoming loculated over time.

A different approach to the treatment of syringomyelia was advocated by Benini and Krayenbühl[18] who reported on the treatment of ventriculoatrial shunting in two patients who had undergone prior cervical laminectomies for drainage of a syrinx. Both patients showed significant amelioration in their symptoms. A subsequent report by Krayenbühl[80] in 1974 revealed that of 22 patients with syringomyelia who underwent ventriculoatrial shunting, 13 improved, two stabilized, and seven deteriorated over the period of observation. Earlier, Conway[35] had reported the case of a patient with syringomyelia and syringobulbia who underwent insertion of a ventriculojugular shunt, as it was thought he would be too poor a risk for posterior fossa exploration. Although follow-up was limited to three months, some improvement was noted in his condition. Foster and Hudgson[51] recognized that ventriculoatrial shunting was less traumatic than Gardner's operation; however, they felt that it was unsatisfactory in dealing with the pathology at the level of the hindbrain and should be reserved for cases of adhesive arachnoiditis at the level of the foramen magnum where the risks of a posterior fossa exploration were unwarranted. The true incidence of hydrocephalus in patients with syringomyelia remains unknown. In a series of

99 patients, Foster and Hudgson[50] noted that seven patients demonstrated findings on plain skull films suggestive of hydrocephalus. Hurth and Sichez[75] noted the presence of hydrocephalus in 19 (30%) of 63 patients with syringomyelia. West and Williams,[168] using a variety of techniques, estimated the size of the lateral ventricles in 80 patients with "idiopathic communicating" syringomyelia; 23 (29%) were found to have varying degrees of hydrocephalus. Williams[174] advocated treating the hydrocephalus *before* the hindbrain abnormality in those patients with severe symptomatic hydrocephalus. For those with communicating syringomyelia and mild ventriculomegaly, good results could be expected from ventricular shunting alone. This was recently confirmed by Milhorat et al,[102] who noted improvement in the preoperative symptoms and simultaneous resolution of the hydrocephalus and accompanying syringomyelia in all seven patients who underwent ventriculoperitoneal shunting, with follow-up ranging from 1.5 to 5 years.

Of interest is a report by Sullivan et al[157] documenting complete resolution of a Chiari I malformation by ventriculoatrial shunting in a patient with pseudotumor cerebri and a lumboperitoneal shunt. The fact that syringomyelia can develop years after placement of a lumboureteral shunt had been previously noted by Fischer et al[49] in 1977 and by Welch et al[167] in 1981, demonstrating that in some cases Chiari I malformations with syringomyelia could be produced iatrogenically.

Given the controversy surrounding the pathogenesis of syringomyelia, it is not surprising that treatment has been equally controversial, with claims of success varying widely from one author to another. Enthusiasm for new operations is generally followed by a more sober realization that the longer patients are followed, the greater the number of failures become evident. Faulhauer and Loew[47] analyzed their long-term results in a group of 28 patients with syringomyelia who were treated by syringostomy, suboccipital craniotomy, ventriculoatrial shunts, or a combination of the above. Although improvement was noted in the first few months and years following the surgical interventions, follow-up averaging four years revealed that improvement was maintained in only four of the 28 patients, with five patients succumbing to complications of their disease during the observation period. They concluded that re-evaluation and long-term follow-up of surgically treated syringomyelia patients were essential for the realistic assessment of each therapeutic intervention. Anderson et al[6] came to similar conclusions after retrospectively reviewing their surgical series of 24 patients treated with a variety of surgical procedures. They noted that there was a severe neurological disability in patients in whom the symptoms had been present for more than two years and that the long-term outlook of posterior fossa surgery was usually poor in patients more than 40 years old; those who underwent laminectomy with either aspiration of the syrinx or syringostomy fared no better, with two-thirds continuing to deteriorate over time. Anderson et al observed that seven of the 20 untreated patients in their series had no further progression in their symptoms for many years following their initial presentation, making interpretation of the results of surgical interventions difficult to compare to an untreated group. This important study underscores the need for an extended period of observation before any conclusions can be made regarding the efficacy of a particular therapeutic intervention.

Although it is often not fully understood why a particular therapeutic intervention might succeed in one person and fail in another, despite the fact that both would seem to have identical lesions, a more complete understanding of the pathophysiology of the abnormal CSF dynamics at the level of the craniovertebral junction and within the syringeal cavity itself, combined with the recent advances in imaging, has enabled surgeons to select a more rational approach to the treatment of this condition.[102] As Williams has astutely pointed out, "it is not, of course, necessary for current theory to be correct for a surgical operation to succeed."[176] Even though they might have proven incorrect, it should be evident from this historical review that theories of pathogenesis have guided to a large degree the choice of surgical procedure, either in whole or in part. It is to be hoped that earlier detection of syringeal cavities might lead to earlier surgical interventions in the course of this disorder before irreversible damage to the spinal cord and brain stem occur.

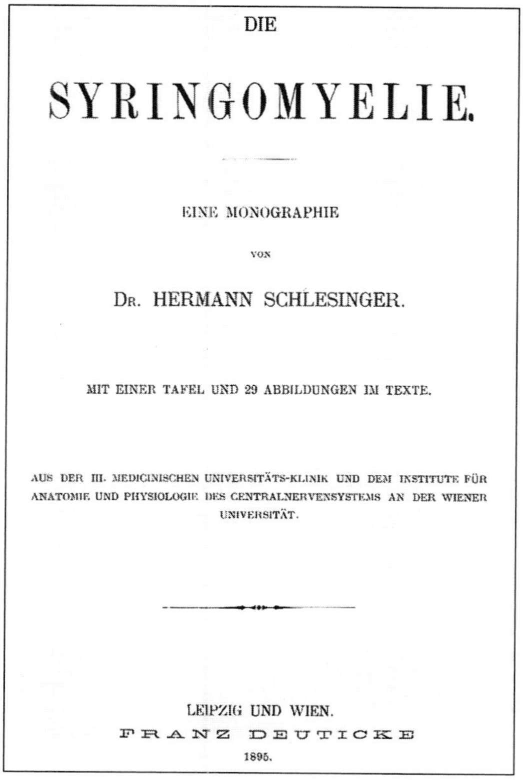
DIE

SYRINGOMYELIE.

EINE MONOGRAPHIE

VON

DR. HERMANN SCHLESINGER.

MIT EINER TAFEL UND 29 ABBILDUNGEN IM TEXTE.

AUS DER III. MEDICINISCHEN UNIVERSITÄTS-KLINIK UND DEM INSTITUTE FÜR ANATOMIE UND PHYSIOLOGIE DES CENTRALNERVENSYSTEMS AN DER WIENER UNIVERSITÄT.

LEIPZIG UND WIEN.
FRANZ DEUTICKE
1895.

Figure 14: Title page of Schlesinger's first monograph, *Die Syringomyelie*, published in 1895. (Reprinted from reference 139)

Conclusion

A little over 100 years ago, Schlesinger[139] published the first monograph on syringomyelia (Figure 14). It comprised 289 pages and contained 526 references. Seven years later, in 1902, the second edition[140] of his work appeared having grown to 611 pages with 1,175 references. As noted above, the number of surgical cases in the early part of the century were relatively few, given the predominance of radiation therapy as the primary therapeutic modality for the treatment of syringomyelia. A recent review[7] found only 193 operative cases prior to 1938. Ballantine and coworkers[9] found a total of 355 reported operations covering the years 1938 to 1971. Seventy years after the second edition of Schlesinger's monograph, the first comprehensive English monograph[14] to be devoted to the subject appeared in 1973 as Volume 1 in a series entitled, *Major Problems in Neurology*. In the foreword to the book, Drake noted that "it appears doubtful that syringomyelia can be regarded as a single entity either from the point of view of clinical presentation, from the viewpoint of pathogenesis, or, most importantly from the standpoint of rational therapy." The same year, Gardner[55] published a monograph entitled, *The Dysraphic States From Syringomyelia to Anencephaly*, in which he attempted to explain the pathogenesis of all dysraphic conditions as resulting from increasing degrees of overdistention of the lumen of the neural tube or of its subarachnoid space, occurring at various stages of embryonic development. Although his theories are no longer tenable, Gardner deserves credit for having stimulated a great deal of interest in the Chiari malformations associated with syringomyelia and is ultimately responsible for having directed attention to the deformity at the level of the hindbrain, rather than the syrinx itself, which had been the focus of attention for the better part of a century.

At a recent workshop in Heidelberg,[41] it was estimated that the number of reported operative cases, extracted from a total of 1,152 papers, had jumped to 3,077 by 1991, a testimony to the significant increase in interest in this relatively uncommon neurological condition. Despite the fact that our knowledge of the anatomy, pathogenesis, and pathophysiology of syringomyelic cavities has increased substantially, no uniformity of thought regarding the optimal management of this condition exists. For this reason alone, an historical appreciation of the theories of pathogenesis and the various modalities of treatment is essential in order that "new" ideas might be placed in their proper context.

Acknowledgement: The author wishes to thank Toby Appel of the Yale History of Medicine Library and Richard Wolfe, Curator of Rare Books and Manuscripts at the Countway Library, Harvard.

REFERENCES

1. Abbe R, Coley WB: Syringomyelia, operation—exploration of cord—withdrawal of fluid—exhibition of patient. **J Nerv Ment Dis 19:**512-520, 1892

2. Aboulker J: La stase veineuse. **Neurochirurgie 25 (Suppl 1):**108-110, 1979

3. Aboulker J: La syringomyélie et les liquides intrarachidiens. **Neurochirurgie 25 (Suppl 1):**1-144, 1979

4. Adams RD, Schatzki R, Scoville WB: The Arnold-Chiari malformation. Diagnosis, demonstration by intraspinal Lipiodol and successful surgical treatment. **N Engl J Med 225:**125-131, 1941

5. Adelstein LJ: The surgical treatment of syringomyelia. **Am J Surg 40:**384-395, 1938

6. Anderson NE, Willoughby EW, Wrightson P: The natural history and the influence of surgical treatment in syringomyelia. **Acta Neurol Scand 71:**472-479, 1985

7. Aschoff A, Kunze S: 100 years syrinx-surgery—a review. **Acta Neurochir 123:**157-159, 1993

8. Ball MJ, Dayan AD: Pathogenesis of syringomyelia. **Lancet 2:**799-801, 1972

9. Ballantine HT, Ojemann RG, Drew JH: Syringohydromyelia, in Krayenbühl H, Maspes PE, Sweet WH (eds): **Progress in Neurological Surgery.** Basel: Karger, 1971, Vol 4, pp 227-245

10. Barbaro NM, Wilson CB, Gutin PH, et al: Surgical treatment of syringomyelia. Favorable results with syringoperitoneal shunting. **J Neurosurg 61:**531-538, 1984

11. Barnett HJ: Syringomyelia associated with spinal arachnoiditis, in Barnett HJM, Foster JB, Hudson P (eds): **Syringomyelia.** London: WB Saunders, 1973, pp 245-259

12. Barnett HJ, Jousse AT, Ball MJ: Pathology and pathogenesis of progressive cystic myelopathy as a late sequel to spinal cord injury, in Barnett HJ, Foster JB, Hudson P (eds): **Syringomyelia.** London: WB Saunders, 1973, pp 261-301

13. Barnett HJM, Botterell EH, Jousse AT, et al: Progressive myelopathy as a sequel to traumatic paraplegia. **Brain 89:**159-174, 1966

14. Barnett HJM, Foster JB, Hudson P (eds): **Syringomyelia.** London: WB Saunders, 1973

15. Bastian HC: On a case of concussion-lesion, with extensive secondary degenerations of the spinal cord, followed by general muscular atrophy. **Med Chir Trans (Series II):**499-542, 1867

16. Batzdorf U: Syringomyelia related to abnormalities at the level of the craniovertebral junction, in Batzdorf U (ed): **Syringomyelia: Current Concepts in Diagnosis and Treatment.** Baltimore, Md: Williams & Wilkins, 1991, pp 163-182

17. Baümler A: Über Höhlenbildungen im Rückenmark. **Dtsch Arch Klin Med 40:**443-543, 1887

18. Benini A, Krayenbühl H: Ein neuer chirurgischer Weg zur Behandlung der Hydro- und Syringomyelie. Embryologische Grundlage und erste Ergebnisse. **Schweiz Med Wochenschr 99:**1137-1142, 1969

19. Bering EA Jr: Choroid plexus and arterial pulsation of cerebrospinal fluid: demonstration of the choroid plexuses as a cerebrospinal fluid pump. **Arch Neurol Psychiatry 73:**165-172, 1955

20. Bertrand G: Dynamic factors in the evolution of syringomyelia and syringobulbia. **Clin Neurosurg 20:**322-333, 1973

21. Bielschowsky M, Unger E: Syringomyelie mit Teratom- und extramedullärer Blastombildung. Zur Kenntnis der Pathogenese der syringomyelie. **J Psychol Neurol 25:**173-218, 1920

22. Biyani A, El Masry WS: Post-traumatic syringomyelia: a review of the literature. **Paraplegia 32:**723-731, 1994

23. Boman K, Iivanainen M: Prognosis of syringomyelia. **Acta Neurol Scand 43:**61-68, 1967

24. Borysowicz J: Results of treatment of syringomyelia with nitrogen mustard. **Polish Med J 6:**728-732, 1967

25. Brunner JC: De Hydrocephalo, sire Hydrope capitis, in Bonneti T (ed): **Sepulchretum. Book I. 2nd ed.** Geneva: Cramer & Perachon, 1700, p 396

26. Bucy PC, Lichtenstein BW: Arnold-Chiari deformity in an adult without obvious cause. **J Neurosurg 2:**245-250, 1945

27. Bullard WN: Syringomyelia: glioma of the spinal cord. Laminectomy. **Med Surg Rep Bost City Hosp 10:**197-207, 1899

28. Camus J, Roussy G: Cavités médullaires et méningites cervicales: étude expérimentale. **Rev Neurol 22:**213-225, 1914

29. Carmel PW, Markesbery WR: Early descriptions of the Arnold-Chiari malformation. The contribution of John Cleland. **J Neurosurg 37:**543-547, 1972

30. Charcot JM, Joffroy A: Deux cas d'atrophie musculaire progressive avec lésions de la substance grise et des faisceaux antérolatéraux de la moelle épinière. **Arch Physiol Norm Pathol (1er série) 2:**354-367, 629-649, 744-760, 1869

31. Chiari H: Über Veränderungen des Kleinhirns, des Pons und der Medulla Oblongata in Folge von Congenitaler Hydrocephalie des Grosshirns. **Denkschr Akad Wiss Wien 63:**71-116, 1896

32. Chiari H: Über Veränderungen des Kleinhirns in Folge von Hydrocephalie des Grosshirns. **Dtsch Med Wochenschr 17:**1172-1175, 1891

33. Chorobski J, Stepien L: On the syndrome of Arnold-Chiari. Report of a case. **J Neurosurg 5:**495-500, 1948

34. Cleland J: Contribution to the study of spina bifida, encephalocele, and anencephalus. **J Anat Physiol 17:**257-291, 1883

35. Conway LW: Hydrodynamic studies in syringomyelia. **J Neurosurg 27:**501-514, 1967

36. Czerny LJ, Heinismann JI: Beitrage zur Pathologie und Röntgentherapie der Syringomyelie. **Z Neurol Psych 125:**573-614, 1930

37. Delherm L, Morel-Kahn M: Treatment of syringomyelia by roentgentherapy. **Am J Surg 9:**302-314, 1930

38. D'Errico A: The surgical treatment of hydrocephalus associated with spina bifida. **Yale J Biol Med 11:**425-430, 1939

39. Dimitroff S: Über Syringomyelie. **Arch Psychiatrie 29:**299-339, 1897

40. Dohrmann GJ: Cervical spinal cord in experimental hydrocephalus. **J Neurosurg 37:**538-542, 1972

41. Donauer E: 100 years syrinx surgery. Proceedings of a workshop, December 13-15, 1991 at Heidelberg.

Acta Neurochir 123:157-225, 1993

42. du Boulay G, Shah SH, Currie JC, et al: The mechanism of hydromyelia in Chiari type I malformations. **Br J Radiol 47:**579-587, 1974

43. Dyste GN, Menezes AH, VanGilder JC: Symptomatic Chiari malformations: an analysis of presentation, management, and long-term outcome. **J Neurosurg 71:**159-168, 1989

44. Ellertsson AB: Syringomyelia and other cystic spinal cord lesions. **Acta Neurol Scand 45:**403-417, 1969

45. Elsberg CA: **The Diagnosis and Treatment of Surgical Diseases of the Spinal Cord and Its Membranes.** Philadelphia, Pa: WB Saunders, 1916

46. Estienne C: **La dissection des parties du corps humain divisée en trois livres.** Paris: Simon de Collines, 1546

47. Faulhauer K, Loew K: The surgical treatment of syringomyelia. Long-term results. **Acta Neurochir 44:** 215-222, 1978

48. Feigin I, Ogata J, Budzilovich G: Syringomyelia: the role of edema in its pathogenesis. **J Neuropathol Exp Neurol 30:**216-232, 1971

49. Fischer EG, Welch K, Shillito J Jr: Syringomyelia following lumboureteral shunting for communicating hydrocephalus. Report of three cases. **J Neurosurg 47:**96-100, 1977

50. Foster JB, Hudgson P: The radiology of communicating syringomyelia, in Barnett HJM, Foster JB, Hudgson P (eds): **Syringomyelia.** London: WB Saunders, 1973, pp 50-63

51. Foster JB, Hudgson P: The surgical treatment of communicating syringomyelia, in Barnett HJM, Foster JB, Hudgson P (eds): **Syringomyelia.** London: WB Saunders, 1973, pp 64-78

52. Frazier CH: Shall syringomyelia be added to the lesions appropriate for surgical intervention? **JAMA 95:**1911-1912, 1930

53. Frazier CH, Rowe SN: The surgical treatment of syringomyelia. **Ann Surg 103:**481-497, 1936

54. Ganière P: Le baron Antoine Portal, Président perpétuel de l'Académie Royale de Médecine. **Bull Acad Natl Med 150:**539-545, 1966

55. Gardner WJ: **The Dysraphic States From Syringomyelia to Anencephaly.** Amsterdam: Excerpta Medica, 1973

56. Gardner WJ: Hydrodynamic mechanism of syringomyelia: its relationship to myelocele. **J Neurol Neurosurg Psychiatry 28:**247-259, 1965

57. Gardner WJ, Angel J: The mechanism of syringomyelia and its surgical correction. **Clin Neurosurg 6:**131-140, 1959

58. Gardner WJ, Bell HS, Poolos PN, et al: Terminal ventriculostomy for syringomyelia. **J Neurosurg 46:**609-617, 1977

59. Gardner WJ, Goodall RJ: The surgical treatment of Arnold-Chiari malformation in adults: an explanation of its mechanism and importance of encephalography in diagnosis. **J Neurosurg 7:** 199-206, 1950

60. Gardner WJ, McMurry FG: "Non-communicating" syringomyelia: a non-existent entity. **Surg Neurol 6:** 251-256, 1976

61. Gerlach W: Ein Fall von kongenitaler Syringomyelie mit intramedullarer Teratombildung. **Dtsche Z Nervenheilkd 5:**271-301, 1894

62. Giese E, Ossinskaja W: Weitere Beobachtungen über die Röntgentherapie der Syringomyelie. **Strahlentherapie 43:**739-748, 1932

63. Goodman PC: The new light: discovery and introduction of the X-ray. **AJR 165:**1041-1045, 1995

64. Gowers WR, Horsley V: A case of tumour of the spinal cord. Removal; recovery. **Med Chir Trans (Series II) 53:**377-428, 1888

65. Grinker RR: **Neurology.** Springfield, Ill: Charles C Thomas, 1934, p 914

66. Gull W: Case of progressive atrophy of the muscles of the hands: enlargement of the ventricle of the cord in the cervical region, with atrophy of the gray matter (hydromyelus). **Guys Hosp Report (3rd series) 8:**244-250, 1862

67. Hall PV, Muller J, Campbell RL: Experimental hydrosyringomyelia, ischemic myelopathy, and syringomyelia. **J Neurosurg 43:**464-470, 1975

68. Hallopeau FH: Contributions à l'étude de la sclérose diffuse péri-épendymaire. **Gaz Med Paris 25:**394, 1870

69. Harris T: On a case of multiple spinal and cerebral tumours (sarcomata), with a contribution to the pathology of syringomyelia. **Brain 8:**447-473,1885

70. Hassin GB: A contribution to the histopathology and histogenesis of syringomyelia. **Arch Neurol Psychiatry 3:**130-146, 1920

71. Haworth EM: The treatment of syringo-myelia by X rays. **Br J Radiol 7:**643-653, 1934

72. Hennenberg R, Koch M: Zur Pathogenese der Syringomyelie und über Hämatomyelie bei Syringomyelie. **Monatsschr Psychiatr Neurol 54:**117-140, 1923

73. Hoffman HJ, Neill J, Crone KR, et al: Hydrosyringomyelia and its management in childhood. **Neurosurgery 21:**347-351, 1987

74. Holmes G: The Goulstonian lectures on spinal injuries of warfare: Part 1. The pathology of acute spinal injuries. **Br Med J 2:**769-774, 1915

75. Hurth M, Sichez J-P: La chirurgie de la charnière cranio-cervicale: étude critique à propos de 63 cas d'hydrosyringomyélie opérés. **Neurochirurgie 25 (Suppl 1):**114-128, 1979

76. Jirásek A: Endomyelographie bei Syringomyelie. **Zentralbl Chir 54:**2447-2452, 1927

77. Joffroy A, Achard: De la myélite cavitaire. **Arch Physiol Norm Pathol (3eme série) 10:**435-472, 1887

78. Jonesco-Sisesti N: **Tumeurs Médullaires Associées à un Processus Syringomyélique.** Paris: Masson, 1929

79. Kirgis HD, Echols DH: Syringo-encephalomyelia. Discussion of related syndromes and pathologic processes, with a report of a case. **J Neurosurg 6:** 368-375, 1949

80. Krayenbühl H: Evaluation of the different surgical approaches in the treatment of syringomyelia. **Clin Neurol Neurosurg 77:**110-128, 1974

81. Laha RK, Malik HG, Langille RA: Post-traumatic syringomyelia. **Surg Neurol 4:**519-522, 1975

82. Langhans T: Über Höhlenbildung im Rückenmark in folge Blutstauung. **Arch Pathol Anat Physiol 85:** 1-25, 1881

83. Léri A: Radiologie, in Marie P (ed): **La Pratique Neurologique.** Paris: Masson, 1911, pp 1163-1190

84. Lesoin F, Petit H, Thomas III CE, et al: Use of the syringoperitoneal shunt in the treatment of syringomyelia. **Surg Neurol 25:**131-136, 1986

85. Levaditi C, Lépine P, Schoen R: Contribution

expérimentale à l'étude étiologique de la syringomyélie. **Bull Acad Med (3eme série) 101:** 669-680, 1929

86. Levy WJ, Mason R, Hahn JF: Chiari malformation presenting in adults: a surgical experience in 127 cases. **Neurosurgery 12:**377-390, 1983

87. Leyden E: Über Hydromyelus und Syringomyelie. **Arch Path Anat Physiol 68:**1-20, 1876

88. Lichtenstein BW: Cervical syringomyelia and syringomyelia-like states associated with Arnold-Chiari deformity and platybasia. **Arch Neurol Psychiatry 49:**881-894, 1943

89. Lichtenstein BW, Zeitlin H: Ganglioneuroma of the spinal cord associated with pseudosyringomyelia: a histologic study. **Arch Neurol Psychiatry 37:** 1356-1370, 1937

90. List CF: Neurologic syndromes accompanying developmental anomalies of occipital bone, atlas and axis. **Arch Neurol Psychiatry 45:**577-616, 1941

91. Logue V: Syringomyelia: a radiodiagnostic and radiotherapeutic saga. **Clin Radiol 22:**2-16, 1971

92. Logue V, Edwards MR: Syringomyelia and its surgical treatment—an analysis of 75 patients. **J Neurol Neurosurg Psychiatry 44:**273-284, 1981

93. Love JG, Olafson RA: Syringomyelia: a look at surgical therapy. **J Neurosurg 24:**714-718, 1966

94. Mackay RP, Favill J: Syringomyelia and intramedullary tumor of the spinal cord. **Arch Neurol Psychiatry 33:**1255-1278, 1935

95. Markow DA, Gorjelik R, Liwschitz S: Über die Röntgentherapie der spinalen Gliose. **Strahlentherapie 45:**349-354, 1932

96. Matsumoto T, Symon L: Surgical management of syringomyelia—current results. **Surg Neurol 32:** 258-265, 1989

97. McConnell AA, Parker HL: A deformity of the hind-brain associated with internal hydrocephalus. Its relation to the Arnold-Chiari malformation. **Brain 61:**415-429, 1938

98. McLaurin RL, Bailey OT, Schurr PH, et al: Myelomalacia and multiple cavitations of spinal cord secondary to adhesive arachnoiditis: an experimental study. **Arch Pathol 57:**138-146, 1954

99. McLean DR, Miller JDR, Allen PBR, et al: Posttraumatic syringomyelia. **J Neurosurg 39:**485-492, 1973

100. Milhorat TH, Capocelli AL Jr, Anzil AP, et al: Pathological basis of spinal cord cavitation in syringomyelia: analysis of 105 autopsy cases. **J Neurosurg 82:**802-812, 1995

101. Milhorat TH, Johnson WD, Miller JI: Syrinx shunt to posterior fossa cisterns (syringocisternostomy) for bypassing obstructions of upper cervical theca. **J Neurosurg 77:**871-874, 1992

102. Milhorat TH, Johnson WD, Miller JI, et al: Surgical treatment of syringomyelia based on magnetic resonance imaging criteria. **Neurosurgery 31:**231-245, 1992

103. Mixter WJ: Discussion of Frazier CH, Rowe SN: The surgical treatment of syringomyelia. **Ann Surg 103:** 497, 1936

104. Morgagni GB (Alexander B, trans): **The Seats and Causes of Disease.** London: Millar and Cadel, 1769 (Letter XII, Article 9:370)

105. Mucenieks P: Über die operative Therapie der Syringomyelie. **Dtsche Z Chir 240:**346-361, 1933

106. Netsky MG: Syringomyelia: a clinicopathological study. **Arch Neurol Psychiatry 70:**741-777, 1953

107. O'Brien FW: Roentgen therapy in syringomyelia. **Radiology 24:**16-21, 1935

108. Ogryzlo MA: The Arnold-Chiari malformation. **Arch Neurol Psychiatry 48:**30-46, 1942

109. Oldfield EH, Muraszko K, Shawker TH, et al: Pathophysiology of syringomyelia associated with Chiari I malformation of the cerebellar tonsils. Implications for diagnosis and treatment. **J Neurosurg 80:**3-15, 1994

110. Ollivier d'Angers CP: **De la Moelle Epinière et de ses Maladies.** Paris: Chez Crevot, 1824

111. Ollivier d'Angers CP: **Traité de la Moelle Epinière et de ses Maladies.** Paris: Chez Crevot, 1827, pp 178-183

112. Ollivier d'Angers CP: **Traité des Maladies de la Moelle Epinière.** Paris: Méquignon-Marvis Père et Fils, 1837

113. Oppel WA: Erfahrungen mit der operativen Behandlung der Syringomyelie nach Poussepp. **Arch Klin Chir 155:**416-434, 1929

114. Oppenheim H: **Lehrbuch der Nervenkrankheiten für Ärzte und Studirende.** ed 2. Berlin: S Karger, 1898

115. Osborne DRS, Vavoulis G, Nashold BS Jr, et al: Late sequelae of spinal cord trauma. Myelographic and surgical correlation. **J Neurosurg 57:**18-23, 1982

116. Padovani R, Cavallo M, Gaist G: Surgical treatment of syringomyelia: favorable results with syringosubarachnoid shunting. **Surg Neurol 32:**173-180, 1989

117. Peerless SJ, Durward QJ: Management of syringomyelia: a pathophysiological approach. **Clin Neurosurg 30:**531-576, 1983

118. Peiper H: Die operative Behandlung der Syringomyelie. **Nervenarzt 4:**436-453, 1931

119. Penfield W, Coburn DF: Arnold-Chiari malformation and its operative treatment. **Arch Neurol Psychiatry 40:**328-336, 1938

120. Philippe C, Oberthür: Classifications des cavités pathologiques intramédullaires. **Rev Neurol 8:** 171-175, 1900

121. Philippon J, Sangla S, Lara-Morales J, et al: Treatment of syringomyelia by syringo-peritoneal shunt. **Acta Neurochir (Suppl) 43:**32-34, 1988

122. Phillips TW, Kindt GW: Syringoperitoneal shunt for syringomyelia: a preliminary report. **Surg Neurol 16:**462-466, 1981

123. Portal A: **Cours d'Anatomie Médicale.** Paris: Beaudoin, 1803, Vol 4, pp 117-118

124. Poser CM: **The Relationship Between Syringomyelia and Neoplasm.** Springfield, Ill: Charles C Thomas, 1956

125. Poussepp L: Traitement opératoire dans deux cas de syringomyélie. Amélioration notable. **Rev Neurol 45:**1171-1179, 1926

126. Rath G: Charles Estienne: Contemporary of Vesalius. **Med Hist 8:**354-359, 1964

127. Raymond F: La syringomyélie. **Rev Generale Clinique Therapeutique 19:**817-818, 1905

128. Rhoton AL Jr: Microsurgery of Arnold-Chiari malformation in adults with and without hydromyelia. **J Neurosurg 45:**473-483, 1976

129. Rossier AB, Foo D, Shillito J, et al: Posttraumatic cervical syringomyelia. Incidence, clinical presentation, electrophysiological studies, syrinx protein and results of conservative and operative treatment.

Brain 108:439-461, 1985

130. Rossier AB, Foo D, Shillito J, et al: Posttraumatic syringomyelia: incidence, clinical presentation, electrophysiological studies, syrinx protein and results of conservative and operative treatment. **Brain 108:** 439-461, 1985

131. Rossier AB, Werner A, Wildi E, et al: Contribution to the study of late cervical syringomyelic syndromes after dorsal or lumbar traumatic paraplegia. **J Neurol Neurosurg Psychiatry** 31:99-105, 1968

132. Rullier DM: Destruction d'une grande partie de la moelle épinière avec contracture des bras, et mobilité parfaite des membres inférieurs. **J Physiol Exp Pathol** 3:173-190, 1823

133. Russell DS, Donald C: Mechanism of internal hydrocephalus in spina bifida. **Brain** 58:203-215, 1935

134. Sahatchieff S: Le traitement de la syringomyélie par rayons X. **Bulletin Officiel de la Société Française d'Electrothérapie et de la Radiologie Médicale.** 1912, p 233

135. Sarnat HB: Embryology and dysgeneses of the posterior fossa, in Batzdorf U (ed): **Syringomyelia: Current Concepts in Diagnosis and Treatment.** Baltimore, Md: Williams & Wilkins, 1991, pp 3-34

136. Schaeffer H: Le traitement opératoire de la syringomyélie. **Presse Med** 40:379-383, 1932

137. Schlesinger EB, Antunes JL, Michelsen WJ, et al: Hydromyelia: clinical presentation and comparison of modalities of treatment. **Neurosurgery 9:** 356-365, 1981

138. Schlesinger H: **Beiträge zur Klinik der Rückenmarks—und Wirbeltumoren.** Jena: Fischer, 1898

139. Schlesinger H: **Die Syringomyelie.** Leipzig/Vienna: Franz Deuticke, 1895

140. Schlesinger H: **Die Syringomyelie.** Leipzig/Vienna: Franz Deuticke, 1902

141. Schultze F: Klinisches und Anatomisches über die Syringomyelie. **Z Klin Med** 13:523-557, 1888

142. Schultze F: Über Spalt, Höhlen und Ghombildung im Rückenmark und in der Medulla oblongata. **Virchows Arch** 87:510-540, 1882

143. Schurch B, Wichmann W, Rossier AB: Post-traumatic syringomyelia (cystic myelopathy): a prospective study of 449 patients with spinal cord injury. **J Neurol Neurosurg Psychiatry** 60:61-67, 1996

144. Schwalbe E, Gredig M: Über Entwicklungsstörungen des Kleinhirns, Hirnstamms und Halsmarks bei Spina bifida (Arnold'sche und Chiari'sche Missbildung). **Beitr Pathol Anat** 40:132-194, 1907

145. Sett P, Crockard HA: The value of magnetic resonance imaging (MRI) in the follow-up management of spinal injury. **Paraplegia** 29:396-410, 1991

146. Sgouros S, Williams B: A critical appraisal of drainage for syringomyelia. **J Neurosurg** 82:1-10, 1995

147. Sicard JA, Forestier J: Méthode radiographique d'exploration de la cavité épidurale par le Lipiodol. **Rev Neurol** 2:1264-1266, 1921

148. Sicard JA, Haguenau J, Mayer C: Lipiodol intraépendymaire chez un syringomyélique opéré. Suites opératoires. **Rev Neurol** 46:418-421, 1926

149. Simon T: Über Syringomyelie und Geschwulstbildung in Rückenmark. **Arch Psychiatr Nervenkrankh** 5:120-163, 1875

150. Simpson JA, Weiner ESC: **The Oxford English Dictionary.** 2nd ed. Oxford: Clarendon Press, 1989, Vol

17, p 494

151. Singounas EG, Karvounis PC: Terminal ventriculostomy in syringomyelia. **Acta Neurochir 46:** 293-295, 1979

152. Squier MV, Lehr RP: Post-traumatic syringomyelia. **J Neurol Neurosurg Psychiatry** 57:1095-1098, 1994

153. Steele GH: The Arnold-Chiari malformation. **Br J Surg** 34:280-282, 1947

154. Stephanus C: **De dissectione partium corporis humani libri tres.** Paris: Simon de Collines, 1545

155. Stilling B: **Neue Untersuchungen über den Bau des Rückenmarks.** Cassel: Verlag von Heinrich Hotop, 1856, pp 4-27

156. Strümpell A: Beiträge zur Pathologie des Rückenmarks. I Spastische Spinalparalysen. **Arch Psychiatr Nervenkrankh** 10:676-717, 1880

157. Sullivan LP, Stears JC, Ringel SP: Resolution of syringomyelia and Chiari I malformation by ventriculoatrial shunting in a patient with pseudotumor cerebri and a lumboperitoneal shunt. **Neurosurgery** 22:744-747, 1988

158. Tamaki K, Lubin AJ: Pathogenesis of syringomyelia: case illustrating the process of cavity formation from embryonic cell rests. **Arch Neurol Psychiatry** 40:748-761, 1938

159. Tator CH, Meguro K, Rowed DW: Favorable results with syringosubarachnoid shunts for treatment of syringomyelia. **J Neurosurg** 56:517-523, 1982

160. Tauber ES, Langworthy OR: A study of syringomyelia and the formation of cavities in the spinal cord. **J Nerv Ment Dis** 81:245-264, 1935

161. van Houweninge Graftdijk CJ: **Over Hydrocephalus.** Leyden: Eduard Ijdo, 1932

162. Vernon JD, Silver JR, Ohry A: Post-traumatic syringomyelia. **Paraplegia** 20:339-364, 1982

163. Vitek J: La ponction dorsale thérapeutique et diagnostique des cavités syringomyéliques. L'endomyélographie au lipiodol injecté sans operation dans les poches syringomyéliques. **Bruxelles Med 9:** 311-313, 1928

164. Vitek J: Nouvelle méthode décompressive et évacuatrice de la cavité syringomyélique par ponction faite à son pôle inférieur. Ponction bipolaire de la cavité syringomyélique. **Presse Med** 40:1507-1508, 1932

165. Wagner FC Jr, Dohrmann GJ, Bucy PC: Histopathology of transitory traumatic paraplegia in the monkey. **J Neurosurg** 35:272-276, 1971

166. Weed LH: **The Development of the Cerebro-Spinal Fluid Spaces in Pig and Man; Contributions to Embryology, 5:14.** Washington, DC: Carnegie Institute of Washington, Publication No 225, 1917, pp 1-116

167. Welch K, Shillito J, Strand R, et al: Chiari I "malformation"—an acquired disorder? **J Neurosurg** 55:604-609, 1981

168. West RJ, Williams B: Radiographic studies of the ventricles in syringomyelia. **Neuroradiology 20:** 5-16, 1980

169. Westberg G: Gas myelography and percutaneous puncture in the diagnosis of spinal cord cysts. **Acta Radiol (Suppl)** 252:1-67, 1966

170. Williams B: A critical appraisal of posterior fossa surgery for communicating syringomyelia. **Brain** 101:223-250, 1978

171. Williams B: The distending force in the production of "communicating syringomyelia." **Lancet 2:**

189-193, 1969

172. Williams B: The distending force in the production of communicating syringomyelia. **Lancet 2:**41-42, 1970 (Letter)

173. Williams B: On the pathogenesis of syringomyelia: a review. **J R Soc Med 73:**798-806, 1980

174. Williams B: Syringomyelia. **Neurosurg Clin North Am 1:**653-685, 1990

175. Williams B, Bentley J: Experimental communicating syringomyelia in dogs after cisternal kaolin injection. Part 1. Morphology. **J Neurol Sci 48:**93-107, 1980

176. Williams B, Fahy G: A critical appraisal of "terminal ventriculostomy" for the treatment of syringomyelia. **J Neurosurg 58:**188-197, 1983

177. Williams B, Page N: Surgical treatment of syringomyelia with syringopleural shunting. **Br J Neurosurg 1:**63-80, 1987

178. Williams B, Terry AF, Jones HWF, et al: Syringomyelia as a sequel to traumatic paraplegia. **Paraplegia 19:**67-80, 1981

179. Wilson SAK: Syringomyelia: syringobulbia, in Bruce AN (ed): **Neurology.** London: Edward Arnold, 1940, p 1404

180. Wisoff JH, Epstein F: Management of hydromyelia. **Neurosurgery 25:**562-571, 1989

181. Woodard JS, Freeman LW: Ischemia of the spinal cord: an experimental study. **J Neurosurg 13:**63-72, 1956

182. Wyburn-Mason R: **The Vascular Abnormalities and Tumours of the Spinal Cord and Its Membranes.** London: H Kimpton, 1943

183. Yamada H, Yokota A, Haratake J, et al: Morphological study of experimental syringomyelia with kaolin-induced hydrocephalus in a canine model. **J Neurosurg 84:**999-1005, 1996

CHAPTER 2

CLASSIFICATION OF THE CHIARI MALFORMATIONS AND SYRINGOMYELIA

NAZIH MOUFARRIJ, MD, AND ISSAM A. AWAD, MD, MSC, FACS

They do certainly give strange and new-fangled names to diseases! — Plato

Stedman's *Medical Dictionary* defines "classification" as a systematic arrangement into classes or groups. Since ancient times, diseases have been classified to facilitate understanding of etiology or prognosis, to clarify pathophysiological mechanisms, or to guide therapeutic intervention. Mostly, such arrangement has reflected current thinking and prevailing theories of disease. Classification has evolved with expanding knowledge so as to accommodate novel concepts and hypotheses, including a more refined and mechanistic definition of individual pathological entities.

During the past decade, a large amount of information has contributed to a rethinking of the classification of the Chiari malformations and syringomyelia.[5,7] This information came from a variety of sources, including magnetic resonance imaging (MRI),[1,8,20,32,35,38,42,48,49,53,56,59,64] cine MRI,[44,62] intraoperative ultrasonography,[5,44] clinical series[4,6,32,35,36,40,42,44,48-51,53,54,56-58,66,68] and case reports,[3,9,21,26,28,29,31,43,55,61,65,69] autopsy and pathological studies,[3,5,33,34,37,52] as well as experimental investigations.[11,14,39] This chapter will attempt to synthesize this material into a practical work-

ing classification of the Chiari malformation and syringomyelia. Although the Chiari malformation is the most common cause of syringomyelia, the two entities may present independently and are often distinct in their clinical manifestations. For the sake of clarity, the two entities will be classified and discussed separately. Proposed classification schemes will attempt to reflect, whenever possible, pathophysiological categorizations and features which have been shown to affect clinical management or prognosis.

THE CHIARI MALFORMATIONS

Conventional Classification

Hans Chiari was the first to classify the various degrees of hindbrain herniation through the foramen magnum, describing the types I, II, and III, which continue to be referred to in current literature.[13,16,17,30] Of note is the presence of intermediary forms among these types. Type IV was later added to Chiari's original classification. The history of the nomenclature of the Chiari malformation and the controversies regarding Julius Arnold's contribution are discussed in detail in a separate chapter of this book.

The type I malformation consists of herniation of the cerebellar tonsils and sometimes part of the medulla below the foramen magnum. Recently, Badie et al[1] demonstrated that patients with a type I malformation had a significantly smaller posterior fossa compared to control subjects. They defined the posterior fossa ratio as the volume of the posterior fossa divided by the volume of the supratentorial area as calculated from MRI. They also found that Chiari I malformation patients with a smaller posterior fossa ratio tended to develop symptoms earlier and respond better to suboccipital decompression than those with a normal posterior fossa ratio.[1]

The type II malformation as described by Chiari included herniation of the cerebellar vermis, the fourth ventricle, a greater part of the medulla, and sometimes part of the pons through the foramen magnum. This type is commonly associated with lumbar myelomeningoceles[21,50,63] and hydrocephalus.

The type III malformation includes herniation of the posterior fossa contents into the high cervical canal and to various degrees into a cervical-occipital meningocele.[45]

The type IV malformation refers to cases with hypoplasia of the cerebellum. Since this is not a hindbrain hernia, it is often dropped from the classification of Chiari malformation and is of historical interest only.

Classification Based on the Presence or Absence of Syringomyelia

The conventional classification described above has the disadvantages of being unable to accommodate intermediary forms (especially between types I and II) and does not consider the presence or absence of syringomyelia, which is important from the standpoint of clinical presentation, management, and outcome.[4,6,7,48,49] The advent of MRI has allowed a superior definition of the pathoanatomical correlates in these cases. Among adult patients with features of Chiari I or II malformation and minimal or no association of myelodysplasia and hydrocephalus, there is an emerging consensus that categorical differences among types I and II may be quite arbitrary.[6,7,27,30,51,53] It remains important to note that Chiari II malformation presents mostly in childhood and may be associated with lumbar myelomeningocele.[17,41,50,63] Earlier clinical presentation is likely due to the extent of hindbrain herniation and/or associated craniospinal dysmorphism, rather than an arbitrary categorization of type I and II malformations.[10] Syringomyelia may develop in Chiari II malformation cases, most notably after repair of myelomeningocele (see below).[50,63]

This information coupled with clinical correlation regarding presentation and outcome allowed the formulation by Pillay et al[47-49] in 1991 of a novel classification of symptomatic Chiari malformation based on the presence or absence of syringomyelia, independent of the degree of hindbrain herniation. They noted that Chiari malformation patients with hindbrain herniation alone typically had a better prognosis than patients with associated syringomyelia and responded better to surgical intervention. These observations have since been confirmed by others.[7]

Acquired Chiari Malformation and Other Less Common Associations

Chiari malformation has been noted to occur after lumboperitoneal shunting, with an incidence on MRI of approximately 70%;[15] more than one-half of these cases are potentially symptomatic.[46] Acquired Chiari malformation has also been reported after multiple lumbar punctures, after shunting of a prepontine arachnoid cyst, in the presence of bilateral chronic subdural hematomas, and *de novo* in an adult without apparent cause as demonstrated on serial MRI.[19,40,56] An association between Chiari malformation and neurofibromatosis was reported in one series as 4%.[8] A genetic basis for Chiari malformation was suggested in an adult triplet with MRI documentation of the malformation, with each member being affected to a variable degree.[10]

The Chiari Malformations: Proposed Comprehensive Classification

The Chiari malformation is defined as a hindbrain herniation without associated mass lesion or hydrocephalus. A comprehensive classification is proposed synthesizing the above categories into a simple but relevant working scheme (Table 1).

Category I would include any Chiari malformation, irrespective of the amount of hindbrain herniation but exclusive of associated lumbar myelomeningocele or occipital-cervical encephalocele. This is further subdivided into congenital and acquired categories with specific clinical associations. The presence or absence of associated syringomyelia is also noted.

Category II would include any Chiari malformation in association with lumbar myelodysplasia.[50,63] This type also may or may not be associated with hydrocephalus or syringomyelia.

Category III would include any Chiari malformation, irrespective of the amount of hindbrain herniation but with associated occipital-cervical encephalocele. It may or may not be associated with syringomyelia.

TABLE 1
PROPOSED COMPREHENSIVE CLASSIFICATION OF THE CHIARI MALFORMATIONS

I. Hindbrain herniation (tonsils ± brain stem) without lumbar myelomeningocele or occipital-cervical encephalocele
   1) congenital
   2) acquired
      a. basal arachnoiditis
      b. lumboperitoneal shunts
      c. multiple lumbar punctures
      d. *de novo*

II. With a lumbar myelomeningocele

III. With an occipital-cervical encephalocele

Each of the above categories is further divided according to the presence or absence of associated syringomyelia.

SYRINGOMYELIA

The term "syringomyelia" is used to indicate the presence of a fluid-filled cavity within the spinal cord. We use this term to include hydromyelia, which traditionally referred to a dilatation of the central canal by cerebrospinal fluid (CSF) that is usually in communication with the fourth ventricle.[68]

The Barnett Pathoetiological Classification

Barnett et al[3] are credited with contributing the first English monograph on syringomyelia in 1973. They concluded their work by proposing a working classification of this disease, and correctly foresaw that their classification would be updated and restructured as new information became available.[5,34,38,48] They classified syringomyelia into five categories as follows:

1. Communicating syringomyelia (syringo-hydromyelia). The term "communicating" was used to indicate communication with the CSF space and not with the fourth ventricle.
   a) With developmental anomalies at the foramen magnum and in the posterior fossa.
   b) Associated with acquired abnormalities at the base of the brain (basal arachnoiditis, posterior fossa tumors, and cysts).[12,31]

2. Syringomyelia as a late sequel to trauma.
   a) Serious spinal cord injury.
   b) Mild to moderate spinal cord injury.

3. Syringomyelia as a sequel to spinal arachnoiditis.

4. Syringomyelia associated with spinal cord tumors.

5. Idiopathic syringomyelia. This variety was thought to be apparently unrelated to any of the above pathoetiological factors. It was usually confined to the spinal cord but rarely extended into the brain stem and was without demonstrable communication with the subarachnoid space or fourth ventricle. It is likely that some of these cases represent a *forme fruste* of syringomyelia in association with Chiari malformation.[48]

The Milhorat Classification According to Magnetic Resonance Imaging Features

By fully utilizing the information provided by MRI in the sagittal and axial planes, as well as at the level of the craniovertebral junction and posterior fossa, Milhorat et al[35,36] proposed a novel classification of syringomyelia with therapeutic implications. They strengthened their classification by studying a large autopsy series and demonstrated good correlation between MRI features and histopathology.[33,34,37,38] A synthesis of their categories is as follows:

1. Central syringomyelia. This typically represents an oval or circular dilatation of the central canal, uniformly enlarged except at its poles and at periodic constrictions produced by webs or septa. The etiological categories of this type of syringomyelia include the Chiari malformation, communicating hydrocephalus, and craniocervical and basilar invagination. The syrinx usually communicates with the fourth ventricle as visualized by MRI (probably equivalent to what was classically termed hydromyelia). There is a strong association with hydrocephalus and an implication of disturbed CSF dynamics.[24,43,68]

2. Central syringomyelia with paracentral extension. The paracentral component of the syrinx is typically found at a pole of the cavity and extends preferentially to the posterolateral quadrant of the spinal cord. The paracentral extensions appear in some cases to reach the pial surface, communicating with the subarachnoid space as seen on MRI. This has been confirmed in cases with postmortem correlation. Etiological correlates include Chiari malformation, basilar invagination, other base-of-skull pathology, trauma, degenerative spinal disease, communicating hydrocephalus, and extramedullary obstructions.[2,4,5,12,23,31-33,38,40,44,51,53,58,61,62,69] The cavities are usually caudal to the obstructive lesion. Like the first category, this is thought to be due to disturbance in CSF dynamics, but without typical communication with the fourth ventricle.

3. Eccentric syringomyelia. By definition, these cavities do not involve the central canal. They are usually the result of spinal cord injury such as trauma, spondylosis, disc herniation, infection, transverse myelitis, infarction, hemorrhage (spontaneous or from a vascular malformation), or radiation necrosis, with resulting myelomalacia.[5,20,29,33,52] The location of the cavity is usually dorsal and lateral to the central canal and in the watershed zone between the anterior and posterior spinal artery territories.

Syringomyelia:
Proposed Comprehensive Classification

A comprehensive classification scheme may be considered, integrating classical pathoetiological concepts and the more novel MRI and pathological information. The following six categories are intended to represent a practical classification with implications regarding surgical management and prognosis (Table 2).

I. Syringomyelia communicating with the fourth ventricle. The communication would be demonstrated by an imaging modality, usually MRI. This category constitutes about 10% of the total cases of syringomyelia, significantly less than previously thought. The cavities are usually of the central type as described by Milhorat et al, and a shunting procedure may be a therapeutic option.[43,58,59] In some of these cases, there also may be blockage to CSF circulation as noted below (i.e., in association with Chiari malformation).

II. Syringomyelia due to blockage of CSF circulation (without fourth ventricular communication). Enough evidence has accumulated to indicate that a block to CSF circulation, anywhere from the basal posterior fossa and caudally, can cause syringomyelia.[2,5,12,24,25,27,28,31,33,47,69] This is likely the most common category of syringomyelia, accounting for at least one-half of the cases. The prime example at the posterior fossa level is the Chiari malformation, although the Chiari malformation may also cause communicating syringomyelia (see above). Other etiological categories include: basal adhesive arachnoiditis (including postinflammatory and posttraumatic) and compressive pathology. Release of adhesions, decompression at the level of blockage, and shunting procedures are associated with variable and usually transient success.

III. Syringomyelia due to spinal cord injury. The mechanisms of injury vary, including postnecrotic cavitation following ischemic injury, posthemorrhagic cavitation, degenerative disease, and posttraumatic myelomalacia.[12,14,18,20,66,69] Focal arachnoiditis may further contribute to cord cavitation.[20] These syringes are typically eccentric, focal (at the level of pathology), and with an associated signal of cord gliosis. This category likely accounts for less than 10% of cases of syringomyelia.

IV. Syringomyelia and spinal dysraphism. Spinal dysraphism may cause syringomyelia via a variety of mechanisms,[12,23,41] including those mentioned under the previous three categories. Identification and treatment of associated dysraphism (including untethering and release of adhesions) likely has the greatest impact on arresting progression of syringomyelia.

V. Syringomyelia due to intramedullary tumors. The fluid in this type of syringomyelia is usually a secretory result of neoplastic cells or is post-hemorrhagic. Unlike CSF, it is yellowish, and proteinaceous. Fluid formation within the cavity may be contributed to by a block to CSF flow (mass effect from the tumor and/or adhesive arachnoiditis) via a mechanism described under the second category above. In one report, the most common tumors associated with syringomyelia were ependymomas and hemangioblastomas.[54] With the advent of MRI with gadolinium enhancement, this category is relatively easily defined through more accurate delineation of the associated neoplasm. The extramedullary intradural and extradural tumors are best considered separately (under the second category above) because they cause syringomyelia by block to CSF flow primarily and because their surgical management is somewhat different.

VI. Idiopathic syringomyelia. This category includes cases not classifiable under any of the above categories.

TABLE 2

Proposed Comprehensive Classification of Syringomyelia

I. Communicating (with the fourth ventricle) as demonstrated by imaging studies

II. Blockage of CSF circulation
  1) at the posterior fossa-craniovertebral junction level
    a. Chiari malformation
      • congenital
      • acquired
    b. basal adhesive arachnoiditis
      • postinfectious
        meningitis
      • chemical
        contrast material
      • from blood in subarachnoid space
        trauma (birth, surgical, other)
        subarachnoid hemorrhage
        intraparenchymal hemorrhage
      • inflammatory
        sarcoid
        after radiation therapy
    c. masses
      • cysts
        arachnoid
        Dandy-Walker
      • infections
        pyogenic abscesses
        tuberculomas
        hydatid
        other
      • inflammatory
        rheumatoid arthritis pannus
      • occipital encephalocele
    d. basilar impression/invagination
    e. meningeal carcinomatosis

  2) at the spinal level
    a. tumors
      • intradural–extramedullary
      • meningeal carcinomatosis
      • extradural
    b. arachnoid cysts
    c. adhesive arachnoiditis (as above)
      • infections
      • from blood in subarachnoid space

      • chemical (contrast material, medications)
      • postoperative
      • traumatic
    d. infectious masses
      • tuberculosis (Pott's disease)
      • hydatid
      • epidural or subdural abscesses

III. Injury to spinal cord tissue (usually eccentric syringomyelia)
  1) trauma
  2) radiation necrosis
  3) infarction
    a. arterial
    b. venous (including dural arteriovenous malformation)
  4) hemorrhage
    a. arteriovenous malformation
    b. tumor
    c. aneurysm
  5) infection
    a. transverse myelitis
    b. intramedullary abscess
    c. syphilis
    d. human immunodeficiency virus
  6) post-inflammatory
    a. transverse myelitis
    b. demyelinating disease
  7) degenerative spinal cord disease
    a. amyotrophic lateral sclerosis
    b. compressive myelopathy (disc disease, canal stenosis)

IV. Dysraphism

V. Intramedullary Tumors
  1) primary
  2) metastatic

VI. Idiopathic syringomyelia
  1) occult block to CSF circulation
  2) *forme fruste* of Chiari malformation (block at craniocervical level or communicating syringomyelia)
  3) other unknown mechanisms

Conclusion

Numerous classifications have been discussed for the Chiari malformations and syringomyelia, reflecting the evolution of understanding of the associated diseases. We have integrated the various schemes into a broad categorization of the two entities, considering pathoetiological, prognostic, and therapeutic implications. These classifications are practical and pragmatic, and necessarily temporary, with evolving pathophysiological concepts and diagnostic and therapeutic possibilities. The individual categories are discussed in subsequent chapters, including the many arguments for and against their respective separate consideration.

References

1. Badie B, Mendoza D, Batzdorf U: Posterior fossa volume and response to suboccipital decompression in patients with Chiari I malformation. **Neurosurgery** 37:214-218, 1995

2. Barnett HJM, Foster JB, Hudgson P (eds): **Syringomyelia.** London: WB Saunders, 1973, pp 30-49

3. Barnett HJM, Rewcastle NB: Syringomyelia and tumors of the nervous system, in Barnett HJM, Foster JB, Hudgson P (eds): **Syringomyelia.** London: WB Saunders, 1973, pp 261-301

4. Batzdorf U: Chiari I malformation with syringomyelia. Evaluation of surgical therapy by magnetic resonance imaging. **J Neurosurg** 68:726-730, 1988

5. Batzdorf U (ed): **Syringomyelia: Current Concepts in Diagnosis and Treatment.** Baltimore, Md: Williams & Wilkins, 1991

6. Bell WO, Charney EB, Bruce DA, et al: Symptomatic Arnold-Chiari malformation: review of experience with 22 cases. **J Neurosurg** 66:812-816, 1987

7. Bindal AK, Dunsker SB, Tew JM Jr: Chiari I malformation: classification and management. **Neurosurgery** 37:1069-1074, 1995

8. Bognanno IR, Edward MK, Lee TA, et al: Cranial MR imaging in neurofibromatosis. **AJR** 151:381-388, 1988

9. Bondurant CP, Oró JJ: Spinal cord injury without radiographic abnormality and Chiari malformation. **J Neurosurg** 79:833-838, 1993

10. Cavender RK, Schmidt JH III: Tonsillar ectopia and Chiari malformations: monozygotic triplets. Case report. **J Neurosurg** 82:497-500, 1995

11. Chakrabortty S, Tamaki N, Ehara K, et al: Experimental syringomyelia in the rabbit: an ultrastructural study of the spinal cord tissue. **Neurosurgery** 35:1112-1120, 1994

12. Chapman PH, Frim DM: Symptomatic syringomyelia following surgery to treat retethering of lipomyelomeningoceles. **J Neurosurg** 82:752-755, 1995

13. Chiari H: Concerning alterations in the cerebellum resulting from cerebral hydrocephalus. **Pediatr Neurosci** 13:3-8, 1987 (translation, classical article; original 1891)

14. Cho KH, Iwasaki Y, Imamura H, et al: Experimental model of posttraumatic syringomyelia: the role of adhesive arachnoiditis in syrinx formation. **J Neurosurg** 80:133-139, 1994

15. Chumas PD, Armstrong DC, Drake JM, et al: Tonsillar herniation: the rule rather than the exception after lumboperitoneal shunting in the pediatric population. **J Neurosurg** 78:568-573, 1993

16. Gardner WJ, Goodall RJ: The surgical treatment of Arnold-Chiari malformation in adults: an explanation of its mechanism and importance of encephalography in diagnosis. **J Neurosurg** 7:199-213, 1950

17. Haines SJ, Berger M: Current treatment of Chiari malformations types I and II: a survey of the Pediatric Section of the American Association of Neurological Surgeons. **Neurosurgery** 28:353-357, 1991

18. Hamada K, Sudoh K, Fukaura H, et al: [An autopsy case of amyotrophic lateral sclerosis associated with cervical syringomyelia.] **No To Shinkei** 46:527-531, 1990 (Jpn)

19. Hassounah MI, Rahm BE: Hindbrain herniation: an unusual occurrence after shunting an intracranial arachnoid cyst. Case report. **J Neurosurg** 81:126-129, 1994

20. Hida K, Iwasaki Y, Imamura H, et al: Posttraumatic syringomyelia: its characteristic magnetic resonance imaging findings and surgical management. **Neurosurgery** 35:886-891, 1994

21. Holiday PO III, Pillsbury D, Kelly DL, et al: Brain stem auditory evoked potential in Arnold-Chiari malformation: possible prognostic value and changes with surgical decompression. **Neurosurgery** 16:48-53, 1985

22. Huang PP, Constantini S: "Acquired" Chiari I malformation. Case report. **J Neurosurg** 80:1099-1102, 1994

23. Iskandar BJ, Oakes WJ, McLaughlin C, et al: Terminal syringohydromyelia and occult spinal dysraphism. **J Neurosurg** 81:513-519, 1994

24. Isu T, Iwasaki Y, Akino M, et al: Hydrosyringomyelia associated with a Chiari I malformation in children and adolescents. **Neurosurgery** 26:591-597, 1990

25. Isu T, Sasaki S, Takamura H, et al: Foramen magnum decompression with removal of the outer layer of the dura as treatment for syringomyelia occurring with Chiari I malformation. **Neurosurgery** 33:845-850, 1993

26. Jack CR Jr, Kokmen E, Onofrio BM: Spontaneous decompression of syringomyelia: magnetic resonance imaging findings. Case report. **J Neurosurg** 74:283-286, 1991

27. Kobayashi T, Ogawa A, Kameyama M, et al: Chiari malformation with compression of the medulla oblongata by the vertebral arteries. Case report. **J Neurosurg** 77:307-309, 1992

28. Kosary IZ, Braham J, Shaked I, et al: Cervical syringomyelia associated with occipital meningioma. **Neurology** 19:1127-1130, 1969

29. Levy R, Rosenblatt S, Russell E: Percutaneous drainage and serial magnetic resonance imaging in the diagnosis of symptomatic post-traumatic syringomyelia: case report and review of the literature. **Neurosurgery** 29:429-434, 1991

30. Levy WJ, Mason LN, Hahn JF: Chiari malformation presenting in adults: a surgical experience in 127 cases. **Neurosurgery** 12:377-390, 1983

31. Lovely TJ, Buchheit WA: Syringomyelia as a postoperative sequela of the resection of a chordoma of the clivus: case report. **Neurosurgery** 28:431-433, 1993

32. Masur H, Oberwittler C: Syringomyelia in Chiari malformation: relation to extent of cerebellar tissue herniation. **Neurosurgery** 33:948-949, 1993 (Letter)

33. Milhorat TH, Capocelli AL Jr, Anzil AP, et al: Pathological basis of spinal cord cavitation in syringomyelia: analysis of 105 autopsy cases. **J Neurosurg** 82:802-812, 1995

34. Milhorat TH, Johnson RW, Milhorat RH, et al: Clinicopathological correlations in syringomyelia using axial magnetic resonance imaging. **Neurosurgery** 37:206-213, 1995

35. Milhorat TH, Johnson WD, Miller JI: Syrinx shunt to posterior fossa cisterns (syringocisternostomy) for bypassing obstructions of upper cervical theca. **J Neurosurg** 77:871-874, 1992

36. Milhorat TH, Johnson WD, Miller JI, et al: Surgical treatment of syringomyelia based on magnetic resonance imaging criteria. **Neurosurgery** 31:231-245, 1992

37. Milhorat TH, Kotzen RM, Anzil AP: Stenosis of central canal of the spinal cord in man: incidence and

pathological findings in 232 autopsy cases. **J Neurosurg 80:**716-722, 1994

38. Milhorat TH, Miller JI, Johnson WD, et al: Anatomical basis of syringomyelia occurring with hindbrain lesions. **Neurosurgery 32:**748-754, 1994

39. Milhorat TH, Nobandegani F, Miller JI, et al: Noncommunicating syringomyelia following occlusion of the central canal in rats. Experimental model and histological findings. **J Neurosurg 78:**274-279, 1993

40. Morioka T, Shono T, Nishio S, et al: Acquired Chiari I malformation and syringomyelia associated with bilateral chronic subdural hematoma. Case report. **J Neurosurg 83:**556-558, 1995

41. Muhonen MG, Menezes AH, Sawin PD, et al: Scoliosis in pediatric Chiari malformations without myelodysplasia. **J Neurosurg 77:**69-77, 1992

42. Newman PK, Terenty TR, Foster JB: Some observations on the pathogenesis of syringomyelia. **J Neurol Neurosurg Psychiatry 44:**964-969, 1981

43. Ogilvy CS, Borges LF: Treatment of symptomatic syringomyelia with a ventriculoperitoneal shunt: a case report with magnetic resonance scan correlation. **Neurosurgery 22:**748-750, 1988

44. Oldfield EH, Muraszko K, Shawker TH, et al: Pathophysiology of syringomyelia associated with Chiari I malformation of the cerebellar tonsils. Implications for diagnosis and treatment. **J Neurosurg 80:**3-15, 1994

45. Pang D, Dias MS: Cervical myelomeningoceles. **Neurosurgery 33:**363-373, 1993

46. Payner TD, Prenger E, Berger TS, et al: Acquired Chiari malformations: incidence, diagnosis and management. **Neurosurgery 34:**429-434, 1994

47. Pillay PK, Awad IA, Hahn JF: Gardner's hydrodynamic theory of syringomyelia revisited. **Cleve Clin J Med 59:**373-380, 1992

48. Pillay PK, Awad IA, Little JR, et al: Surgical management of syringomyelia: a five year experience in the era of magnetic resonance imaging. **Neurol Res 13:** 3-9, 1991

49. Pillay PK, Awad IA, Little JR, et al: Symptomatic Chiari malformation in adults: a new classification based on magnetic resonance imaging with clinical and prognostic significance. **Neurosurgery 28:** 639-645, 1991

50. Pollack IF, Pang D, Albright AL, et al: Outcome following hindbrain decompression of symptomatic Chiari malformations in children previously treated with myelomeningocele closure and shunts. **J Neurosurg 77:**881-888, 1992

51. Raftopoulos C, Sauchez A, Matos C, et al: Hydrosyringomyelia–Chiari I complex. Prospective evaluation of a modified foramen magnum decompression procedure: Preliminary results. **Surg Neurol 39:** 162-169, 1993

52. Reddy KKV, Del Bigio MR, Sutherland GR: Ultrastructure of the human posttraumatic syrinx. **J Neurosurg 71:**239-243, 1989

53. Sahuquillo J, Rubio E, Poca MA, et al: Posterior fossa reconstruction, a surgical technique for the treatment of Chiari I malformation and Chiari I/syringomyelia complex. Preliminary results and magnetic resonance imaging quantitative assessment of hindbrain migration. **Neurosurgery 35:** 874-885, 1994

54. Samii M, Klekamp J: Surgical results of 100 intramedullary tumors in relation to accompanying syringomyelia. **Neurosurgery 35:**865-873, 1994.

55. Santoro A, Delfini R, Innocenzi G, et al : Spontaneous drainage of syringomyelia. Report of two cases. **J Neurosurg 79:**132-134, 1993.

56. Sathi S, Stieg PE: Acquired Chiari I malformation after multiple lumbar punctures: Case report. **Neurosurgery 32:**306-309, 1993.

57. Sgouros S, Williams B: A critical appraisal of drainage in syringomyelia. **J Neurosurg 82:**1-10, 1995.

58. Stovner LJ, Rinck P: Syringomyelia in Chiari malformation: relation to extent of cerebellar tissue herniation. **Neurosurgery 31:**913-917, 1992

59. Sullivan LP, Stears JC, Ringel SP: Resolution of syringomyelia and Chiari I malformation by ventriculoatrial shunting in a patient with pseudotumor cerebri and a lumboperitoneal shunt. **Neurosurgery 22:** 744-747, 1988

60. Tachibana S, Iida H, Yada K: Significance of positive Queckenstedt test in patients with syringomyelia with Arnold-Chiari malformations. **J Neurosurg 76:** 67-71, 1992

61. Tokoro K, Chiba Y, Yagishita S, et al: Cordectomy for syringobulbo-myelia with sleep apnea secondary to a spinal extramedullary tumor: case report. **Neurosurgery 24:**118-124, 1989

62. Tominaga T, Koshu K, Ogawa A: Transoral decompression evaluated by cine-mode magnetic resonance imaging: a case of basilar impression accompanied by Chiari malformation. **Neurosurgery 28:**883-885, 1991

63. Vandertop WP, Asai A, Hoffman HJ, et al: Surgical decompression for symptomatic Chiari II malformation in neonates with myelomeningocele. **J Neurosurg 77:**541-544, 1992

64. Vaquero J, Martinez R, Arias A: Syringomyelia-Chiari complex: magnetic resonance imaging and clinical evaluation of surgical treatment. **J Neurosurg 73:** 64-68, 1990

65. Vengsarkar US, Panchal VG, Tripathi PD et al: Percutaneous thecoperitoneal shunt. Report of three cases. **J Neurosurg 74:**827-831, 1991

66. Williams B: Difficult labour as a cause of communicating syringomyelia. **Lancet 2:**51-53, 1977

67. Williams B: LP shunting in cases of Chiari malformation. **J Neurosurg 71:**950-951, 1989 (Letter)

68. Wisoff JH, Epstein F: Management of hydromyelia. **Neurosurgery 25:**562-571, 1989

69. Yu HC, Mosley IF: Syringomyelia and cervical spondylosis: a clinicoradiological investigation. **Neuroradiology 29:**143-151, 1987

CHAPTER 3

PATHOGENESIS AND DEVELOPMENT THEORIES

ULRICH BATZDORF, MD

The development of hydrosyringomyelia related to abnormalities at the craniovertebral junction is a complex process that at this time is still incompletely understood. The types of abnormalities at the craniocervical junction seen in conjunction with hydrosyringomyelia can be grouped into several different categories: abnormalities of the bony skeleton; the presence of abnormal soft tissue masses, including neoplasms and inflammatory masses; and displaced but essentially normal neural structures and membranous structures of various types. The large series compiled by Williams[32] attests to the varied etiological factors. It is beyond the scope of this chapter to address factors influencing the development of bony abnormalities, neoplasms, inflammatory masses, or membranes of inflammatory or posthemorrhagic origin at the craniocervical junction. The common features relevant to development of syringohydromyelia will, however, be discussed. Syringomyelia may occur in relation to abnormalities at the craniovertebral junction (Table 1) and, as a consequence of abnormalities at spinal levels, remote from the skull base (Table 2).

As is evident from Williams' review,[32] over 70% of etiological factors related to the development of hydrosyringomyelia, hereafter referred to as syringomyelia, are in the group referred to as hindbrain herniation or Chiari malformation and represent displaced but normal neural structures (Table 1).

TABLE 1

ETIOLOGICAL CATEGORIES FOR SYRINGOMYELIA-RELATED ABNORMALITIES AT THE CRANIOVERTEBRAL JUNCTION

A. Bony abnormalities*
   Small posterior fossa
   Platybasia
   Basilar invagination
   Assimilation of atlas

B. Soft tissue masses of abnormal nature
   Tumors (e.g., meningioma at foramen magnum)
   Inflammatory masses

C. Neural tissue
   Cerebellar tonsils and vermis (e.g., hindbrain herniation and "Chiari malformation")

D. Membranous abnormalities
   Rhombic roof
   Arachnoid cysts
   Posthemorrhagic membranes
   Postinflammatory membranes
   Vascularized membranes

* Other skeletal abnormalities, such as scoliosis and Klippel-Feil anomalies, have a frequent association with syringomyelia but do not have a clear etiological relationship.

TABLE 2

ETIOLOGICAL CATEGORIES FOR PRIMARY SPINAL SYRINGOMYELIA

A. Arachnoid scarring related to spinal trauma

B. Arachnoid scarring related to meningeal inflammation

C. Arachnoid scarring related to surgical trauma

D. Subarachnoid space stenosis due to spinal neoplasm or vascular malformation

E. Subarachnoid space stenosis, with possible scarring, related to disc and osteophytic disease

F. Idiopathic (?)

The discussion of current concepts of pathophysiology of syringohydromyelia will focus on three different aspects of this complex problem: 1) the development of hindbrain herniation; 2) the development of syringomyelia in relation to abnormalities at the craniovertebral junction; and 3) the mechanisms of extension and expansion of syringomyelic cavities.

DEVELOPMENT OF HINDBRAIN HERNIATION

Hindbrain herniation may develop in children or adults as a result of excessive drainage of cerebrospinal fluid (CSF) from the subarachnoid space below the level of the foramen magnum.[13] This type of "acquired Chiari malformation" or hindbrain herniation is not infrequently seen in children undergoing lumboperitoneal shunting for a variety of indications,[8] as well as in adults with abnormal drainage or leakage of CSF from the spinal theca. Factors that appear to play a role in the development of tonsillar descent under these circumstances include the compliance of juvenile neural tissue, making it more possible for the cerebellar tonsils to be compressed and molded through the foramen magnum. The rate of fluid drainage, or leakage into surrounding soft tissues, also would appear to be important. In some patients with acquired hindbrain herniation, a syrinx cavity may then develop.[23] The tonsillar descent and syrinx formation appear to be reversible when the overdrainage problem has been corrected. It is tempting to postulate that a similar mechanism might apply to the development of the majority of cases of hindbrain herniation seen in clinical practice, but an overdrainage mechanism has not been demonstrated for the large number of patients with hindbrain descent and syringomyelia. A related situation might exist in infants with meningoceles or myelomeningoceles. A large number of these patients have Chiari II abnormalities. However, in these infants hindbrain herniation persists after closure of the midline defect. There is a growing tendency to regard Chiari II abnormalities as a different entity from the Chiari I type; the Chiari II abnormalities may be more truly a "malformation."[6,26,27] Van Hoytema and van den Berg[28] postulated that the posterior medullary velum remains intact in children with Chiari II malformations.

Historically, it was believed that hydrocephalus was the initiating "force" that *pushed* the contents of the posterior fossa through the foramen magnum. This was Chiari's concept,[7] based on his original observations of 24 autopsy cases. An opposing concept was that the contents of the posterior fossa were *pulled* through the foramen magnum in situations in which the spinal cord was anchored, or tethered (e.g., an infant with meningocele). It was postulated that the spinal cord cannot ascend in normal fashion as axial growth takes place, thus exerting downward traction on the brain stem.[18,24] Differential growth of spine and spinal cord, with a spillover of neural elements (akin to a mushroom) beyond the posterior fossa, was also suggested.[25] These concepts had initial appeal, but with more experience, it became clear that hydrocephalus is present in only approximately 10% of patients with a Chiari I abnormalities and thus would not account for the majority of adults or adolescents presenting with hindbrain herniation.[29] Similarly, hindbrain descent is not seen in the majority of patients with the tethered cord syndrome, including adults who present with symptoms of tethered cord. In theory, downward traction would have occurred over the course of many years in such patients, but hindbrain herniation generally does not accompany the adult tethered cord syndrome.

An embryological cause of hindbrain herniation was suggested by Patten,[22] who theorized that there was local tissue overgrowth, and by Daniel and Strich,[10] who attributed descent of the hindbrain through the foramen magnum to failure of formation of the normal pontine flexures in embryonic life.

Gardner[14] attributed tonsillar descent to the "water-hammer" effect of arterial pulsations transmitted to the CSF, the tonsils being forced downward when the outlet foramina of the fourth ventricle are inadequately opened due to persistence of the rhombic roof.

Pressure gradient theories were first advanced by Emery and MacKenzie,[11] although the source of the pressure differential was not clearly defined. Williams[34] established experimentally that a pressure differential exists after the tonsils have descended and that this pressure differential favors progressive tonsillar descent. He termed this cranial-spinal pressure dissociation. Venous distention within the spinal canal was considered the major source of the pressure changes.

The possible etiological role of a relatively small posterior fossa in patients with Chiari I abnormalities is not entirely clear. Several studies have shown that the posterior fossa is relatively small in patients with this abnormality.[4,19] Such an underlying skeletal disproportion could be genetically determined, as suggested by the small number of familial cases of Chiari I abnormalities; birth trauma cited by Williams[30] also might play a role in skeletal development of the skull, although Williams considered trauma more in terms of molding of the cranium during parturition and local tissue edema and hemorrhage of the tonsils initiating the protrusion of the cerebellar tonsils through the foramen magnum.

DEVELOPMENT OF SYRINGOMYELIA IN RELATION TO ABNORMALITIES AT THE CRANIOVERTEBRAL JUNCTION

Chiari,[7] in his 1895 publication, postulated that syringomyelia represents persistence of a physiological state of embryonic hydromyelia, along with hydrocephalus. The criticism of this concept, based on the relatively low incidence of hydrocephalus (10%) by modern imaging techniques, has already been noted.[29] Gardner and Angel[15] theorized that patients with syringomyelia had a persistent opening of the central canal at the obex and that CSF pulsations, in the presence of inadequate outlet foramina of the fourth ventricle, forced fluid into the central canal. His recommendation that the obex opening be plugged was based on this theory. Current studies reveal that few patients (approximately 10%) with syringomyelia and Chiari I abnormality have maintained an opening at the obex.[29] Milhorat et al,[20] on the other hand, postulated that intercurrent ependymitis of the central canal ependyma produced an obstruction to "normal" upward flow of CSF in the central canal, resulting in distention of the central canal. Such a pattern of "normal" CSF flow in the central canal, however, has not been demonstrated in man to date, but CSF production by ependymal cells of the central canal has been suggested.[9]

The possibility that a syrinx cavity may develop from posttraumatic hematomyelia has been cited as a possible mechanism to explain the formation of posttraumatic syringomyelia. Arachnoid scarring at the site of injury, however, seems the more likely association. Patients may develop posttraumatic syringomyelia after relatively minor spine injuries.[17]

Current thinking favors some form of transparenchymal fluid migration. Ball and Dayan[5] proposed fluid migration along the Virchow-Robin spaces of the spinal cord in the face of an obstruction at the foramen magnum and suggested that such fluid then ruptured secondarily into the remnants of the central canal. Aboulker[1] proposed transparenchymal migration of CSF along the course of the dorsal roots, a suggestion based on the observation, subsequently confirmed many times, that water-soluble contrast medium migrates from the subarachnoid space into an existing syringomyelic cavity.[3] This constitutes the basis for obtaining six-hour delayed computed tomography scans to establish the diagnosis of syringomyelia. This observation on imaging studies does not favor a specific route of transparenchymal fluid migration. Oldfield et al[21] believe that the systolic pressure waves of CSF may force fluid into the cord along perivascular and interstitial spaces when there is a par-

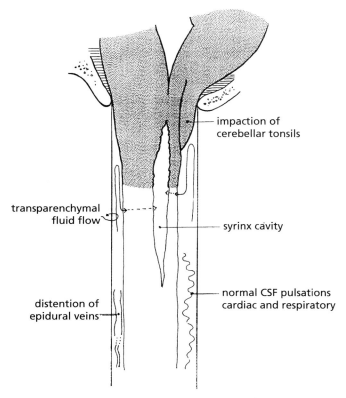

Figure 1: Diagrammatic representation of postulated mechanisms of syrinx filling.

tial obstruction at the foramen magnum due to tonsillar impaction. Experimental evidence in rats supports the concept of fluid flow from the subarachnoid space into the spinal cord parenchyma[16] and central canal.[27] The forces that drive fluid appear to be enhanced by the partial flow obstruction (e.g., tonsils and scar) common to various types of syringomyelia (Figure 1).

The mechanism and route of this fluid transport which results in syrinx cavity formation have not been elucidated to date. The observation of water-soluble contrast medium migration into an *existing* syringomyelic cavity is, however, not necessarily equivalent to *establishing* a syrinx cavity when none was previously present. The mechanism, however, might be similar.

From the broadest perspective, a partial obstruction or constriction of the subarachnoid space appears to be the pathophysiological abnormality common to all forms of syringomy-

elia. Cranial-spinal, or spinal-spinal, pressure dissociation results from an inability to achieve near-instantaneous pressure equilibration across this subarachnoid constriction, thus interfering with normal and continuous pulsations of CSF that take place in response to the cardiac cycle and respirations.

MECHANISM OF EXTENSION AND EXPANSION OF SYRINGOMYELIC CAVITIES

Gardner[14] envisioned that CSF entering the central canal at the obex would dissect into the spinal cord in progressive fashion, propelled by the arterially generated water-hammer pulse. Subsequently, the lack of continuity of syringomyelic cavities with the fourth ventricle became well recognized.[29] Apparent segmentation of syringomyelic cavities into separate compartments is not infrequently recognized in magnetic resonance images and would be difficult to explain by Gardner's theory.

Ball and Dayan[5] postulated ongoing transparenchymal fluid migration toward the central canal, which would presumably result in a progressive increase or accumulation of fluid within the syrinx cavity.

Williams[31,33] developed the concept that fluid within the syrinx cavity dissects in an axial direction under the influence of pressure differentials that are generated by epidural venous distention in the presence of a partially blocked CSF system at the craniovertebral junction. This prevents the normal near-instantaneous pressure equilibration throughout the system. The concept appears valid to date, and offers an explanation for the instances in which patients have documented neurological progression of symptoms following a coughing spell, a situation which would forcefully propel the fluid within an intramedullary cyst in an upward direction.

The concept of cranial-spinal pressure dissociation, confirmed by Williams[34] on the basis of experimental evidence in man, remains a valuable working concept in our current thinking about syringomyelia. A mechanism of cranial-spinal pressure dissociation can be postulated for syringomyelia related to abnormalities at the craniovertebral junction, irrespective of the specific etiology of the pressure dissociation.

Newer noninvasive techniques of evaluating CSF flow, such as cardiac-gated magnetic resonance imaging,[2,12] may provide us with at least some answers to the many remaining questions relating to the development and progression of hydrosyringomyelia.

REFERENCES

1. Aboulker J: La syringomyélie et les liquides intra-rachidiens. Neurochirurgie 25 (Suppl 1):9-144, 1979
2. Armonda RA, Citrin CM, Foley KT, et al: Quantitative cine-mode magnetic resonance imaging of Chiari I malformations: an analysis of cerebrospinal fluid dynamics. Neurosurgery 35:214-224, 1994
3. Aubin ML, Vignaud J, Jardin C, et al: Computed tomography in 75 clinical cases of syringomyelia. AJNR 2:119-204, 1981
4. Badie B, Mendoza D, Batzdorf U: Posterior fossa volume and response to suboccipital decompression in patients with Chiari I malformation. Neurosurgery 37:214-218, 1995
5. Ball MJ, Dayan AD: Pathogenesis of syringomyelia. Lancet 2:799-801, 1972
6. Carmel PW: The Chiari malformations and syringomyelia, in Hoffman HJ, Epstein F (eds): Disorders of the Developing Nervous System: Diagnosis and Treatment. Boston, Mass: Blackwell Scientific, 1986
7. Chiari H: Über Veränderungen des Kleinhirns, des Pons und der Medulla Oblongata in Folge von congenitaler Hydrocephalie des Grosshirns. Denkschr Akad Wiss Wien 63:71-116, 1895
8. Chumas PD, Kulkarni AV, Drake JM, et al: Lumbo-peritoneal shunting: a retrospective study in the pediatric population. Neurosurgery 32:376-383, 1993
9. Cornil L, Mosinger M: Sur les processus proliferatifs de l'ependyme médullaire (rapports avec les tumeurs intramédullaires et la syringomyélia). Rev Neurol 1:749-754, 1933
10. Daniel PM, Strich SJ: Some observations on the congenital deformity of the central nervous system known as the Arnold-Chiari malformation. J Neuropathol Exp Neurol 17:255-266, 1958
11. Emery JL, MacKenzie N: Medullo-cervical dislocation deformity (Chiari II deformity) related to neurospinal dysraphism (meningomyelocele). Brain 96:155-162, 1973
12. Enzmann DR: Imaging of syringomyelia, in Batzdorf U (ed): Syringomyelia: Current Concepts in Diagnosis and Treatment. Baltimore, Md: Williams & Wilkins, 1991, pp 116-139
13. Fischer EG, Welch K, Shillito J Jr: Syringomyelia following lumboureteral shunting for communicating hydrocephalus. Report of three cases. J Neurosurg 47:96-100, 1977
14. Gardner WJ: The Dysraphic States From Syringomyelia to Anencephaly. Amsterdam: Excerpta Medica, 1973
15. Gardner WJ, Angel J: The mechanism of syringomyelia and its surgical correction. Clin Neurosurg 6:131-140, 1959
16. Ikata T, Masaki K, Kashiwaguchi S: Clinical and experimental studies on permeability of tracers in normal spinal cord and syringomyelia. Spine 13:737-741, 1988
17. La Haye PA, Batzdorf U: Posttraumatic syringomyelia. West J Med 148:657-663, 1988
18. Lichtenstein BW: Distant neuroanatomic complications of spina bifida (spinal dysraphism). Hydrocephalus, Arnold-Chiari deformity, stenosis of the aqueduct of Sylvius; etc.; pathogenesis and pathology. Arch Neurol Psychiatry 47:195-214, 1942
19. Marin-Padilla M, Marin-Padilla TM: Morphogenesis of experimentally induced Arnold-Chiari malformation. J Neurol Sci 50:29-55, 1981
20. Milhorat TH, Kotzen RM, Anzil AP: Stenosis of central canal of spinal cord in man: incidence and pathological findings in 232 autopsy cases. J Neurosurg 80:716-722, 1994
21. Oldfield EH, Muraszko K, Shawker TH, et al: Pathophysiology of syringomyelia associated with Chiari I malformation of the cerebellar tonsils. Implications for diagnosis and treatment. J Neurosurg 80:3-15, 1994
22. Patten BM: Embryological stages in the establishing

of myeloschisis with spina bifida. **Am J Anat 93:** 365-395, 1953

23. Payner T, Prenger E, Berger TS, et al: Acquired Chiari malformations: incidence, diagnosis and management. **Neurosurgery 34:**429-434, 1994

24. Penfield W, Coburn DF: Arnold Chiari malformation and its operative treatment. **Arch Neurol Psychiatry 40:**328-336, 1938

25. Roth M: Cranio-cervical growth collision: another explanation of the Arnold-Chiari malformation and of basilar impression. **Neuroradiology 28:**187-194, 1986

26. Ruge JR, Masciopinto J, Storrs BB, et al: Anatomical progression of the Chiari II malformation. **Childs Nerv Sys 8:**86-91, 1992

27. Stoodley MA, Jones NR, Brown CJ: Evidence for rapid fluid flow from the subarachnoid space into the spinal cord central canal in the rat. **Brain Res 707:**155-164, 1996

28. van Hoytema GJ, van den Berg R: Embryological studies of the posterior fossa in connection with Arnold Chiari malformation. **Dev Med Child Neurol (Suppl)** 11:61-76, 1966

29. West RJ, Williams B: Radiographic studies of the ventricles in syringomyelia. **Neuroradiology 20:** 5-16, 1980

30. Williams B: Difficult labour as a cause of communicating syringomyelia. **Lancet 2:**51-53, 1977

31. Williams B: On the pathogenesis of syringomyelia: a review. **J R Soc Med 73:**798-806, 1980

32. Williams B: Pathogenesis of syringomyelia, in Batzdorf U (ed): **Syringomyelia: Current Concepts in Diagnosis and Treatment.** Baltimore, Md: Williams & Wilkins, 1991, pp 59-90

33. Williams B: Progress in syringomyelia. **Neurol Res 8:**130-145, 1986

34. Williams B: Simultaneous cerebral and spinal fluid pressure recording. 2. Cerebrospinal dissociation with lesions at the foramen magnum. **Acta Neurochir 59:**123-142, 1981

CHAPTER 4

IMAGING OF SYRINGOMYELIA AND THE CHIARI MALFORMATIONS

MARI SCHENK, MD, AND PAUL M. RUGGIERI, MD

CHIARI I MALFORMATION

Type I Chiari malformation is a hindbrain malformation characterized by downward displacement of the cerebellar tonsils through the foramen magnum into the cervical canal. The tonsils are often asymmetric in position and occasionally only one tonsil is displaced. Classically, the fourth ventricle and medulla are normal in position; however, there may be minimal caudal displacement of the medulla and mild angulation of the cervicomedullary junction (Figure 1).[12,36] In these cases, the radiographic distinction between Chiari I and Chiari II malformations is less clear. Generally, the differentiation is made by the absence of a history of myelomeningocele and lack of supratentorial anomalies in Chiari I patients.[11,15] Cervical syringohydromyelia in Chiari I is common, occurring in 30% to 50% of patients. Ventriculomegaly has been reported in up to 20% of patients, but is usually mild.[26]

Prior to the introduction of magnetic resonance imaging (MRI), radiographic evaluation of the craniocervical junction consisted of myelography followed by computed tomography (CT). MRI has facilitated the diagnosis of Chiari I malformation by permitting direct sagittal imaging of the craniocervical junction and is now the procedure of choice for pre- and postoperative evaluation. Imaging consists of multiplanar views of the brain which include

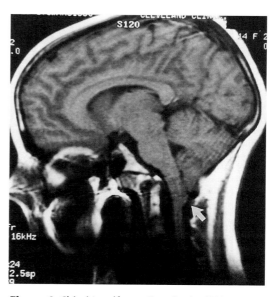

Figure 1: Chiari I malformation. Sagittal T1-weighted MRI. There is mild caudal extension of the medulla resulting in a cervicomedullary kink *(arrow)*. Note the normal size and position of the fourth ventricle.

the craniocervical junction. Tonsillar position is easily identified on a sagittal short repetition time (TR), short echo time (TE) (T1-weighted) sequence and is measured from the inferior aspect of the foramen magnum to the tonsillar tip (Figure 2A).[24] The inferior aspect of the foramen magnum is defined by a line connecting

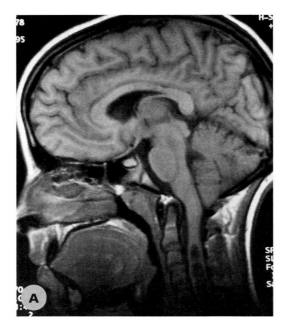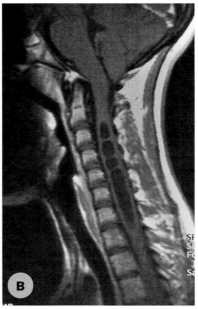

Figure 2: Chiari I malformation. **A)** Sagittal short TR, short TE, T1-weighted MRI demonstrating caudal extension of the tonsil below the foramen magnum. The tonsil exhibits the typical triangular or pegged shape. **B)** Sagittal T1-weighted surface coil examination of the cervical spine in the same patient. A cervical syrinx distends the cord. Multiple thin, fibroglial bands within the syrinx result in a septated appearance.

the cortex (seen as lack of signal) of the inferior aspect of the clivus (basion) and the cortex overlying the ventral aspect of the exoccipital bone (opisthion). Surface coil imaging of the cervical spine (sagittal and axial T1-weighted images) should be performed to evaluate for a cervical syrinx cavity in patients with a Chiari I malformation (Figure 2B). If the syrinx cavity extends caudad to the field of view, a separate examination of the thoracic spine should be performed as well to define the full extent of the central syrinx cavity.

Tonsillar Position

The widespread use of MRI has revealed a spectrum of minor downward displacement of the tonsils ("tonsillar ectopia") and Chiari I malformations. The degree of downward displacement considered abnormal is somewhat controversial. Several quantitative studies of tonsillar position with MRI have been performed in which "normal" was based on lack of sympto-

matology. In 1985, Aboullez et al[1] found that in 82 normal controls, the tonsils did not extend more than 3 mm below the foramen magnum while 13 symptomatic Chiari I patients had tonsillar descent of at least 5 mm. Perhaps more importantly, the tonsils had a pointed configuration in all of the latter cases. The authors concluded that ectopia of the cerebellar tonsils up to 3 mm is normal, between 3 and 5 mm is borderline, and greater than 5 mm is "clearly pathologic." Barkovich et al[3] in 1986 studied 200 asymptomatic patients and 25 symptomatic Chiari I patients. No patient with less than 3 mm of ectopia was symptomatic. If 3 mm below the foramen magnum is taken as the lowest normal tonsillar position, their sensitivity was 96% and specificity was 99.5% for distinguishing normal patients from those with Chiari I malformation. Mikulis et al[24] in 1992 evaluated tonsillar position in 221 asymptomatic patients and found a trend toward tonsillar ascent with increased age. Utilizing distances based on two standard deviations from the mean, the authors suggested the following criteria for abnormal tonsillar posi-

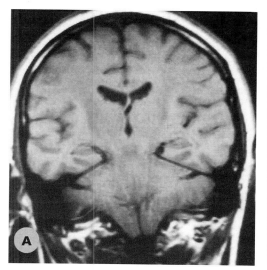
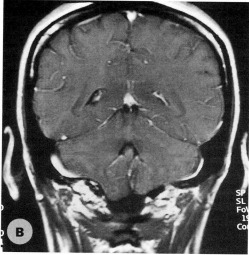

Figure 3: Chiari I malformation. **A)** Mild tonsillar ectopia. Coronal T1-weighted MRI after contrast enhancement in an asymptomatic patient. Note that the right tonsil is only slightly ectopic and maintains a normal rounded configuration. Asymmetric tonsillar position is not uncommon. **B)** Coronal T1-weighted image showing the typical pointed appearance of the tonsils in a patient with Chiari I malformation.

tion: first decade, 6 mm; second and third decades, 5 mm; fourth to eighth decades, 4 mm; and ninth decade, 3 mm.

With the more widespread use of MRI, it has become evident that many patients with Chiari I radiographically are clinically asymptomatic. In 1992, Elster and Chen[13] correlated symptoms with MRI findings and observed that herniations greater than 12 mm were invariably symptomatic. However, approximately 30% of patients with tonsils 5-10 mm below the foramen magnum were asymptomatic. While it is possible that some of these patients may eventually develop symptoms, the findings imply that many Chiari I malformations are incidentally discovered and of little clinical significance. Thus, radiographic findings in combination with the individual clinical assessment are necessary for proper diagnosis.

In general, the radiographic diagnosis of Chiari I malformation is made by a combination of the assessment of tonsillar displacement, tonsillar configuration, and the resultant compression of the cervicomedullary junction at the level of the foramen magnum.[1,24,26] Tonsils that retain a normal rounded configuration and project less than 3 mm below the foramen magnum

are considered to be within the normal range (Figure 3A). A patient with Chiari I malformation will have tonsillar herniation of 3 mm or greater and the tonsils will appear confined or pegged in shape (Figure 3B). Additional criteria for diagnosis include absence of the stigmata of a Chiari II malformation (myelomeningocele, supratentorial anomalies) or elevated intracranial pressure (mass lesion, cerebral edema).

Associated Anomalies

Osseous anomalies of the skull base and spine are associated with Chiari I malformations. The most common skeletal anomalies are atlanto-occipital assimilation, fused cervical vertebrae, and basilar invagination. In general, these findings are readily delineated on conventional radiographs. However, basilar invagination, present in up to 25% of patients, can be identified on midline sagittal T1-weighted MRI. When present, more than one-third of the dens will project above a line drawn between the dorsal margin of the hard palate and the opisthion (Chamberlain's line). Sagittal T1-weighted images also demonstrate fused cervical vertebrae. Fused segments typically are foreshortened in their anterior-to-posterior dimension and frequently a thin, horizontal, hypointense line can be seen between the segments, which represents the rudimentary disc space.

ACQUIRED CHIARI MALFORMATION

The acquired Chiari malformation has been reported in patients with communicating hydrocephalus who have been treated with lumboperitoneal shunts[8,34,41] and has also been seen in a patient following multiple lumbar punctures.[33,38] Although the pathogenesis is uncertain, a negative pressure gradient created by drainage of cerebrospinal fluid (CSF) through the shunt or through a dural tear may result in a reversible downward "pulling" force on the tonsils.[41] MRI has demonstrated low-lying cerebellar tonsils in patients with normal tonsillar position documented prior to shunting. This acquired descent of the cerebellar tonsils is radiographically indistinguishable from true Chiari I malformations. In many patients, these acquired Chiari malformations have suddenly become symptomatic postoperatively, with subsequent relief of symptoms following conversion to a ventriculoperitoneal shunt or posterior fossa decompression. The corresponding MRI studies have demonstrated reversal of the tonsillar herniation in previously symptomatic patients following removal of the lumbar shunt.[34,41]

CHIARI II MALFORMATION

Type II Chiari malformation is a complex malformation involving the hindbrain, spinal cord, and mesodermal structures of the skull and spine. The spectrum of abnormalities described in Chiari II patients is wide and it is unusual to see all of the stigmata in an individual. Moreover, the degree of deformity can vary from one patient to another. Essentially all patients have a myelomeningocele and hydrocephalus, and a small posterior fossa is almost always present. The incidence of other findings is more variable. MRI is the procedure of choice for radiographic evaluation of Chiari II patients since it

allows a detailed, multiplanar anatomical evaluation of the entire spectrum of abnormalities.

Cervicomedullary Junction

The hindbrain deformity is characterized by downward displacement of the inferior cerebellar vermis, fourth ventricle, and medulla through an enlarged foramen magnum into the upper cervical canal. Occasionally, the pons may herniate as well. The so-called "cascade of herniations" is difficult to reliably detect by CT,[30] but is clearly demonstrated on MRI.[12,43] The spatial relationships of the hindbrain deformity and caudal extent of the herniations are best appreciated on sagittal T1-weighted (short TR, short TE) images.

The degree of deformity of the cervicomedullary junction is quite variable. The medulla may descend only a short distance into the cervical canal, remaining in vertical alignment with the inferiorly displaced cervical cord. With further descent of the medulla, the downward excursion of the cervical cord becomes limited by the dentate ligaments, causing the medulla to buckle posterior to the cord. The end result is a Z-shaped cervicomedullary "kink." The medulla, then, extends down dorsal to the upper cervical cord, forming a "spur" of tissue with its inferior tip usually between C2 and C4. Rarely, the spur may extend as low as the upper thoracic level.[22] Emery and McKenzie[14] classified the spectrum of pathology into five major groups with increasing degrees of severity. The number in parentheses indicates the percent of occurrence in their study.

Group 1 (4%): The medulla and fourth ventricle do not extend below the level of the foramen magnum. There is mild caudal displacement of the cervical cord with ascending upper cervical nerve roots.

Group 2 (26%): The medulla and fourth ventricle descend vertically, in line with and above the displaced cervical cord. The fourth ventricle leads directly into the central canal of the cervical spinal cord.

Group 3 (26%): Mild buckling of the medulla dorsal to the cervical cord is present, so there is less than 5 mm of overlap of the medulla and the cord. Because of this buckling, the fourth ventricle lies partially behind the cord and the central canal arises from the anterior surface of the fourth ventricle.

Group 4 (23%): Severe buckling of the medulla with greater than 5 mm overlap of the medulla and cord.

Group 5 (21%): Severe buckling of the medulla is associated with a sac-like process or diverticulum of the dorsal surface of the fourth ventricle. The diverticulum protrudes caudad to the kink behind the cervical cord and may contain choroid plexus.

The length of the medullary kink depends, in part, on the length of the upper cervical dentate ligaments. That is, short dentate ligaments anchor the cervical cord relatively high in position, resulting in a longer medullary kink.

Along with the medulla, the fourth ventricle descends below the foramen magnum, stretching from the posterior fossa down into the upper cervical canal. The result is a fourth ventricle that is low in position, elongated, and sagittally flattened. A slit-like appearance is typical and is best depicted on sagittal MRI, although it may be recognized on CT as absence or flattening of the fourth ventricle (anterior-to-posterior dimension) in a patient with a small posterior fossa.[29] If the fourth ventricle is enlarged or even "normal" in size in a patient with a Chiari II malformation, the possibility of shunt malfunction or entrapment of the fourth ventricle should be considered.[10,29] Isolation of the fourth ventricle can result from aqueductal narrowing and diminished fourth ventricular outflow in patients with Chiari II malformation who have been previously shunted. Newer MRI techniques that evaluate CSF flow can facilitate this diagnosis by demonstrating lack of normal flow in the aqueduct and foramen of Magendie.[37]

The Chiari II cerebellum protrudes into the cervical canal as part of the "cascade of herniations" posterior to the medulla and fourth ventricle (Figure 4).[27] The medial aspects of the cerebellar hemispheres extend below the enlarged foramen magnum, with the majority of cerebellar tissue residing at or appearing to rest upon the posterior arch of C1, whose sagittal diameter is smaller than the enlarged foramen magnum. Typically, only the nodulus, uvula, and pyramis of the vermis (designated the "peg" or "tail") extend below C1. The length of this tail is variable and does not correlate with the

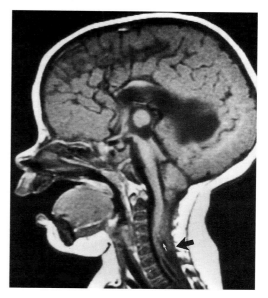

Figure 4: Chiari II malformation. "Cascade of herniations" is visible on a sagittal T1-weighted MRI. There is herniation of the medulla, fourth ventricle, and vermis into the cervical canal. The fourth ventricle is elongated and narrowed. The vermian "peg" *(large black arrow)* extends below the medullary spur *(small white arrow)*. Note the small posterior fossa, the nearly vertical course of the tentorium, partial agenesis of the corpus callosum, and cord syrinx.

length of the medullary spur. In 75% of cases, it terminates above the level of the spur; in 25%, the vermian tail extends below the medulla, dorsal to the cervical cord.[35] At pathology, there is often atrophy and dysplasia within the tail.[27] Accordingly, on MRI the tail is thin and elongated and may be low in signal intensity relative to the cord on T1-weighted sequences.[10] In approximately 2% of patients with Chiari II malformation, only the cerebellar tonsils extend below the level of the foramen magnum. A history of a myelomeningocele or the presence of supratentorial anomalies distinguishes these patients from those with Chiari I malformation. The overlapping herniations (medulla, fourth ventricle, and cerebellum) crowd into the upper cervical canal, causing anterior displacement and compression of the more ventral structure. Typically, the maximum degree of compression occurs at the foramen magnum and the posterior arch of C1.[27,35]

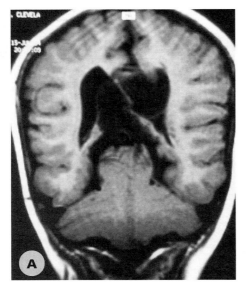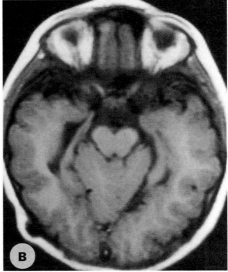

Figure 5: Chiari II malformation with hypoplastic tentorium. **A)** Coronal T1-weighted MRI. The superior cerebellum protrudes upward through a widened incisura, "towering" above the hypoplastic tentorium. **B)** Axial T1-weighted image showing the typical heart-shaped configuration of the cerebellum which extends upward through the widened incisura and wraps around lateral to the brain stem.

Posterior Fossa

In Chiari II patients, the tentorium is hypoplastic and inserts low on the occipital bone. The result is a small posterior fossa, low position of the dural sinuses and torcular herophili, and a wide incisura.[31,35] The spatially confined cerebellar hemispheres tend to extend anterolaterally into the prepontine and premedullary cisterns, partially wrapping around the brain stem. Naidich et al[28] refer to this as a "triple peak" appearance on axial imaging in which the midline brain stem is flanked between two cerebellar margins. The cerebellum is usually flattened superiorly by the low inserting tentorium or, less frequently, protrudes up through the widened tentorial incisura resulting in a "towering" cerebellum. The latter is best appreciated on coronal MRI and is more commonly seen following decompression of the lateral ventricles (Figure 5A).[11] On axial images, the "towering" cerebellum will have a bullet- or heart-shaped configuration (Figure 5B).[31]

Supratentorial Compartment

In addition to hindbrain deformity, patients with Chiari II malformation usually have supratentorial anomalies as well. As mentioned previously, hydrocephalus is almost always present. The degree of hydrocephalus, however, can be quite variable and may not appear until after closure of the myelomeningocele.[29] Often, the atria and occipital horns are disproportionately enlarged relative to the remainder of the lateral ventricles (colpocephaly), which persists even after shunting (Figure 6). Following shunting, axial images also commonly demonstrate enlargement of the posterior interhemispheric fissure as well as a diamond-shaped cistern posterior to the third ventricle, representing the confluence of the superior vermian, ambient wing, and velum interpositum cisterns. This enlargement results, in part, from inward collapse of the atria and occipital horns following decompression.[12,29,43] When hydrocephalus is present, the third ventricle is usually only mildly

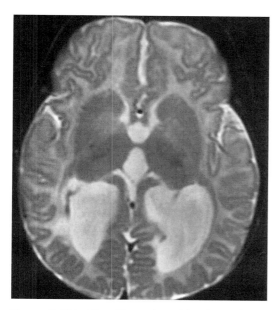

Figure 6: Chiari II malformation with colpocephaly. Axial T2-weighted MRI showing that the atria and occipital horns of the lateral ventricles are disproportionately enlarged compared to the frontal horns.

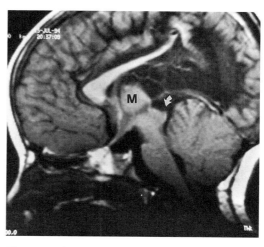

Figure 7: Chiari II malformation with supratentorial anomalies. Sagittal T1-weighted MRI showing a hypoplastic corpus callosum (absent splenium), beaked tectum (curved arrow), and an enlarged massa intermedia (M). Also note the posterior scalloping of the basiocciput.

dilated (a distinguishing feature from isolated aqueductal stenosis) so that the walls remain parallel or biconcave.[29] When they are biconcave, the inward bowing is typically maximal at the site of an enlarged massa intermedia.

A spectrum of other anomalies may also be seen in this group of patients. Stenogyria is an anomalous gyral pattern, particularly prominent in the medial occipital region, in which the gyri (of normal cortical thickness) are small and closely spaced together.[43] Abnormalities of the corpus callosum have been described in up to 80% of these patients and are best appreciated on the midline sagittal image. Most commonly, the splenium is hypoplastic or absent altogether. The tectum may be displaced superiorly by the cerebellum, which in combination with posterior and inferior elongation of the tectum results in a "beaked" appearance (Figure 7).[43] Lastly, in patients with Chiari II malformation the falx is usually hypoplastic or fenestrated. As a result, the medial hemispheric gyri may interdigitate across the midline, resulting in focal obliteration or a "zigzag" appearance of the in-

terhemispheric fissure on axial images.[30] The septum pellucidum may also be absent or fenestrated.[29]

Skull and Spine

Bony changes involving the cranium and spine are frequently observed in Chiari II patients. Prior to 6 months of age, scalloping of the inner and outer tables of the membranous calvarium may be evident on plain films or CT.[30] This is referred to as a lacunar skull (lückenschädel) and is most striking at birth, but generally disappears after approximately 6 months. It represents a mesodermal dysplasia and is not caused by pressure effects relating to hydrocephalus; consequently, the resolution is not temporally related to shunting. Additional skull findings often identified on CT include scalloping of the petrous pyramids and basiocciput (but not basisphenoid).[30,45] Normally, the posterior surface of the petrous pyramids is convex posteriorly. In Chiari II patients, this bony margin may be flattened (10%) or concave

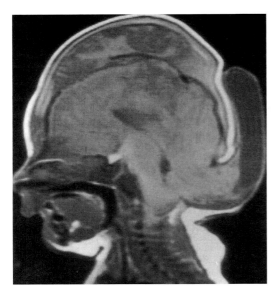

Figure 8: Chiari III malformation. Sagittal T1-weighted MRI demonstrating a low occipital/ high cervical encephalocele with herniation of cerebellar tissue through the bone defect.

posteriorly (80%) while the petrous ridges and jugular tubercles are generally spared. Concavity of the anterior wall of the upper cervical canal may also occur, typically extending from the C1 to C3 levels. This results in widening of the anterior cervical subarachnoid space so that the cervical cord may appear relatively dorsal in position. This should not be mistaken for a ventral arachnoid cyst.[10] Although the cause of the petrous pyramid and cervical concavity is uncertain, unlike the lacunar skull, it persists (and is observed more frequently) in older patients and thus may be a pressure-related phenomenon rather than a mesodermal dysplasia.[7,10,12,43,45]

CHIARI III MALFORMATION

In the type III Chiari malformation, there is a low occipital and/or high cervical encephalocele in combination with features of Chiari II. The bony defect is in continuity with the foramen magnum (Figure 8). Typically, the encephalocele contains variable amounts of dysplastic cerebellar and occipital tissue and, occasionally, the pons and medulla. The occipital horns may extend into the encephalocele and can be disproportionately enlarged, probably secondary to constriction at the skull defect. Anomalies of the deep venous system and dural sinuses are frequent. Preoperatively, the role of MRI is to establish the contents of the encephalocele; specifically, to determine the amount of solid tissue, the degree of ventricular extension, and the position of the brain stem. MRI does not reliably identify anomalous venous drainage.[7]

SYRINGOMYELIA

Syringomyelia is a pathological condition characterized by the formation of a longitudinally oriented CSF cavity within the cord. It occurs in association with congenital malformations, trauma, inflammation, intramedullary tumor, and compressive lesions, but is at times idiopathic. Congenital syringomyelia is most common and is found in association with both Chiari I and Chiari II malformations. In Chiari I malformation, syrinx cavities occur in approximately 30%-50% of patients and are typically within the cervical cord.[33] Usually, the C1 segment of the cord is spared, although occasionally the cervical syrinx may extend above the foramen magnum into the brain stem (syringobulbia). Size is quite variable so that cavitation may extend from the upper cervical cord to the conus with associated cord expansion or may involve only a very short segment of a normal-sized cord.[26] Skip areas of syrinx may also occur. In patients with Chiari II malformation, concurrent syringohydromyelia occurs in approximately 45% to 95% and may be anywhere in the spinal cord, although it is most often thoracic.[27] Of note is that when the cord is tethered in patients with Chiari II, there may be mild dilatation of the distal-most aspect of the central canal within the conus (the terminal ventricle), which is likely of no clinical consequence.

Conventional Radiographs

The role of conventional radiographs in syringomyelia is the detection of associated entities or the identification of an etiology such as posttraumatic syringomyelia. Rarely, direct evidence of a large syrinx can be seen as an increased anterior-to-posterior diameter of the spinal canal secondary to pressure effects. Well recognized is the association of syringomyelia with a neuropathic shoulder joint or Klippel-Feil syndrome, both of which are readily delineated on conventional radiographs. Yet, the most common plain film finding is, in fact, scoliosis. Increasingly recognized is that scoliosis may be the initial presenting sign in children with syringomyelia, including Chiari I-associated syringomyelia.[23] MRI has been advocated in children with radiographic or clinical features atypical for an idiopathic scoliosis which may signal underlying intraspinal pathology, including a convex left thoracic curve, early onset, rapid progression, or neurological signs and symptoms.[4,6,9,20] Following treatment of the syrinx, the scoliosis has been reported to stabilize or even improve.[11,25]

CT Myelography

Intrathecal contrast is needed in combination with CT to consistently identify syrinx cavities and tonsillar position.[18,21] A syrinx is identified by delayed accumulation of water-soluble contrast medium within the cord, which is seen in the majority of cases by 4 hours postinjection. However, in a few cases, uptake into the syrinx cavity may not be visualized until 12 or 24 hours postinjection. Thus, if there is a high clinical suspicion of syrinx and none is detected at 4 hours, additional delayed scans should be obtained. There are several limitations of CT myelography, including: a significant cumulative radiation dose, especially if the entire cervical and thoracic spine needs to be imaged to define the rostral and caudal extents of the syrinx; a potential for false positive examinations, since uptake of contrast medium can occur in an area of myelomalacia, mimicking a posttraumatic syrinx;[19] and a reported high false-negative rate (27%) when compared to MRI.[42] Particularly difficult to identify on CT myelography are small syrinx cavities in an atrophic or normal-sized cord. The use of CT myelography, therefore, should be limited to patients who cannot undergo MRI examinations or in whom metal artifact results in inadequate MRI.

Magnetic Resonance Imaging

MRI, with its high contrast resolution and multiplanar capabilities, allows accurate identification, characterization, and postoperative assessment of syringomyelia and is clearly the diagnostic modality of choice. Attention to scan parameters, however, is necessary for optimal visualization of syrinx cavities. Thin section 3-mm sagittal and 5-mm axial images of the spine should be obtained to limit partial volume effects, allowing optimal visualization of even small syrinx cavities. In addition to slice thickness, attention must be given to matrix size and field of view in order to minimize an artifact referred to as Gibbs or truncation artifact, which can result in the false appearance of a syrinx on sagittal images. The artifact occurs at high-contrast linear interfaces within the spinal canal (bright CSF-low signal intensity cord interface) and is most prominent on large field-of-view, low spatial resolution, T2-weighted images. On T2-weighted images (bright CSF), it is recognized as a bright band of high signal extending vertically within the entire length of the visualized cord, paralleling the ventral surface of the cord (Figure 9). This artifact is usually less conspicuous (and of lower signal intensity) on T1-weighted images due to the smaller contrast difference between the low signal intensity CSF and cord. By limiting the field of view and increasing the imaging matrix (i.e., 256 × 256 instead of 128 × 256), the artifact can be reduced. The trade-off is an increase in the scan time with the associated increased likelihood of patient motion. Finally, surface coils should be utilized in order to increase signal to noise, thus improving image quality.

T1-weighted images best delineate cord and syrinx morphology. Sagittal and axial planes define the rostral and caudal extents of the syrinx and identify the presence of fibroglial septations. Axial images are especially useful in detecting the eccentricity and multiplicity of cavities and in determining the size of the cord and the degree of cord thinning around the syrinx (Figure 10C and D). Axial images are also

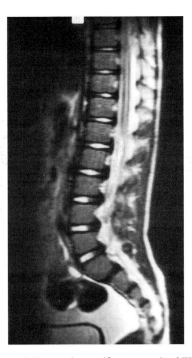

Figure 9: Truncation artifact on sagittal T2-weighted MRI. The linear band of high signal within the cord represents truncation artifact and results in the false appearance of a syrinx. The artifact is prominent because of the low spatial resolution (128 × 256; i.e., 126 phase-encoding steps) of the image.

more sensitive in the detection of small syrinx cavities, particularly in patients with scoliosis. On T1-weighted images, a syrinx appears fusiform in shape, has well-defined margins, and is uniformly low in signal intensity, paralleling CSF (Figure 10A). Slight differences in signal intensity of CSF in the cavity versus the spinal subarachnoid space can occur, relating to differences in the pulsatility of the fluid.[15] In general, the larger the size and the greater the turbulence within the syrinx, the lower is the signal intensity of its fluid. A sagittal T1-weighted sequence should include the craniocervical junction in order to identify the presence of a Chiari I malformation. If a Chiari malformation is present, T1-weighted images are generally sufficient for diagnosis and surgical planning.

While T1-weighted sequences provide morphological detail, T2-weighted sequences best evaluate for pathological change within the cord that can be associated with syringomyelia, such as myelomalacia (posttraumatic syrinx), gliosis (simple syrinx), or tumor. The long TR pulse sequence is usually performed as a dual echo in which the first echo is a long TR, short TE sequence referred to as the intermediate-weighted, balanced, or spin-density image, and the second echo is a long TR, long TE T2-weighted

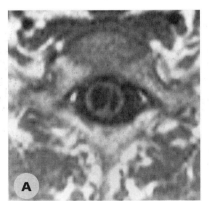

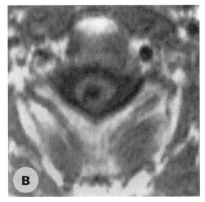

Figure 10: MRI appearance of a syrinx before **(A-D)** and after **(E and F)** shunting. **A** and **B)** Sagittal T1-weighted spin-echo and T2-weighted fast spin-echo sequences demonstrating the typical appearance of a syrinx. The syrinx has well-defined margins and is isointense to CSF **(A).** Multiple areas of flow void (dark signal) are present within the cavity, indicating pulsatile flow **(B).**

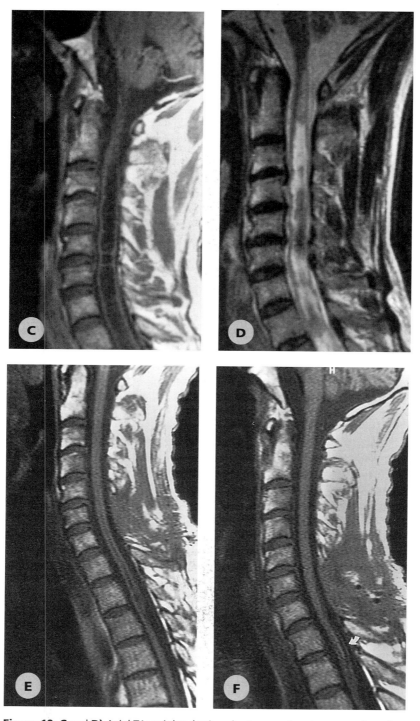

Figure 10: C and **D)** Axial T1-weighted spin-echo images showing expansion of the cord by the cavity. The linear band within the syrinx represents a fibroglial septation. **E** and **F)** Sagittal T1-weighted spin-echo images obtained following shunting. The syrinx cavity is now collapsed. The shunt tube appears as a linear area of low signal intensity *(arrow)* coursing into the inferior aspect of the collapsed syrinx at T2-3.

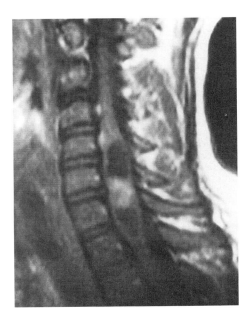

Figure 11: Cervical cord astrocytoma. Contrast-enhanced sagittal T1-weighted image of the cervical spine. A syrinx cavity enlarges the cord between C5 and T1 and there is enhancement of a tumor nidus within the cavity.

image. The first echo (intermediate-weighted) is especially valuable in distinguishing a posttraumatic syrinx from myelomalacia. Both will be high in signal on the T2-weighted sequence; however, on the intermediate-weighted image, a posttraumatic syrinx remains isointense to CSF, while posttraumatic myelomalacia is increased in signal relative to both CSF and normal cord. On T2-weighted images, high signal can be seen within the cord adjacent to a syrinx cavity in which the differential considerations are gliosis adjacent to a benign syrinx or intramedullary tumor with an associated syrinx.[15] In most instances, differentiation is made by determination of associated mass effect (i.e., tumor should focally enlarge the cord while gliosis should not). Differentiation is facilitated by the administration of an intravenous paramagnetic contrast medium (gadolinium), which causes the tumor, but not gliosis, to enhance.[39]

Ideally, the addition of gadolinium-enhanced scans to the examination should be tailored to the specific disease process. Its role is in the characterization of the syrinx cavity when the underlying cause is unclear (idiopathic syrinx) or when tumor is suspected. Thus, in the absence of a Chiari malformation or obvious evidence of trauma, gadolinium helps discriminate a benign syrinx from a syrinx associated with tumor. Specifically, a small tumor nidus may not be apparent on a noncontrast examination, mimicking a benign syrinx, but may show enhancement following contrast administration. Even when tumor is evident on T2-weighted images, the addition of a T1-weighted scan with contrast medium can increase the conspicuousness of tumor and help discriminate the more solid from cystic portions (Figure 11).

Ultrasound

In adults, the use of ultrasound in evaluation of the spine is limited due to its inability to image through ossified bony structures. However, high-resolution ultrasound (7.5 MHz transducer) may be utilized in the operative setting following laminectomy for localization and optimal placement of shunt tubes.[42] The normal cord can be visualized with ultrasound as a uniformly hypoechoic structure with a hyperechoic ventral and dorsal surface. A syrinx cavity is easily identified as a sharply marginated, anechoic cavity within the cord substance. By identifying the widest area and most superficial point of the syrinx, the catheter can be entered into the cavity with minimal myotomy. The course of the shunt catheter can then be followed to verify placement in a location that does not impinge on normal cord tissue. Following placement, the adequacy of drainage (and absence of loculations) can also be assessed.

Dynamic Imaging

Newer dynamic MRI techniques have been developed that can evaluate normal and abnormal CSF flow within the spine. It is hoped that CSF flow studies implemented with routine spin-echo imaging of the spine can improve specificity and possibly have an impact on patient management in patients with syringomyelia. For example, the presence of prominent flow in a hydromyelic cavity of a symptomatic patient preoperatively may help predict the success of shunting. Additionally, studying flow patterns may help in understanding the mechanism of formation and growth of these cavities.

The same phenomena that cause CSF flow artifact on routine spin-echo images can be exploited to evaluate CSF motion in the spinal canal. On T2-weighted sequences without flow compensation, the effect of pulsatile flow can be seen as areas of signal void (black) within the high signal intensity CSF, although their presence is not a constant (Figure 10B). MR phase imaging is a more reliable technique, which is sensitive to slow flow and has the capability of quantification.[15,37] It is a gradient-echo sequence which utilizes bipolar gradients to encode velocity along a preselected direction (e.g., rostrocaudal and caudorostral flow in the sagittal plane). Magnetic spins moving along the direction of the gradients acquire a phase shift that is proportionate to their velocity. This phase shift is encoded in terms of velocity and direction along the gradient. Caudal motion is depicted in shades of white, cranial motion in shades of black, and no flow (stationary tissue) is gray. To obtain a cine format, the cardiac cycle is divided into multiple frames. The sequence is synchronized to the cardiac cycle (peripheral pulse or cardiac gating) so that images are obtained in the same plane for each frame across the cardiac cycle. These are then displayed in a closed loop cine format so that variation in velocity and direction can be studied over time.

Normal patterns of brain motion and CSF flow have been identified. During systole, the sequential caudal-to-rostral flow of blood into the intracranial arterial compartment results in the sequential expansion of the brain parenchyma. This, in turn, appears to pump CSF out of the ventricular system. Systolic expansion of the hemispheres also compresses the subarachnoid space, leading to caudal flow in the basal cisterns. Intracranial CSF motion in combination with downward movement of the brain stem during systole then transmits CSF pulsations into the spinal canal.[16,17] Thus, caudal flow occurs normally during systole in the basal cisterns and in the spinal subarachnoid space. Flow is most rapid in the cervical and upper

thoracic regions and decreases more inferiorly. Following cardiac diastole, CSF motion reverses, flowing rostrally in the spinal canal. Flow has been found to be most prominent in wider subarachnoid spaces (ventral to the cervical cord) and somewhat compartmentalized by nerve roots and dentate ligaments.[37]

MR phase-contrast imaging has demonstrated pulsatile fluid motion in syrinx cavities in synchrony with the adjacent subarachnoid space. The identification of pulsatile flow appears to be related more to the size of the cavity than to the etiology. Flow is seen in congenital, large posttraumatic, and benign syrinx cavities above intramedullary tumors (but not in tumoral cysts or cystic myelomalacia).[37] Moreover, large cavities generally demonstrate prominent intraluminal flow while small syrinx cavities (less than two vertebral segments) may not show any flow. Following decompression, syrinx flow decreases as the size of the cavity decreases and may be eliminated with near complete collapse of the syrinx.

SYRINGOMYELIA AND THE CHIARI I MALFORMATION

Dynamic Imaging

Despite the lack of a single unifying theory regarding the pathogenesis of syringomyelia, common to all theories is the presence of abnormal CSF motion. As data and experience continue to be collected and technological capabilities continue to advance, phase-contrast imaging will hopefully add new insight into the mechanism of syrinx formation. Early studies in patients with Chiari I malformation have demonstrated abnormal dynamics at the foramen magnum. Specifically, Quencer et al[37] in 1990 observed CSF flow ventrally, but absent flow dorsally in Chiari I patients. Wolpert et al[44] in 1994 identified abnormal pulsatile downward movement of the tonsils during systole, with velocities 10 times normal. As recently as 1994, Oldfield et al,[32] utilizing both phase-contrast MRI and intraoperative ultrasound, made several observations. MR images demonstrated only limited flow during systole or diastole across the foramen magnum, but prominent

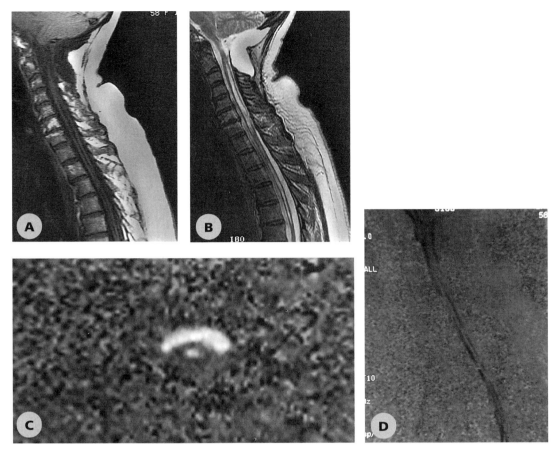

Figure 12: Postoperative evaluation in a patient with a Chiari I malformation and cervicothoracic syrinx following foramen magnum decompression. Sagittal T1-weighted spin-echo **(A)** and sagittal T2-weighted fast spin-echo **(B)** MRI sequences demonstrating a residual syrinx cavity that contains pulsatile flow seen as low signal (flow void) within the syrinx on the T2-weighted image. Also note pulsatile CSF flow (low signal) in the anterior subarachnoid space. A large postoperative pseudomeningocele *(arrow)* is present. **C** and **D)** Images from a phase-contrast CSF flow study in the same patient. The axial image **(C)** shows caudal flow (high signal) in both the anterior subarachnoid space and within the syrinx. The sagittal image **(D)** demonstrates rostral flow (low signal) anterior and posterior to the cervicomedullary junction, within the anterior subarachnoid space, and within the syrinx.

and synchronous CSF flow in the spinal subarachnoid space and syrinx cavity. Ultrasound demonstrated pulsatile downward motion of the tonsils, which was synchronous with pulsatile contraction of the syrinx wall, both of which decreased or disappeared following opening of the dura. Based upon their observations, the authors proposed the following mechanism of syrinx formation. The tonsils plug the normal flow of CSF at the foramen magnum, partially isolating the CSF space of the spinal canal. Rapid downward movement of the tonsils causes a systolic pressure wave, which forces

CSF into perivascular and interstitial spaces of the cord, resulting in formation and propagation of a syrinx cavity.

Postoperative Evaluation

MRI is useful postoperatively for the purpose of evaluating the adequacy of decompression at the foramen magnum and of syrinx cavities, particularly when symptoms recur or are progressive.[2,5,15,40,42] Following foramen magnum decompression, CSF should be identified anterior to the cervicomedullary junction and posterior to the tonsils on sagittal T1-weighted images (Figure 12A). Occasionally, a change in the configuration of the tonsils from a pointed to a more rounded appearance will also be seen.[36] Postoperative MRI can also verify collapse of the syrinx, which is often gradual over several months.[5] Accordingly, syrinx flow will decrease on CSF dynamic studies as the size of the cavity decreases and may be eliminated with near collapse of the cavity (Figure 10E and F). In cases in which the cavity is shunted directly, the catheter position can be identified as a tubular area of low signal extending into the cord and syrinx. This is often best appreciated on T2-weighted or gradient-echo images. Recurrence of the syrinx due to shunt malfunction or loculations within the cavity can be seen as an increase in size of either the entire extent (shunt malfunction) or a portion (loculation) of the syrinx. Also, flow studies may show a return or increase in pulsatile flow as the size of the syrinx increases (Figure 12B-D).

REFERENCES

1. Aboullez AO, Sartor K, Geyer CA, et al: Position of cerebellar tonsils in the normal population and in patients with Chiari malformation: a quantitative approach with MR imaging. **J Comput Assist Tomogr 9**:1033-1036, 1985
2. Barkovich AJ, Sherman JL, Citrin CM, et al: MR of postoperative syringomyelia. **AJNR 8**:319-327, 1987
3. Barkovich AJ, Wippold FJ, Sherman JL, et al: Significance of cerebellar tonsillar position on MR. **AJNR 7**: 795-799, 1986
4. Barnes PD, Brody JD, Jaramillo D, et al: Atypical idiopathic scoliosis: MR imaging evaluation. **Radiology 186**:247-253, 1993
5. Batzdorf U: Chiari I malformation with syringomyelia. Evaluation of surgical therapy by magnetic resonance imaging. **J Neurosurg 68**:726-730, 1988
6. Bradley WG: Flow phenomena, in Stark DD, Bradley WG (eds): **Magnetic Resonance Imaging.** 2nd ed. St Louis, Mo: Mosby Year Book, 1992, pp 287-290
7. Castillo M, Quencer RA, Dominquez R: Chiari III malformation: imaging features. **AJNR 13**:107-113, 1992
8. Chumas PD, Armstrong DC, Drake JM, et al: Tonsillar herniation: the rule rather than the exception after lumboperitoneal shunting in the pediatric population. **J Neurosurg 78**:568-573, 1993
9. Coomrad RW, Richardson WJ, Oakes WJ: Left thoracic curves can be different. **Orthop Trans IX**: 128-129, 1985
10. Curnes JT, Oakes WJ, Boyko OB: MR imaging of hindbrain deformity in Chiari II patients with and without symptoms of brainstem compression. **AJNR 10**:293-302, 1989
11. Dyste GN, Menezes AH, VanGilder JC: Symptomatic Chiari malformations. An analysis of presentation, management, and long-term outcome. **J Neurosurg 71**:159-168, 1989
12. El Gammal T, Mark EK, Brooks BS: MR imaging of Chiari II malformation. **AJR 150**:163-170, 1988
13. Elster AD, Chen MY: Chiari I malformations: clinical and radiologic reappraisal. **Radiology 183**:347-353, 1992
14. Emery JL, MacKenzie N: Medullo-cervical dislocation deformity (Chiari II deformity) related to neurospinal dysraphism (myelomeningocele). **Brain 96**: 155-162, 1973
15. Enzmann DR: Imaging of syringomyelia, in Batzdorf U (ed): **Syringomyelia: Current Concepts in Diagnosis and Treatment.** Baltimore, Md: Williams & Wilkins, 1991, pp 116-139
16. Enzmann DR, Pelc NJ: Brain motion: measurement with phase-contrast MR imaging. **Radiology 185**: 653-660, 1992
17. Enzmann DR, Pelc NJ: Normal flow patterns of intracranial and spinal cerebrospinal fluid defined with phase-contrast cine MR imaging. **Radiology 178**: 467-474, 1991
18. Forbes WSC, Isherwood I: Computed tomography in syringomyelia and the associated Arnold-Chiari type I malformation. **Neuroradiology 15**:73-78, 1978
19. Kochan JP, Quencer RM: Imaging of cystic and cavitary lesions of the spinal cord and canal, in Modic MT (ed): **The Radiologic Clinics of North America.** Philadelphia, Pa: WB Saunders, 1974, pp 457-472
20. Lewonowski K, King JD, Nelson ND: Routine use of magnetic resonance imaging in idiopathic scoliosis patients less than eleven years of age. **Spine 17**: S109-S116, 1992
21. Li KC, Chui MC: Conventional and CT metrizamide myelography in Arnold-Chiari I malformation and syringomyelia. **AJNR 8**:11-17, 1987
22. MacKenzie NG, Emery JL: Deformities of the cervical cord in children with neurospinal dysraphism. **Dev Med Child Neurol 25 (Suppl)**:58-61, 1971
23. Madsen JR, Scott RM: Chiari malformations, syringomyelia, and intramedullary spinal cord tumors. **Curr Opin Neurol Neurosurg 6**:559-563, 1993
24. Mikulis DJ, Diaz O, Egglin TK, et al: Variance of the position of the cerebellar tonsils with age: preliminary report. **Radiology 183**:725-728, 1992
25. Muhonen MG, Menezes AH, Sawin PD, et al: Scoliosis in pediatric Chiari malformations without myelodysplasia. **J Neurosurg 77**:69-77, 1992
26. Naidich TP: Chiari malformations, in Weinberg PE (ed): **Neuroradiology Test and Syllabus, Part 1.** Virginia: The American College of Radiology, 1990, pp 205-225
27. Naidich TP, McLone DG, Fulling KH: The Chiari II malformation: Part IV. The hindbrain deformity. **Neuroradiology 25**:179-197, 1983
28. Naidich TP, Pudlowski RM, Naidich JB: Computed tomographic signs of Chiari II malformation. II: Midbrain and cerebellum. **Radiology 134**:391-398, 1980
29. Naidich TP, Pudlowski RM, Naidich JB: Computed tomographic signs of the Chiari II malformation. III: Ventricles and cisterns. **Radiology 134**:657-663, 1980
30. Naidich TP, Pudlowski RM, Naidich JB, et al: Computed tomographic signs of the Chiari II malforma-

tion. I: Skull and dural partitions. **Radiology 134:** 65-71, 1980

31. Naidich TP, Zimmerman RA: Common congenital malformations of the brain, in Brant-Zawadzki M, Norman D (eds): **Magnetic Resonance Imaging of the Central Nervous System.** New York, NY: Raven Press, 1987, pp 131-150

32. Oldfield EH, Muraszko K, Shawker TH, et al: Pathophysiology of syringomyelia associated with Chiari I malformation of the cerebellar tonsils. Implications for diagnosis and treatment. **J Neurosurg 80:**3-15, 1994

33. Pannullo SC, Reich JB, Krol G: MRI changes in intracranial hypotension. **Neurology 43:**919-926, 1993

34. Payner TD, Prenger E, Berger TS, et al: Acquired Chiari malformations: incidence, diagnosis, and management. **Neurosurgery 34:**429-434, 1994

35. Peach B: Arnold-Chiari malformation. Anatomic features of 20 cases. **Arch Neurol 12:**613-621, 1965

36. Pillay PK, Awad IA, Little JR, et al: Symptomatic Chiari malformation in adults: a new classification based on magnetic resonance imaging with clinical and prognostic significance. **Neurosurgery 28:** 639-645, 1991

37. Quencer RM, Donovan Post MJ, Hinks RS: Cine MR in the evaluation of normal and abnormal CSF flow: intracranial and intraspinal studies. **Neuroradiology** 32:371-391, 1990

38. Sathi S, Stieg PE: "Acquired" Chiari I malformation after multiple lumbar punctures: case report. **Neurosurgery 32:**306-309, 1993

39. Sze G, Krol G, Zimmerman RD, et al: Intramedullary disease of the spine: diagnosis using gadolinium-DTPA-enhanced MR imaging. **AJR 151:**1193-1204, 1986

40. Vaquero J, Martínez R, Arias A: Syringomyelia-Chiari complex: magnetic resonance imaging and clinical evaluation of surgical treatment. **J Neurosurg 73:** 64-68, 1990

41. Welch K, Shillito J, Strand R, et al: Chiari I "malformation"—an acquired disorder? **J Neurosurg 55:** 604-609, 1982

42. Wilberger JE Jr, Maroon JC, Prostko ER, et al: Magnetic resonance imaging and intraoperative neurosonography in syringomyelia. **Neurosurgery 20:** 599-605, 1987

43. Wolpert SM, Anderson M, Scott RM, et al: Chiari II malformation: MR imaging evaluation. **AJR 149:** 1033-1042, 1987

44. Wolpert SM, Bhadelia RA, Bogdan AR, et al: Chiari I malformations: assessment with phase-contrast velocity MR. **AJNR 15:**1299-1308, 1994

45. Yu HC, Deck MDF: The clivus deformity of the Arnold-Chiari malformation. **Radiology 101:** 613-615, 1971

CHAPTER 5

THE CHIARI I MALFORMATION

R. PATRICK JACOB, MD, AND ALBERT L. RHOTON, JR., MD

The diagnosis of the Chiari malformation refers to a group of congenital, and occasionally acquired, hindbrain abnormalities that are characterized by caudal displacement of portions of the cerebellum through the foramen magnum. They are frequently associated with other findings, including caudal displacement of the medulla and/or fourth ventricle, hydrocephalus, midbrain abnormalities, cerebellar abnormalities, and myelodysplasias. In his series of such patients, Chiari categorized these patients into four different groups.[8,9] With several refinements, this classification scheme continues to be used.

Chiari I malformations have the hallmark finding of cerebellar tonsils ectopically located below the level of the foramen magnum.[6,15] This exists as a continuum. The degree of displacement of the tonsils varies from a few millimeters to the mid-cervical spine. In severe cases, the medulla and fourth ventricle may also be caudally displaced. Characteristically, these patients present during adolescence or early adulthood. In one-third to three-quarters of patients with a Chiari malformation, there is also a hydromyelic cavity in the spinal cord, most often in the cervical region. The term "hydromyelia" refers to the dilatation of the ependymal-lined central canal of the spinal cord, which can directly communicate with the fourth ventricle through the obex. The term

"syringomyelia" refers to a cyst within the spinal cord that is separate from the central canal and does not communicate with the fourth ventricle.[35] The terms are frequently used interchangeably, and occasionally as syringohydromyelia. Syringobulbia refers to a cystic cavity within the brain stem.

Chiari II malformations comprise a more severe group of abnormalities that are characterized by caudal displacement of the cerebellar tonsils and vermis below the foramen magnum. In many instances, the fourth ventricle is aberrant in position as well. Frequently observed with this abnormality are "beaking" of the tectal plate (fusion of the collicular plate) kinking of the brain stem, as well as hindbrain and tentorial abnormalities. The type II malformation occurs almost exclusively in patients with other myelodysplasias, especially myelomeningoceles.[20] Hydrocephalus is present in nearly all of these patients.

Chiari III malformations are also associated with the caudal displacement of the cerebellar tonsils and vermis into the cervical spinal canal along with the brain stem. The fourth ventricle is caudally displaced as well. Brain stem abnormalities similar to the type II malformation are usually observed, although they may be more severe in degree. This abnormality is characteristically associated with a cervical myelomeningocele.[14]

PATHOGENESIS

A discussion of the modern theories describing the etiology of the congenital Chiari malformations begins with Gardner's work.[13] The "hydrodynamic theory" relates the development of tonsillar herniation and other dysraphic states to disordered embryogenesis in and around the fetal hindbrain.[14] The initial insult is the failure of pathways for cerebrospinal fluid (CSF) egress from the embryological fourth ventricle to open normally at the foramina of Luschka and Magendie. This blockage at the normal exits of the fourth ventricle results in increased pressure. The cerebellar tonsils migrate caudally in response to this pressure gradient, causing the hallmark finding of crowding of the foramen magnum. This elevated pressure can also be transmitted through the obex to the spinal cord and continued pressure allows for persistence or dilatation of the central canal of the spinal cord, resulting in the formation of a hydromyelic cavity. Arterial pulsation and Valsalva maneuvers are believed to be the driving forces for the progressive enlargement of these cysts.

This theory does not completely explain spinal conditions such as syringomyelic cysts that do not communicate with the fourth ventricle. Syringomyelia associated with a Chiari I malformation is the most common cystic lesion of the spinal cord. In many cases, the cysts are not in communication with the spinal cord. In an effort to explain this phenomenon, Williams[37-39] advanced a theory based on pressure differential between the intraspinal and intracranial compartments.

The process begins with a Valsalva maneuver, which distends the epidural venous complex, creating a pressure wave. This drives CSF intracranially. Because of the size of the intracranial space and its compliance, there is typically little resistance to this inward flow. As the intraspinal pressure drops back toward baseline, in the normal state, there should be unrestricted flow of fluid from the cranial compartment into the spinal subarachnoid space. However, in the individual with a Chiari malformation there is an impedance to this caudal flow of CSF. This may be due to arachnoidal adhesions around the foramen magnum or to outlet obstruction at the fourth ventricle. It is this pressure differential of a two-compartment hydrodynamic system which impels the cerebellar tonsils down from the higher pressure intracranial compartment into the foramen magnum and the lower pressure spinal compartment.

These observations were supported clinically by Williams,[37,38] who measured CSF pressures in the intracranial and intraspinal compartments in both asymptomatic and symptomatic individuals. In symptomatic individuals, the pressure gradient across these two compartments persisted longer than in asymptomatic patients. These findings are also consistent with the reports of acquired Chiari malformations in adults who have undergone lumboperitoneal shunting procedures.[23,36] In these cases, the pressure gradient is iatrogenic, and interestingly is reversible with removal of the spinal shunt. Similar findings of a significant pressure gradient have been reported in patients with Chiari malformations during cervical flexion.[33] The flexion results in dynamic compression of the foramen magnum and obstruction of CSF outflow.

Oldfield further advanced the description of the pathophysiology with phase-contrast cine magnetic resonance imaging (MRI).[21,33] This imaging technique elegantly demonstrated the downward movement of CSF during systole. This pressure wave caused abrupt downward herniation of the cerebellar tonsils into the foramen magnum. Postoperative studies, after decompression and duraplasty, confirmed the absence of this pathological fluid movement and of the cerebellar tonsils. Additionally, CSF pulsations were observed within the syrinx cavity, even if it was discontinuous with the fourth ventricle.

CLINICAL PRESENTATION

Chiari I malformations usually present in young adults (average age 29 years); however, the age range at presentation is quite wide, extending into the geriatric population. Less than one-third of patients present in the pediatric age group.[12] Presenting symptoms are listed in Table 1. The most common symptom is pain. Headache, neck pain, and arm pain are the most common complaints. Leg pain is less com-

TABLE 1

PRESENTING SYMPTOMS IN
PATIENTS WITH CHIARI I MALFORMATION*

Headache/neck pain	61%
Arm/hand numbness	60%
Dysesthesia/paresthesia	55%
Upper extremity weakness	44%
Leg weakness/gait difficulty	39%

* Data adapted from Pillay,[26] Piper,[27] and Batzdorf.[4]

TABLE 2

PREOPERATIVE PHYSICAL FINDINGS IN
PATIENTS WITH CHIARI I MALFORMATION*

Sensory deficit	74%
Weakness/atrophy	61%
Spasticity	43%
Cranial neuropathy	24%

* Data adapted from Pillay,[26] Piper,[27] and Batzdorf.[4]

mon. The second most common symptom is that of upper extremity weakness, although the lower extremities or all four limbs may be symptomatic. Sensory loss is present in approximately three-quarters of patients. As with the motor complaints, sensory complaints are more commonly located in the upper extremities. Approximately one-quarter to one-half of patients have complaints of ataxia or loss of balance. Between 10% and 25% of patients present with lower cranial nerve complaints. Hoarseness, changes in voice quality, or difficulty in swallowing are the leading cranial nerve complaints. Other symptoms can, on occasion, include visual disturbance, syncope, or sphincter disturbance.[42]

Common physical findings are presented in Table 2. On neurological examination, up to 80% of the symptomatic patients have muscle weakness, muscle wasting, or reflex changes. The neurological findings parallel the patients' complaints, with the upper extremities more impaired than the lower extremities. Muscle atrophy is most frequently observed in the hands or shoulder girdle. The "syringomyelic cord syndrome" is frequently identified, with weakness or wasting and hyporeflexia in the arms and hands and hyperreflexia in the legs.[30] This combination of findings is caused by the loss of the alpha motor neuron pools locally in the cervical region, with damage to the descending long tracts resulting in a lower motor neuron loss in the arms and hands, with upper motor neuron dysfunction in the legs. The sensory loss most commonly encountered is decreased sensation to pain and temperature. The pattern of loss may not always be symmetrical.

Cranial nerve testing may reveal abnormalities in 15% to 25% of symptomatic patients. A decreased gag reflex is the most common cranial nerve abnormality. Vertigo, diplopia, dysphagia, dysarthria, and facial numbness are also observed in a small percentage of patients. The presence of syringobulbia increases the likelihood of brain stem or cranial nerve findings.

These symptoms and signs have been grouped by various authors into categories by anatomical location. Paul et al[22] denoted three principal groups: foramen magnum compression, central cord syndrome, and cerebellar syndrome. Patients in the foramen magnum group had a combination of motor and sensory deficits along with ataxia and lower cranial neuropathies. Headache was also a common complaint in this group. The central cord syndrome patients were symptomatic with typical dissociated sensory loss, upper extremity weakness/wasting, and long tract signs. Patients in the third group presented with primary symptoms of ataxia and/or nystagmus. Saez et al[31] reported findings supporting this division of patients into groups, but also described groups of patients who were principally symptomatic with spasticity, and bulbar palsies as well.

ASSOCIATED CONDITIONS

Congenital Chiari malformations can frequently be associated with a number of other spinal, craniovertebral junction, and cranial abnormalities. The most common companion finding in the presence of a Chiari I malformation is that of a cervical or cervicothoracic syrinx. The symptomatic presence of the cystic cavity within the cervical spinal cord often contributes substantially to the clinical presentation of the patient. Its presence is associated with some of the more disabling neurological deficits seen in this group of malformations.[26] As previously discussed, the exact mechanism of syrinx formation distant from the fourth ventricle remains controversial. It is essential to be aware of the presence, size, and location of an associated syrinx cavity in order to understand the patient's symptomatic presentation of treatment.

Scoliosis is present in one-half to three-quarters of patients with Chiari malformations.[27] The finding is more common in patients with syringomyelia due to imbalance of the spinal axial musculature, as a result of the spinal cord abnormality. Chiari malformation/syringomyelia should be considered in patients who present with scoliosis characterized by rapid progression of the spinal curvature, a left thoracic curvature, or significant pain.[19] Any neurological deficit in the setting of scoliosis requires thorough evaluation. Correction of the Chiari malformation/syringomyelia is an essential step for satisfactory long-term management of the scoliosis.

Skull base congenital abnormalities are also frequently observed in patients with Chiari malformations.[12] Basilar invagination, also observed with Chiari malformations, not infrequently aggravates the bulbar symptomology via ventral medullary compression. The effect of the reduction of the diameter of the foramen magnum becomes clinically symptomatic when the normal distance of 35 mm is reduced to approximately 19 mm.[10,18] This combination of dorsal cervicomedullary compression from impacted cerebellar tonsils and ventral brain stem compression from the odontoid process requires careful consideration with preoperative imaging studies and the selection of the optimal operative approach. In addition, craniovertebral junction motion segment abnormalities can compound the primary pathophysiology by the addition of pathological motion.

The Klippel-Feil syndrome is a congenital abnormality that results in segmentation anomalies of the cervical spine. These can include congenital fusions, hemivertebrae, and spina bifida occulta.[16] This congenital fusion typically results in compensatory exaggerated motion above or below the fused segments. At the occipitocervical junction or C1-2, this can result in dynamic compression of the neural elements or a pannus resulting in ventral compression. These abnormalities must be carefully considered when a decompression is planned, because resultant spinal instability may cause disastrous postoperative neurological deterioration.

NEUROIMAGING

MRI has become the imaging technique of choice to diagnose Chiari malformations (Figures 1 and 2).[2,32] It is accurate, specific, and noninvasive. In the exceptional case when MRI cannot be performed, computed tomography (CT)-myelography/cisternography with formatted reconstructions can provide sufficient diagnostic information.[17] In a number of cases, MRI alone may not be sufficient to clearly define the anatomy at the skull base or bony abnormalities in the cervical spine. The combination of MRI and reformatted CT can define accurately the surgical anatomy and aid in surgical planning.

MRI is exquisitely sensitive to defining the location of the caudal structures of the cerebellum. The spectrum ranges from clearly normal tonsillar position to clearly diagnostic position associated with the Chiari malformation. Patients in whom the Chiari malformation is subtle or borderline can on occasion present a diagnostic dilemma. Barkovich et al[2] examined 200 normal subjects and found that cerebellar tonsils varied from 8 mm above to 5 mm below the foramen magnum. In patients with clinical syndromes consistent with Chiari malformations, the range was from 3 to 29 mm below the foramen magnum. The diagnosis was very secure in patients with more than 5 mm of tonsillar descent. In borderline cases, additional information may be obtained by identifying the position of the obex of the fourth ventricle and the nucleus gracilis on a thin-section MRI.

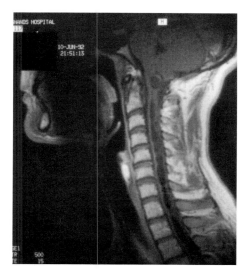

Figure 1: Preoperative sagittal MRI of a man aged 34 years presenting with headache, bilateral hand numbness, and wasting of the hand intrinsic muscles. The scan demonstrates the characteristic finding, of a Chiari I malformation with crowding of the foramen magnum and herniation of the cerebellar tonsils down below the foramen magnum. There is a large syringomyelic cyst present in the entire spinal cord, extending from the caudal medulla down into the thoracic spine.

Quisling et al[28] demonstrated that these structures do not lie below the plane of the foramen magnum in normal subjects.

Often, MRI is among the first diagnostic studies ordered for patients complaining of nontraumatic headaches or craniocervical pain, especially if a neurological abnormality is identified on examination. Careful evaluation of the information visualized on MRI will indicate the need for further imaging studies. If the MRI demonstrates the presence of associated diagnoses, such as scoliosis, basilar invagination, congenital fusions, or Klippel-Feil abnormality, further imaging should be pursued. Plain spine radiographs help to define the bony anatomy and should be supplemented with dynamic flexion-extension views of the cervical spine if instability is suspected clinically or by MRI. CT with multiplanar reconstruction can be very helpful to define anatomy, particularly at the skull base and craniovertebral junction. This is especially so in cases of basilar invagination where ventral decompression is required.

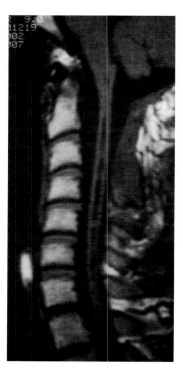
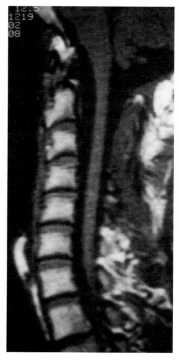

Figure 2: Postoperative sagittal MRI of the same patient as Figure 1 following suboccipital craniectomy and cervical laminectomy. A syringosubarachnoid shunt was placed through a paper-thin dorsal root entry zone myelotomy at C2. A generous duraplasty was used for closure. The MRI demonstrates wide decompression of the foramen magnum with significant reduction in the size of the syrinx. The patient had improvement in complaints of headache and paresthesias, but continues to have some hand weakness. No new deficits have been noted.

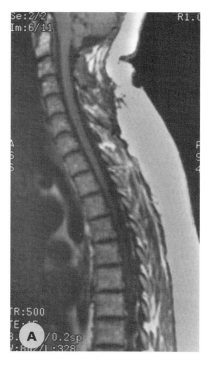
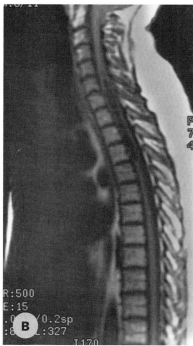

Figure 3: Preoperative sagittal MRI of a woman aged 36 years presenting with headache, hand numbness, and spasticity. **A)** MRI of the posterior fossa reveals the common findings of a type I malformation, with herniation of the cerebellar tonsils down to the mid-body of C2 and an area of flow void suggestive of a large dural venous lake. **B)** The lower cervical and thoracic spinal cord is seen to better advantage. A large syringomyelic cyst is demonstrated which does not communicate with the obex, extending from the mid-cervical region into the upper thoracic region.

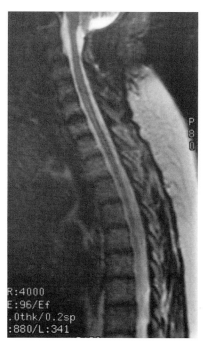

Figure 4: Postoperative sagittal MRI of the same patient as Figure 3, obtained 3 months after suboccipital craniectomy, upper cervical laminectomy, and duraplasty. No surgery was done directly on the cyst. Note that the syrinx had essentially collapsed with adequate decompression of the foramen magnum.

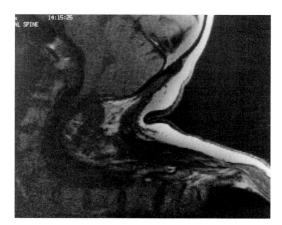

Figure 5: Sagittal MRI following reoperation showing platybasia and a swan-neck deformity associated with a type I malformation. The patient had a progressive myelopathy with difficulty swallowing. She required external skeletal traction for preoperative spinal realignment prior to foramen magnum decompression and occipitothoracic fusion and instrumentation.

SURGICAL TREATMENT

There has been much debate and discussion over the preferred treatment for patients with symptomatic Chiari malformation. The surgical plan should be appropriately tailored to suit the case-specific anatomy and pathology (Figures 3 and 4). Ventral compression should be dealt with via ventral approaches and dorsal compression via a dorsal approach. The important goals center around decompression of the craniocervical segment and the opening of the CSF pathways. Additionally, procedures should not leave the spine mechanically unstable or place functional neural elements at great risk.

Ventral Approaches

If MRI demonstrates findings of basilar invagination or compressive ventral pannus, ventral decompression of the foramen magnum and brain stem is indicated (Figures 5 to 9). If ventral decompression is considered, the preoperative evaluation should include a careful evaluation of craniocervical stability and, if necessary, CT to delineate the bony anatomy. If basilar

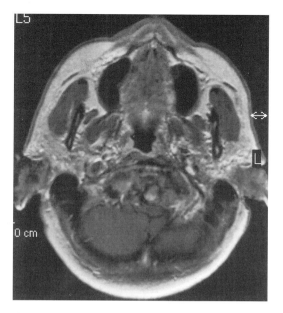

Figure 6: Preoperative sagittal MRI showing a complex type I malformation in a woman aged 67 years who presented with neck pain, hoarseness, repeated episodes of aspiration, and hand numbness. The patient has findings of Chiari I abnormality with tonsillar herniation and crowding of the foramen magnum ventricle. Additionally, there is basilar invagination with the odontoid process compressing the ventral surface of the medulla. A Klippel-Feil abnormality is also demonstrated, with congenital fusion of C2-7 and assimilation of the atlas to the occiput.

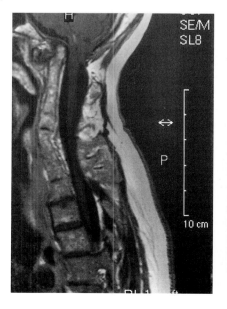

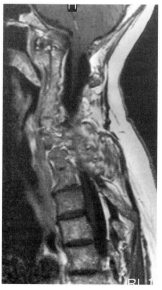

Figure 7: Axial MRI showing the craniocervical junction of the same patient as Figure 6. The ventral compression of the medulla by the odontoid is evident. This degree of ventral compression can only be relieved via a transoral approach.

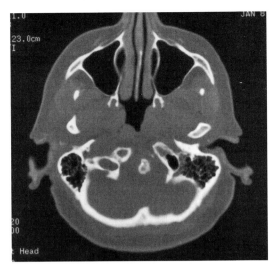

Figure 8: Preoperative axial CT scan of the same patient as Figure 6 showing the bony abnormality with the odontoid process well within the foramen magnum, compressing the brain stem.

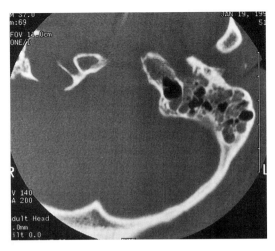

Figure 9: Postoperative CT scan of the same patient as Figure 6 showing resection of the odontoid peg and ventral decompression of the brain stem via a transoral route. This was followed by a posterior foramen magnum decompression, duraplasty, and occipitocervical instrumentation and fusion.

invagination is noted, preoperative cervical traction for reduction of the abnormality should be considered. If the deformity can be successfully reduced, dorsal decompression and duraplasty, along with craniocervical instrumentation and fusion, are required to accomplish the goals of foramen magnum decompression and occipitocervical stabilization. For fixed ventral abnormalities, ventral decompression is clearly indicated as an adjunct to the standard dorsal procedure.

Ventral transoral approaches do not address the fourth ventricular outlet obstruction or impacted cerebellar tonsils observed with Chiari malformations. Therefore, this approach is usually combined with a dorsal procedure. This combined approach renders the C1-2 segment, and very likely the craniocervical junction, mechanically unstable in 75% of patients.[11] When planning a combined ventral and dorsal decompression with suboccipital craniectomy and duraplasty, cervical instability must be anticipated. Dorsal craniocervical fusion can be accomplished with Luque type instrumentation and sublaminar wire fixation, extending from the mid-cervical spine to the occiput. Ventral decompression alone, in the absence of pre-

existing mechanical instability, as in rheumatoid arthritis, renders the C1-2 segment unstable in approximately 50%-60% of the cases.

Dorsal Approaches

The traditional and most common procedure for the treatment of a Chiari malformation is via a dorsal approach. Many variations of this technique have been reported. The primary goals of nearly all of these procedures are the decompression of the foramen magnum/cervicomedullary junction, expansion of the subarachnoid space, and the creation of a CSF pathway that reduces syrinx formation tendencies.[24,25]

Selection of a particular procedure must be individualized. Patients with a syringomyelic clinical presentation are at greater neurological risk than those who present with headache. Accordingly, differences in surgical planning are appropriate.[26] The preoperative planning should take into account the presence and severity of any neurological deficit.

As part of the decompression for patients with a Chiari malformation, a suboccipital craniectomy is performed, enlarging the foramen magnum to 35-40 mm in diameter. This should attempt to enlarge all dorsal dimensions of the foramen magnum, taking care to not disrupt the atlanto-occipital joints. The cervical laminectomy should include C1 and most if not all of C2. The laminectomy in all cases must be carried to below the most caudal extent of the herniated tonsils in order to ensure adequate decompression. The dural opening is performed with particular attention paid to careful hemostasis. The dural incision is carried up to the craniocervical junction where the incision extends rostrolaterally in a "Y" shape. All constricting bands of arachnoid should be released as part of the decompression.[7] With microsurgical technique, the cerebellar tonsils are separated, allowing access to the obex and CSF egress from the fourth ventricle. The use of a Silastic shunt tube from the ventricle to the subarachnoid space is controversial. Excellent results have been reported with and without its use.[3] Dural closure is then obtained with the use of a dural graft or a fascia lata patch, in order to enlarge the subarachnoid space locally.

There are several variations of this procedure that have been published, including plugging of the obex, syrinx shunting procedures, cyst marsupialization, and terminal ventriculostomies. For the most part, these procedures are performed in combination with a foramen magnum decompression and duraplasty. Thus, it is very difficult to establish retrospectively whether the combination of procedures affords additional clinical benefit. These techniques have been proposed for the treatment of the associated syringomyelia and did not primarily address the hindbrain abnormality specific to the Chiari malformation. Many authors recommend suboccipital craniectomy, upper cervical laminectomy, lysis of arachnoidal adhesion, opening of the fourth ventricle, and duraplasty as the initial surgical treatment.[5]

In those patients who worsen after surgery, consideration should be given to reoperation. Repeat imaging studies should be obtained to assess the adequacy of foramen magnum decompression. If the decompression and duraplasty are found to be generous, attention should be directed to the syrinx (syrinx enlargement). Additionally, dynamic cervical spine radiographs should be obtained to evaluate for possible instability. If clinical worsening indicates reoperation, several options are available. If syringomyelic cord syndrome symptoms progress or the syrinx cavity is noted to be enlarging on serial imaging studies, shunting of the cyst cavity and/or plugging of the obex may be incorporated into a reoperative procedure.[34] When considering myelotomy for placement of a shunt tube, the risk of increased neurological deficit must be considered. The incision should be placed over the thinnest aspect of the spinal cord in order to minimize neural injury. This was shown by Rhoton[29] to be at the dorsal root entry zone. Placement of the shunt tube should also be guided by the patient's preoperative deficits in an effort to minimize the risk to neurological function.

If the arachnoid is heavily scarred, as in the case of multiple reoperations, syringosubarachnoid shunt placement may be difficult. In this situation, several options are available for distal shunt placement, including the pleural or peritoneal spaces.[1,41] Terminal ventriculostomy has been retrospectively evaluated by Williams and Fahy[40] and found to be of little benefit, even in reoperation.

OUTCOME

The literature regarding retrospective reviews of patients with Chiari I malformations who have undergone operation spans several decades and differing imaging techniques, with multiple surgical techniques in the hands of many surgeons. As a result, absolute statements are difficult to make. However, several findings are well established. Furthermore, with increased understanding of the pathophysiology, results continue to improve.

Most large series report an improvement in motor strength in 50%-85% of cases.[12,18-21,23,26,29,31,35] However, once muscle atrophy has occurred, there is little hope of improvement in strength. Headache and suboccipital pain are improved in 60%-80% of patients. Dysesthetic pain syndromes are frequently helped even though sensory function does not return. Sensory symptoms appear to have less likelihood for improvement, with most patients being unchanged after surgery. As a group, those patients with a syringomyelic cord syndrome on presentation have a less favorable chance for improvement than those with foramen magnum or cerebellar presentations. As with many other neurological disorders, preoperative neurological status and level of function are highly correlated with postoperative function.

REFERENCES

1. Barbaro NM, Wilson CB, Gutin PH, et al: Surgical treatment of syringomyelia. Favorable results with syringoperitoneal shunting. **J Neurosurg 61:**531-538, 1984

2. Barkovich AJ, Wippold FJ, Sherman JL, et al: Significance of cerebellar tonsillar position on MR. **AJNR 7:**795-799,1986

3. Batzdorf U: Chiari I malformation with syringomyelia. Evaluation of surgical therapy by magnetic resonance imaging. **J Neurosurg 68:**726-730, 1988

4. Batzdorf U: Syringomyelia, Chiari malformation and hydromyelia, in Youmans JR (ed): **Neurological Surgery,** 4th ed. Philadelphia, Pa: WB Saunders, 1996, pp 1090-1105

5. Batzdorf U: Syringomyelia related to abnormalities at the level of the craniocervical junction, in Batzdorf U (ed): **Syringomyelia: Current Concepts in Diagnosis and Treatment.** Baltimore, Md: Williams & Wilkins, 1991, pp 163-182

6. Cameron AH: Malformations of the neuro-spinal axis, urogenital tract and foregut in spina bifida attributable to disturbances of the blastopore. **J Pathol Bacteriol 73:**213-221, 1957

7. Carmel PW: Management of the Chiari malformations in childhood. **Clin Neurosurg 30:**385-406, 1983

8. Chiari H: Concerning alterations in the cerebellum resulting from cerebral hydrocephalus. **Pediatr Neurosci 13:**3-8, 1987 (translation, classical article, original 1891)

9. Chiari H: Über die Pathogenese der Sogennanten Syringomyelie. **Z Hielkunde 9:**307-336, 1888

10. De Barros MC, Farias W, Ataíde L, et al: Basilar impression and Arnold-Chiari malformation. A study of 66 cases. **J Neurol Neurosurg Psychiatry 31:**596-650, 1968

11. Dickman CA, Locantro J, Fessler RG: The influence of transoral odontoid resection on stability of the craniovertebral junction. **J Neurosurg 77:**525-530, 1992

12. Dyste GN, Menezes AH, VanGilder JC: Symptomatic Chiari malformations. An analysis of presentation, management, and long-term outcome. **J Neurosurg 71:**159-168, 1989

13. Gardner WJ: Hydrodynamic mechanism of syringomyelia: its relationship to myelocele. **J Neurol Neurosurg Psychiatry 28:**247-259, 1965

14. Gardner WJ, Angel J: The mechanism of syringomyelia and its surgical correction. **Clin Neurosurg 6:**131-140, 1959

15. Gilbert JN, Jones KL, Rorke LB, et al: Central nervous system anomalies associated with meningomye-

16. Hensinger RN, Lang JE, MacEwen GD: Klippel-Feil syndrome. A constellation of associated anomalies. **J Bone Joint Surg (Am) 56:**1246-1253, 1974

17. Hochman MS, Kobetz SA, Sneider SE, et al: Adult Arnold-Chiari malformation type I demonstrated by CT metrizamide myelography. **Surg Neurol 16:**467-468, 1981

18. Menezes AH, VanGilder JC: Anomalies of the craniovertebral junction, in Youmans JR (ed): **Neurological Surgery: A Comprehensive Reference Guide to the Diagnosis and Management of Neurosurgical Problems,** 3rd ed. Philadelphia, Pa: WB Saunders, 1990, pp 1359-1420

19. Muhonen MG, Menezes AH, Sawin PD, et al: Scoliosis in pediatric Chiari malformations without myelodysplasia. **J Neurosurg 77:**69-77, 1992

20. Oakes WJ: Chiari malformation, hydromyelia, and syringomyelia, in Wilkins RH, Rengachary SS (eds): **Neurosurgery.** New York, NY: McGraw-Hill, 1995, pp 2102-2124

21. Oldfield EH, Muraszko K, Shawker TH, et al: Pathophysiology of syringomyelia associated with Chiari I malformation of the cerebellar tonsils. Implications for diagnosis and treatment. **J Neurosurg 80:**3-15, 1994

22. Paul KS, Lye RH, Strang FA, et al: Arnold-Chiari malformation. Review of 71 cases. **J Neurosurg 58:**183-187, 1983

23. Payner TD, Prenger E, Berger TS, et al: Acquired Chiari malformations: incidence, diagnosis, and management. **Neurosurgery 34:**429-434, 1994

24. Penfield W, Coburn DF: Arnold-Chiari malformation and its operative treatment. **Arch Neurol Psychiatry 40:**328-336, 1938

25. Phillips TW, Kindt GW: Syringoperitoneal shunt for syringomyelia: a preliminary report. **Surg Neurol 16:**462-466, 1981

26. Pillay PK, Awad IA, Little JR, et al: Symptomatic Chiari malformation in adults: a new classification based on magnetic resonance imaging with clinical and prognostic significance. **Neurosurgery 28:**639-645, 1991

27. Piper JG, Menezes AH: Chiari malformation in the adult, in Menezes AH, Sonntag VKH (eds): **Principles of Spinal Surgery.** New York, NY: McGraw-Hill, 1996, pp 379-397

28. Quisling RG, Quisling SG, Mickle JP: Obex/nucleus gracilis position: its role as a marker for the cervicomedullary junction. **J Pediatr Neurosurg 19:**143-150, 1993

29. Rhoton AL Jr: Microsurgery of Arnold-Chiari malformation in adults with and without hydromyelia. **J Neurosurg 45:**473-483, 1976

30. Rhoton AL Jr, Fessler RG: Surgical treatment of Chiari malformation and hydromyelia in adults, in Wilson CB (ed): **Neurosurgical Procedures. Personal Approaches to Classic Operations.** Baltimore, Md: Williams & Wilkins, 1992, pp 169-187

31. Saez RJ, Onofrio BM, Yanagihara T: Experience with Arnold-Chiari malformation, 1960 to 1970. **J Neurosurg 45:**416-422, 1976

32. Spetzler RF, Zabramski JM, Kaufman B: Clinical role

of magnetic resonance imaging in the neurosurgical patient. **Neurosurgery 16:**511-524, 1985

33. Tachibana S, Iida H, Yada K: Significance of positive Queckenstedt test in patients with syringomyelia associated with Arnold-Chiari malformations. **J Neurosurg 76:**67-71, 1992

34. Tator CH, Meguro K, Rowed DW: Favorable results with syringosubarachnoid shunts for treatment of syringomyelia. **J Neurosurg 56:**517-523, 1982

35. Vaquero J, Martinez R, Arias A: Syringomyelia-Chiari complex: magnetic resonance imaging and clinical evaluation of surgical treatment. **J Neurosurg 73:**64-68, 1990

36. Welch K, Shillito J, Strand R, et al: Chiari I "malformation"—an acquired disorder? **J Neurosurg 55:**604-609, 1981

37. Williams B: On the pathogenesis of syringomyelia: a review. **J R Soc Med 73:**798-806, 1980

38. Williams B: Simultaneous cerebral and spinal fluid pressure recording: 1. Technique, physiology, and normal results. **Acta Neurochir 58:**167-185, 1981

39. Williams B: Simultaneous cerebral and spinal fluid pressure recordings. 2. Cerebrospinal dissociation with lesions at the foramen magnum. **Acta Neurochir 59:**123-142, 1981

40. Williams B, Fahy G: A critical apprasial of "terminal ventriculostomy" for the treatment of syringomyelia. **J Neurosurg 58:**188-197, 1983

41. Williams B, Page N: Surgical treatment of syringomyelia with syringopleural shunting. **Br J Neurosurg 1:**63-80, 1987

42. Zager EL, Ojemann RG, Poletti CE: Acute presentations of syringomyelia. Report of three cases. **J Neurosurg 72:**133-138, 1990

CHAPTER 6

THE CHIARI II MALFORMATION OF THE HINDBRAIN AND THE ASSOCIATED HYDROMYELIA

DAVID G. MCLONE, MD, PHD

The Chiari II malformation of the hindbrain is almost invariably associated with a myelomeningocele.[3-5,13] This complex hindbrain malformation is the principal cause of death in children with myelomeningocele, despite surgical intervention and aggressive medical management.[12,23] The precise cause of the clinical manifestations of the Chiari II malformation may relate to the dysplasia of the brain stem and intrinsic "wiring" defects in the human newborn and to progressive hydrocephalus and/or hindbrain compression in the infant or older child.

Previous theories of the Chiari II malformation have described the cause of the malformation in structural and mechanical terms. In the Chiari II hindbrain malformation, the cerebellar vermis is displaced downward below the foramen magnum into the cervical canal (Figure 1); the brain stem is elongated, kinked, and displaced into the cervical canal; the fourth ventricle is elongated and displaced below the foramen magnum; and the superior cerebellum lies above the opening in the dysplastic low-lying tentorium (Figure 2).

Approximately 20% of children with myelomeningocele develop symptoms of hindbrain, cranial nerve, and spinal cord compression. The majority of clinical manifestations of Chiari II malformation occur in infancy, usually before the age of 3 months.[1] In addition to the typical hindbrain abnormalities, multiple cerebral anomalies also occur.

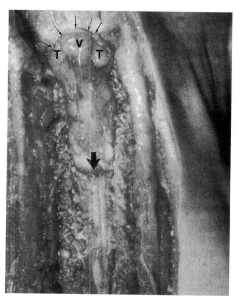

Figure 1: Postmortem examination of a child with a myelomeningocele and the Chiari II malformation. Note the cerebellar vermis (V) and tonsils (T) herniating through the foramen (*small arrows*). The medullary kink is located well into the cervical canal (*arrow*).

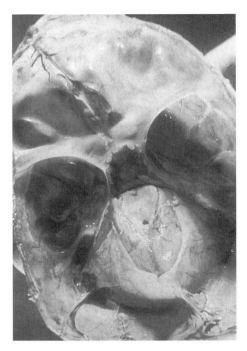

Figure 2: The superior cerebellum bulges through the dysplastic tentorium up into the middle fossa. Note how remarkably small the posterior fossa is.

DEVELOPMENTAL DEFECTS

The author has studied the initial developmental defects of the Chiari II malformation in the embryos of mutant mice with a genetically abnormal neurulation. The delayed Splotch (Spd/Spd) mouse embryo with a sacral neural tube defect was used. At selected time points in the progression of Chiari II malformation, cellular events were studied by light microscopy and electron microscopy. On the basis of these studies, it is suggested that: 1) a series of interrelated time-dependent defects occur in the development of the primitive ventricular system; and 2) defects in or the mistiming of these events result in the Chiari II malformation and the associated pan-central nervous system (CNS) anomalies. A unified theory of the cause of Chiari II malformation of the hindbrain and of the associated pan-CNS anomalies has resulted.[22] This theory examines the cell biology and the developmental neurobiology of the brain and emphasizes the developmental sequence and consequences of six key events:

1) The neural folds fail to neurulate completely, leaving a dorsal myeloschisis. This abnormal neurulation is a prerequisite for later development of the Chiari II malformation.

2) Failure of correct timing of apposition of the walls of the spinal cord with consequent failure to transiently occlude the spinal neurocele (or excessive drainage of "ventricular" cerebrospinal fluid (CSF) through the neural tube defect after the neurocele reopens).

3) This leads to failure to maintain distention of the primitive ventricular system because fluid escapes out through the neural tube defect.

4) The lack of distention of the rhombencephalic vesicle alters the inductive effect of pressure and volume on the surrounding mesenchyme and on the endochondral bone formation, thereby resulting in a small posterior fossa. Consequently, the development of the cerebellum and the brain stem within a small posterior fossa leads to: a) upward herniation, resulting in an enlarged incisural opening and a dysplastic tentorium, and to b) downward herniation, resulting in a large foramen magnum and caudal displacement of the cerebellar vermis and brain stem into the cervical segments.

5) Failure to maintain distention of the primitive ventricular system supratentorially leads to: a) close approximation of the thalami with consequently a small third ventricle and a large massa intermedia; b) inadequate support for the radial glial cells that direct the normal outward migration of neuroblasts with consequent migration defects; and c) failure to maintain the normal radial pattern of collagen formation and ossification in the developing calvarium, leading to lückenschädel.

6) Hydrocephalus is secondary to maldevelopment of the CSF pathway in the posterior fossa.

Neurulation Defect

A defect in neurulation is an *a priori* feature of the Chiari II malformation. In the author's experimental model, the rhombencephalic roof is frequently collapsed, which indicates that the primitive ventricular system was not distended.

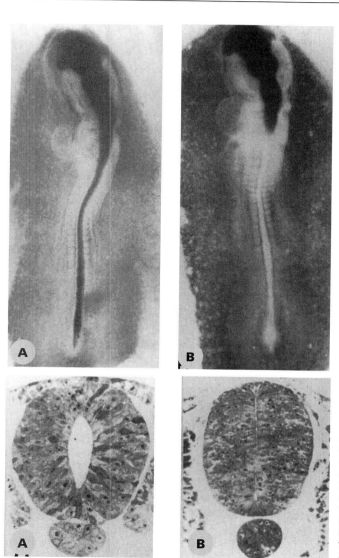

Figure 3: Occlusion of the neurocele (central canal of the embryo) of the chick embryo. **A)** Dye was injected into the cephalic vesicles (embryonic ventricles) and flows into the entire neurocele. **B)** The neurocele closes and dye is excluded from the caudal neurocele (embryonic spinal cord). (Reprinted with permission from Desmond ME, Schoenwolf GC: Timing and positioning of occlusion of the spinal neurocele in the chick embryo. *J Comp Neurol 235*:479-487, 1985)

Failure to Occlude the Spinal Neurocele Transiently

The neurocele is the name given to the central cavity of the developing CNS. Normally, there is transient occlusion of the spinal neurocele as a result of a transient apposition of the medial walls of the embryonic spinal cord during cord and brain development in humans,[7,26,31] mice,[16] and chicks[8,32,38-40] (Figure 3). This normal, transient occlusion appears to be necessary in order to retain CSF within the developing brain and to expand the primitive ventricular system.

Nondistention or collapse of the primitive ventricular system could also result from incomplete occlusion of the spinal neurocele, too short a period of occlusion of the spinal neurocele, or excessive drainage of CSF out of the neural tube defect after reopening of the occluded spinal neurocele. A spectrum of such anomalies should be anticipated.

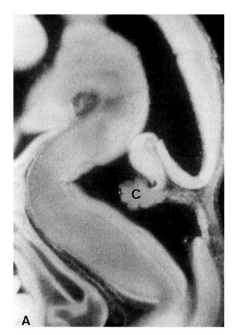
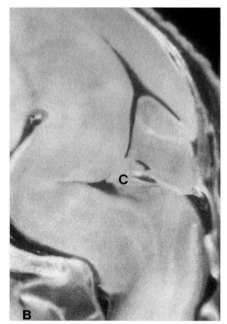

Figure 4: A) The developing posterior fossa of a normal mouse. The neural tube has closed, the rhombencephalic vesicle (embryonic fourth ventricle) is distended, and the cerebellum (C) is blossoming into this space. **B)** A mouse embryo of the same age but with a myelomeningocele, open neural tube. Note the crowded posterior fossa and the already compressed developing cerebellum (C).

Failure to Maintain Distention of the Primitive Ventricular System

Because the neural tube does not close properly and because occlusion of the spinal neurocele is abnormal, CSF escapes down the central canal of the neural tube into the amniotic cavity. Therefore, the primitive ventricular system decompresses and collapses.

Expansion of the primitive ventricular system appears to be required in order to provide the mechanical support for outward migration of neuroblasts and for expansion of the surrounding mesenchyme of the developing cranial vault, permitting it to condense into cartilage or into bone of a size appropriate to future growth. The distention of the rhombencephalic vesicle appears to be required to anticipate the future growth of the cerebellum and to provide sufficient room for it to develop. In human embryos at 35 days gestation, for example, the posterior fossa has formed cartilage and has a fixed volume, even though the cerebellar hemispheres are just beginning to develop from the rhombic lips. Failure of the primitive cranial ventricular system to distend results in a posterior fossa that is too small to accommodate the future growth of the cerebellum.

Development of Chiari II Malformation

Initially, the effect of this lack of distention on the developing hindbrain appears minimal. However, the failure of distention of the rhombencephalic ventricle leaves the basal cranial mesoderm without the inductive force necessary for the normal development of the posterior fossa and its contents, especially the future growth of the cerebellum (Figure 4).[6,15] At the time in which occlusion of the spinal neurocele

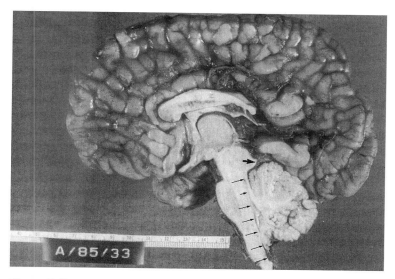

Figure 5: Demonstration of the small third ventricle with a large massa intermedia. Note the floor of the third ventricle is very short and the optic chiasm and mammillary bodies are almost together. Also note the beaked collicular plate *(large arrow)* and the elongated fourth ventricle *(small arrows).*

should normally occur, the mesenchyme surrounding the rhombencephalon contains no collagen. It is made up of widely dispersed cells with large extracellular spaces. Therefore, the mesenchyme is pliable and responds easily to distention by the underlying neural mass.

In Chiari II patients, the volume of the posterior fossa is determined by a nondistended rhombencephalon. Within days, the mesenchyme surrounding the partially collapsed rhombencephalic vesicle condenses. Collagen and cartilage subsequently form, and endochondral bone formation begins. The clivus develops abnormally,[45] and the foramen magnum is large. The volume of the posterior fossa is then fixed and is inadequate.[20] The tentorium is left low and deficient; consequently, the pontine flexure cannot form. Growth of the brain displaces the junction of the brain stem and spinal cord below the foramen magnum, resulting in the angle of the brain stem being altered. It is also likely that the lack of expansion of the rhombencephalic ventricle influences brain stem development, producing disorganization of the cranial nerve nuclei and of their afferent and efferent connections.

Mechanical Effects of Failure to Distend the Third and Lateral Ventricles

Mechanical forces are known to exert intrinsic effects on cellular synthesis; for example, compression and tension are factors in the induction of calcification and bone formation.[25] As a result of failure of the development of the primitive ventricular system, a transcranial disorganization occurs, leading to diverse malformations. The third ventricle fails to distend, so the thalami remain approximated and in contact to form a large massa intermedia (Figure 5). The lateral ventricles fail to distend and thereby fail to support the developing telencephalon. The lack of support for the developing telencephalic hemispheres results in gray matter heterotopia, disorganization of future cerebral gyri, and dysgenesis of the corpus callosum. In experimental animals,[6,16] the developing cerebral cortex becomes disorganized if the fluid is vented from the telencephalic ventricles. Mechanical support by the primitive ventricle appears to be essential to development of normal organization of the cerebral cortex.

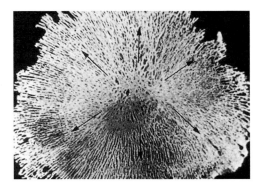

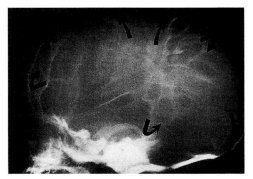

Figure 6: The developing parietal plate of a human fetus. Note the radial ossifying bundles of collagen (*arrows*). With the Chiari II malformation, the bundles are not drawn out over the expanding brain and turn back on themselves.

Normal development of the membranous skull requires distention of the underlying neural mass (i.e., the developing brain and ventricular system). The skull develops from centers in each cranial plate. As the brain expands, collagen bundles are drawn out from those centers in an orderly radial fashion, much like the uniform expansion of the surface of an inflating balloon. As the radial expansion proceeds, the collagen bundles ossify (Figure 6). In children born with a myelomeningocele, the collagen bundles form whorls and coils instead of radial lines. The fibrous tissue between these whorls has varying thicknesses. Ossification of the disorganized collagen mat produces the lückenschädel skull, which is almost invariably seen in patients with myelomeningocele. Late in gestation or postnatally, developing hydrocephalus and/or normal growth and expansion of the neural mass remodels the skull plates, so the lückenschädel skull disappears.

Hydrocephalus

There is increasing evidence that the extracellular matrix and the cellular activity of the cerebrospinal outflow pathway are influenced by time-dependent inductive factors.[17,41] A series of morphogenetic and biochemical events yield a functional outflow pathway. The cause of hydrocephalus in patients with the Chiari II malformation may be variable.[10] An obstruction of the outlets of the fourth ventricle,[37] a blockage at the cerebral aqueduct,[19] obliteration of the subarachnoid space at the level of the foramen magnum by the herniated hindbrain with caudal displacement of the outlets of the fourth ventricle,[14] and/or obstruction at the level of the dysplastic tentorium may block outflow of CSF and, consequently, may contribute to the hydrocephalus.

Between 1975 and 1979, 100 consecutive newborns with myelomeningocele were operated upon and followed prospectively. Review of these 100 children born with a myelomeningocele and undergoing treatment revealed that in 25% of the newborns the head circumference was less than the fifth percentile at birth.[24] Only after closure of the newborn's back did the head circumference increase rapidly. As crowding progresses in the posterior fossa, CSF outflow from the fourth ventricle is occluded. This is especially true at the level of the large incisural opening at the deficient tentorium, where a block is most often seen in the newborn.[10] Consequently, hydrocephalus is likely to be secondary to mistimed developmental steps in the development of the ventricular system. The hydrocephalus is the *result* of the Chiari II hindbrain malformation and the associated pan-CNS anomaly. In a second trimester fetus with a myelomeningocele, the Chiari II malformation of the hindbrain is severe but there is no evidence of hydrocephalus (Figure 7). Hydrocephalus is not the cause of the malformation.

THE UNIFIED THEORY

The author's unified theory incorporates the observation of Padget[33] and Padget and Lindenberg[34] that leakage of CSF is one factor in the cause of a small posterior fossa and emphasizes the role of distention of the embryonic and fetal

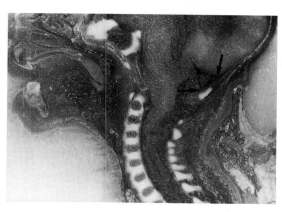

Figure 7: A second trimester spontaneously aborted fetus with a myelomeningocele demonstrates a remarkably small posterior fossa with herniation of hindbrain structures into the upper cervical canal. Note the torcula of the venous sinuses is at the edge of the foramen magnum (*arrows*).

ventricular system in normal cerebral development.[7,26,31] The theory identifies the neural tube defect and the defective occlusion of the spinal neurocele as the developmental factors that cause the Chiari II malformation and the inter-related cerebral and skull anomalies. The Chiari II malformation and lückenschädel are the result of altered inductive pressure on the surrounding mesenchyme, whereas the cerebral anomalies (e.g., dysgenesis of the corpus callosum, large massa intermedia, cortical heterotopia, and polygyria) are the result of lack of distention of the developing telencephalic vesicles. Thus, Chiari II malformation is a result of a series of interrelated time-dependent defects in the development of the ventricular system, which leads to multiple anomalies in the developing brain.

HINDBRAIN DYSFUNCTION

The Chiari II hindbrain malformation[2] continues to be the major cause of death in children with myelomeningocele.[13] Almost all children with myelomeningocele have occasional problems referable to this hindbrain anomaly. In the author's initial series of 100 patients, 32% had significant sequelae of hindbrain dysfunction.

In 13%, the problems were severe and led to repeated hospitalization and surgical procedures to treat or manage the sequelae. One child was born with vocal cord paralysis; the other 12 developed problems in the neonatal period. Eleven of the 13 ultimately died. Of the 32 children with significant sequelae of hindbrain dysfunction, four underwent posterior fossa and cervical decompression because of progressive apnea. Two of these four died; one still requires a tracheostomy, and one has recovered. Of the remaining 28, nine have died. Of the 19 survivors, one has required a tracheostomy and 18 have recovered. The overall mortality rate of 34% in this group is not significantly different from that reported in series in which all children had cervical decompression. Therefore, the natural history of hindbrain dysfunction would appear to be one of gradual improvement over time in those patients who survive the acute problems. Whether posterior fossa and cervical decompression in the neonate alter the course of this disease remains open to question. Several papers have reported benefit from early detection of hindbrain problems and immediate cervical decompression of the Chiari II malformation.[42-45] Because it is difficult to identify which infant will recover spontaneously from stridor due to vocal cord paresis, many authors believe that decompression is indicated for every patient with type II malformation. In all studies, it is agreed that shunt placement or revision is indicated first; however, disagreement arises about what is the next step. Two-thirds recover fully spontaneously and any surgical procedure must produce better results. The surgeon must also weigh the risks and potential benefits to the newborn. There seems to be more agreement about decompression in children who are beyond the neonatal period. Neuroradiological evaluation with magnetic resonance imaging (MRI)[27-29] and brain stem evoked potentials may enable the clinician to identify these children and to anticipate their problems.

HYDROMYELIA

The link between the open neurocele and the Chiari II malformation persists into postnatal life. Abnormal fluid dynamics of hydrocephalus

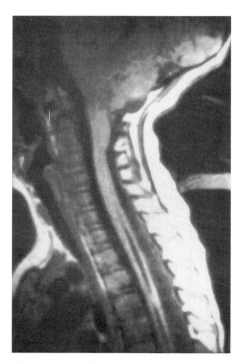

Figure 8: MRI of a child with a Chiari II malformation and an open central canal of the spinal cord.

and cerebellar anomalies at the foramen magnum predispose these individuals to develop hydromyelia. Most children with spina bifida have an obvious open central canal visible on MRI. Although hydromyelia is unusual in the newborn or the unshunted child, it contributes significant morbidity with advancing age to about one-half of the children with a myelomeningocele.

Exactly how the type II malformation causes hydromyelia is not clear. Obviously, most causes have in common an abnormality at the craniovertebral junction. Because hydromyelia is rare in the newborn or in the absence of hydrocephalus, abnormal CSF dynamics are certainly involved. It is likely that this process is initiated by a shunt malfunction, leading to dilatation of the central canal which does not decompress with revision of the cranial shunt.

The term "hydromyelia" is used here to denote a CSF-filled dilatation of the central canal within the spinal cord. Records of 1,195 patients from the Multidisciplinary Spina Bifida Clinic at the Children's Memorial Hospital in Chicago were reviewed to determine the incidence of symptomatic hydromyelia, the pattern of the canal abnormalities, and the treatments that have been found to be effective. Not all 1,195 children in the author's clinic underwent routine MRI. Therefore, in the majority of cases, MRI was obtained for symptomatic children. It is assumed that there is a treatable cause for all deterioration in children with spina bifida.

The combination of hindbrain herniation, hydrocephalus, and caudal spinal cord abnormality in children with a myelomeningocele often leads to hydromyelia. Because the Chiari II malformation involves herniation of the posterior fossa contents, the flow of CSF toward the reabsorption sites is obstructed in several places. This is further complicated in some by arachnoiditis and decrease in reabsorption due to inflammation in the subarachnoid space from leakage of amniotic debris into the subarachnoid spaces prior to birth. Additionally, the spinal cords of these children are tethered to the myelomeningocele closure site, which can lead to spinal cord dysfunction, atrophy, and possibly central canal abnormalities (Figure 8).

Based on the hypothesis that anomalies of the CSF dynamics are the principle mechanisms of hydromyelia in children with a myelomeningocele, a treatment strategy to deal with this problem has been in place in our institution for the past seven years. In the presence of hydrocephalus and hydromyelia, the initial goal is optimal drainage of the ventricular system with a ventriculoperitoneal (VP) shunt.[21,43] If this fails, a decision must be made based on the patient's symptoms between performing a posterior cervical decompression, placing a hydromyelia-pleural shunt, and releasing a tethered cord. In patients with cranial nerve or cervical symptoms, a posterior cervical decompression procedure was performed. In patients with symptoms of scoliosis or lower extremity involvement, a tethered cord release was also often performed. In patients in whom these treatments failed, or who had severe holocord hydromyelia, a hydromyelia-pleural shunt was placed.

In the past seven years, MRI was obtained for every patient with neurological deterioration, including symptoms of scoliosis, upper or lower extremity weakness, increased spasticity, sensory changes, and/or deterioration in bladder or bowel function. MRI of the spine was obtained in a total of 231 children with myelomeningocele and the associated Chiari II malformation. Abnormalities of the central canal were found in 103 of the 231 children with spina bifida.

Following a retrospective review of the MRI scans, the pattern of central canal involvement was categorized into three types: 1) dystrophic cord and enlarged canal due to dysplasia or atrophy (Figures 8 and 9); 2) holocord hydromyelia (Figure 10); and 3) segmental hydromyelia (Figure 11). A "dystrophic cord" is a small spinal cord with an open central canal. The appearance is as if the cord was not fully developed or atrophic as in hydrocephalus *ex vacuo.*

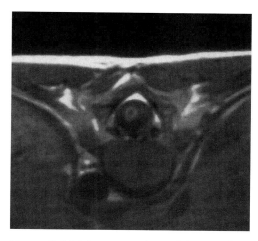

Figure 9: MRI, transverse view, of the spinal cord of a child with a Chiari II malformation demonstrating a small cord with a large central canal. It is not clear whether this commonly seen spinal cord in these children is the result of atrophy or dysplasia.

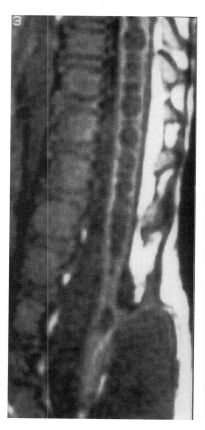
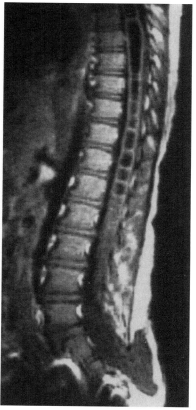

Figure 10: MRI of two children with holocord hydromyelia. Note the "haustra-like" pattern of the cavity.

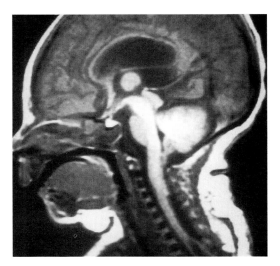

Figure 11: MRI of a child with a Chiari II malformation and a segment of the upper thoracic cord with hydromyelia.

TREATMENT PROCEDURES

Following evaluation of the shunt, children with holocord hydromyelia were treated with hydromyelia-pleural shunting and/or posterior cervical decompression. Ventriculoperitoneal shunt revisions were always performed first when indicated.

EVALUATION OF MRI DATA

In 231 children with a myelomeningocele, nearly 50% (112) had a central canal abnormality. The 112 children were divided between segmental hydromyelia (41 children), holocord hydromyelia (39), and dystrophic cord (32).

Of the 41 patients with segmental hydromyelia, 13 had cervical cavitations and 28 had thoracic or lumbar cavities. The 39 patients with holocord hydromyelia were further divided into two groups: those with moderate hydromyelia (11 children) and those with severe holocord hydromyelia (28). The patients with severe holocord hydromyelia had distended spinal cords due to dramatically enlarged central canals with thinned parenchyma, often with "haustra-like" septations. The patients with moderate hydromyelia had smaller central canals with a diameter less than one-half the diameter of the cord.

The patients with dystrophic cords had very thin spinal cords, in some cases one-third the size of normal, with central canals that were visible on sagittal and axial MRI.

EVALUATION OF SURGICAL OUTCOMES

Only the 80 children with holocord or segmental hydromyelia were included in the outcome analysis (Table 1). Of these, 40 underwent surgery for the treatment of hydromyelia (24 with severe holocord hydromyelia and 16 with segmental hydromyelia).

Patients With Severe Holocord Hydromyelia

Fourteen of the 24 children with severe holocord hydromyelia found by computed tomography (CT) or shunt tap criteria to have nonfunctioning shunts underwent VP shunt revision as their initial treatment. Of these 14, five children had improvement of symptoms and nine did not. Of the nine who did not improve with shunt revision, seven responded to hydromyelia-pleural shunt placement. Two of the nine had posterior cervical decompression procedures, but this procedure failed in both and hydromyelia shunts or stents were required for relief of symptoms.

In 10 of the 24 patients with severe holocord hydromyelia, CT or shunt tap criteria revealed a functioning shunt; posterior cervical decompressions were performed in six of these children because they had symptoms of upper extremity or cranial nerve origin. Four of the six improved, one did not improve and required a hydromyelia-pleural shunt, and one became worse. Four of these 10 children had a tethered cord release because of symptoms of scoliosis or lower extremity dysfunction and all improved.

Patients With Segmental Hydromyelia

Of 41 patients with segmental hydromyelia, 13 had cervical and 28 had thoracolumbar

TABLE 1

REVIEW OF 80 CHILDREN WITH SEGMENTAL OR
HOLOCHORD HYDROMYELIA

	Surgically Treated	No Surgical Treatment	Total
Holochord hydromyelia			39
moderate hydromyelia	0	11	11
severe hydromyelia	24	4	28
Segmental hydromyelia			41
cervical	5	8	13
thoracolumbar	11	17	28

hydromyelia. Five of the 13 patients with cervical hydromyelia were symptomatic and required surgery. Three improved with tethered cord release, one improved with posterior cervical decompression, and one patient failed VP shunt revision and hydromyelia fenestration. Eleven of the 28 patients with thoracolumbar hydromyelia required surgery. Seven improved after initial tethered cord release; the remaining four patients failed VP revision, and then improved with tethered cord release.

Overall Results

Ventriculoperitoneal shunt revisions failed in nine (64%) of 14 patients with severe holocord hydromyelia; in all nine cases, placement of hydromyelia-pleural shunts was successful in improving symptoms. In the 10 children with functioning shunts, holocord hydromyelia, and symptoms of upper extremity or cranial nerve dysfunction, posterior fossa decompression was performed in six patients, with improvement of symptoms in four. One patient became significantly worse, and one required placement of a hydromyelia-pleural shunt. The majority of children (14 of 16) with symptomatic cervical or thoracolumbar hydromyelia improved with tethered cord release and none improved with VP shunt revision.

This retrospective study was carried out to determine what produced the best results and to arrive at a sequence that represents optimal management. After categorizing the children with myelomeningocele into segmental and holocord hydromyelia, the author found that different treatments were effective in these two subsets of patients. Patients with holocord hydromyelia responded to CSF diversion treatments such as VP shunt revision, hydromyelia-pleural shunt, or posterior fossa decompression. Patients with segmental hydromyelia, where there was no radiographic continuity between the fourth ventricle and the hydromyelia cavity, responded to tethered cord release.

In cases of severe holocord hydromyelia, there is communication of CSF with the ventricular system and the preferred first treatment is revision of the VP shunt. Two studies have demonstrated that the ventricular system is in continuity with the central canal in children with myelomeningocele.[21,44] In the mouse, embryo contrast-injected into the mesencephalic vesicle fills the central canal of the spinal cord. It has also been demonstrated in hydrocephalic mice that, once the hydrocephalus is initiated, the central canal dilates[18] (Figure 12). Therefore, a functioning VP shunt may divert CSF from accumulating in the spinal cord central canal and prevent the development of hydromyelia. If the ventricular shunt is not working at a pressure low enough to reduce the central canal volume, placement of a hydromyelia-pleural shunt for effective treatment is required.

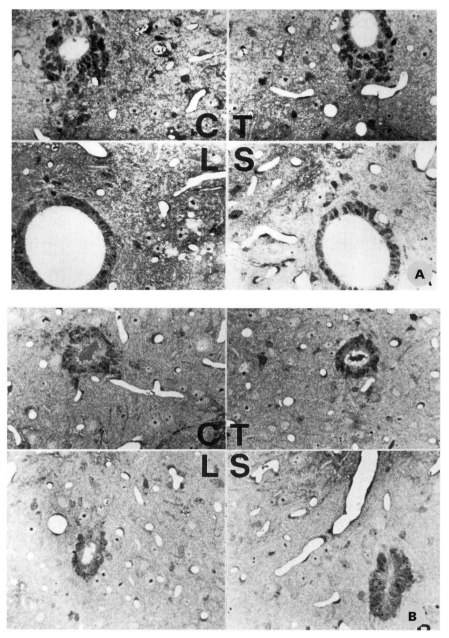

Figure 12: Cross sections of light micrographs of the spinal cords in hydrocephalic mice. **A** demonstrates active hydrocephalus and **B** demonstrates the view after hydrocephalus was decompressed. C = cervical, T = thoracic, L = lumbar, S = sacral.

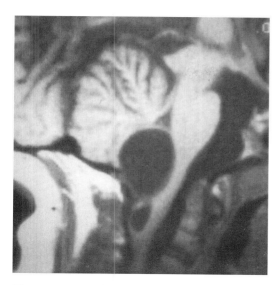

Figure 13: MRI of a child with the Chiari II malformation and hydro-syringobulbia.

Children with new cranial nerve deficits, hindbrain symptoms, and upper extremity involvement should be considered for posterior cervical decompression after establishing that the VP shunt is functioning optimally. Occasionally, the hydromyelia may extend into the bulb and cause hindbrain dysfunction (Figure 13).

In patients with segmental hydromyelia, release of the tethered cord is an effective treatment to improve and arrest progressive deterioration. In some cases, the segmental hydromyelia also improved or disappeared; this may, in some instances, be due to the fact that during tethered cord release, a terminal ventriculostomy was also performed. In these patients, VP shunt revision did not improve symptoms and there was an apparent radiographic discontinuity between the hydromyelia cavity and the fourth ventricle. The mechanism of hydromyelia cavity enlargement may be a function of pulsatile pressure waves forcing CSF into the cord through perivascular and interstitial spaces,[30] rather than through a patent obex.

CONCLUSION

The Chiari II malformation and the often-associated hydromyelia cause significant prob-lems throughout life for the individual born with a myelomeningocele. This birth defect also presents a major management challenge to the neurosurgeon. Life-long jeopardy of deterioration requires observation by a multidisciplinary team of physicians familiar with the nuances of this complex anomaly.

REFERENCES

1. Bell WO, Charney EB, Bruce DA, et al: Symptomatic Arnold-Chiari malformation: review of experience with 22 cases. **J Neurosurg 66:**812-816, 1987
2. Carmel PW: The Arnold-Chiari malformation, in McLaurin RL, Epstein F (eds): **Pediatric Neurosurgery: Surgery of the Developing Nervous System.** New York, NY: Grune & Stratton, 1982, pp 61-77
3. Chiari H: Uber Veränderungen des Kleinhirns, des Pons und der Medulla oblongata in Folge von congenitaler Hydrocephalie des Grosshirns. **Denkschr Akad Wiss Wien 63:**71-116, 1895
4. Chiari H: Uber Veränderungen des Kleinhirns in Folge von Hydrocephalie des Grosshirns. **Dtsch Med Wochenschr 17:**1172-1175, 1891
5. Cleland J: Contribution to the study of spina bifida, encephalocele, and anencephalus. **J Anat Physiol 17:** 257-292, 1883
6. Coulombre AJ, Coulombre JL: The role of mechanical factors in brain morphogenesis. **Anat Rec 130:** 289-290, 1958 (Abstract)
7. Desmond ME: Description of the occlusion of the spinal cord lumen in the early human embryos. **Anat Rec 204:**89-93, 1982
8. Desmond ME, Jacobson AG: Embryonic brain enlargement requires cerebrospinal fluid pressure. **Dev Biol 57:**188-198, 1977
9. Desmond ME, Schoenwolf GC: Timing and positioning of occlusion of the spinal neurocele in the chick embryo. **J Comp Neurol 235:**479-487, 1985
10. French BN: Midline fusion defects of formation, in Youmans JR (ed): **Neurological Surgery.** 2nd ed. Philadelphia, Pa: WB Saunders, 1982, Vol 3, pp 1236-1380
11. Hoffman HJ, Hendrick EB, Humphreys RP: Manifestations and management of Arnold-Chiari malformations in patients with myelomeningocele. **Childs Brain 1:**255-259, 1975
12. Hoffman HJ, Neill J, Crone KR, et al: Hydrosyringomyelia and its management in childhood. **Neurosurgery 21:**347-351, 1987
13. Holinger PC, Holinger LD, Reichert TJ, et al: Respirator obstruction and apnea in infants with bilateral abductor vocal cord paralysis, meningomyelocele, hydrocephalus, and Arnold-Chiari malformation. **J Pediatr 92:**368-373, 1978
14. Ingraham FD, Scott HW Jr: Spina bifida and cranium bifidum. V. The Arnold-Chiari malformation: a study of 20 cases. **N Engl J Med 229:**108-114, 1943
15. Jelínek R, Pexieder T: Pressure of the CSF and the morphogenesis of the CNS. I. Chick embryo. **Folia Morphol 18:**102-110, 1970

16. Kaufman MH: Occlusion of the neural lumen in early mouse embryos analysed by light and electron microscopy. **J Embryol Exp Morphol 78:**211-228, 1983

17. Knepper PA, McLone DG: Glycosaminoglycans and outflow pathways of the eye and brain. **Pediatr Neurosci 12:**240-251, 1985

18. Kuwamura K, McLone DG, Raimondi AJ: The central (spinal) canal in congenital murine hydrocephalus: morphological and physiological aspects. **Childs Brain 4:**216-234, 1978

19. Lichtenstein BW: Distant neuroanatomic complications of spina bifida (spinal dysraphism): hydrocephalus, Arnold-Chiari deformity, stenosis of the aqueduct of sylvius, etc. Pathogenesis and pathology. **Arch Neurol Psychiatry 47:**195-214, 1942

20. McLone DG: The subarachnoid space: a review. **Childs Brain 6:**113-130, 1980

21. McLone DG, Herman JM, Gabrieli AP, et al: Tethered cord as a cause of scoliosis in children with a myelomeningocele. **Pediatr Neurosurg 16:**8-13, 1991

22. McLone DG, Knepper PA: The cause of Chiari II malformation: a unified theory. **Pediatr Neurosci 15:**1-12, 1989

23. McLone DG, Naidich TP: Myelomeningocele: outcome and late complications, in McLaurin RL, et al (eds): **Pediatric Neurosurgery.** 2nd ed. Philadelphia, Pa: WB Saunders, 1989, pp 53-70

24. McLone DG, Raimondi AJ, Sommers MW: The results of early treatment of 100 consecutive newborns with myelomeningocele. Proceedings of the VII Congress of European Society for Paediatric Neurosurgery. **Z Kinderchir 2:**115-117, 1981

25. Moss ML: Functional anatomy of cranial synostosis. **Childs Brain 1:**22-33, 1975

26. Müller F, O'Rahilly R: The development of the human brain from a closed neural tube at stage 13. **Anat Embryol 177:**203-224, 1988

27. Naidich TP, Publowski RM, Naidich JB, et al: Computed tomographic signs of the Chiari II malformation. Part I: Skull and dural partitions. **Radiology 134:**65-71, 1980

28. Naidich TP, Publowski RM, Naidich JB: Computed tomographic signs of Chiari II malformation. Part II: Midbrain and cerebellum. **Radiology 134:** 391-398, 1980

29. Naidich TP, Publowski RM, Naidich JB: Computed tomographic signs of Chiari II malformation. Part III: Ventricles and cisterns. **Radiology 134:**657-663, 1980

30. Oldfield EH, Muraszko K, Shawker TH, et al: Pathophysiology of syringomyelia associated with Chiari I malformation of the cerebellar tonsils. Implications for diagnosis and treatment. **J Neurosurg 80:**3-15, 1994

31. O'Rahilly R, Gardner E: The initial development of the human brain. **Acta Anat 104:**123-133, 1979

32. Pacheco MA, Marks RW, Schoenwolf GC, et al: Quantification of the initial phases of rapid brain enlargement in the chick embryo. **Am J Anat 175:** 403-411, 1986

33. Padget DH: Development of so-called dysraphism: with embryologic evidence of clinical Arnold-Chiari and Dandy-Walker malformations. **Johns Hopkins Med J 130:**127-165, 1972

34. Padget DH, Lindenberg R: Inverse cerebellum morphogenetically related to Dandy-Walker and Arnold-Chiari syndromes: bizarre malformed brain with occipital encephalocele. **Johns Hopkins Med J 131:**228-246, 1972

35. Park TS, Hoffman HJ, Hendrick EB, et al: Experience with surgical decompression of the Arnold-Chiari malformation in young infants with myelomeningocele. **Neurosurgery 13:**147-152, 1983

36. Pollack IF, Kinnunen D, Albright AL: The effect of early craniocervical decompression on functional outcome in neonates and young infants with myelodysplasia and symptomatic Chiari II malformations: results from a prospective series. **Neurosurgery 38:**703-710, 1996

37. Russell DS, Donald C: The mechanism of internal hydrocephalus in spina bifida. **Brain 58:**203-215, 1935

38. Schoenwolf GC, Desmond ME: Descriptive studies of occlusion and reopening of the spinal canal of the early chick embryo. **Anat Rec 209:**251-263, 1984

39. Schoenwolf GC, Desmond ME: Neural tube occlusion precedes rapid brain enlargement. **J Exp Zool 230:**405-407, 1984

40. Schoenwolf GC, Desmond ME: Timing and positioning of reopening of the occluded spinal neurocele in the chick embryo. **J Comp Neurol 246:** 459-466, 1986

41. Vanden Hoek TL, Goossens W, Knepper PA: Fluorescence labeled lectins, glycoconjugates, and the development of the mouse AOP. **Invest Ophthalmol Visual Sci 28:**451-458, 1987

42. Vandertop WP, Asai A, Hoffman HJ, et al: Surgical decompression for symptomatic Chiari II malformation in neonates with myelomeningocele. **J Neurosurg 77:**541-544, 1992

43. Wisoff JH: Hydromyelia: a critical review. **Childs Nerv Syst 4:**1-8, 1988

44. Wisoff JH, Epstein F: Management of hydromyelia. **Neurosurgery 25:**562-571, 1989

45. Yu HC, Deck MDF: The clivus deformity of the Arnold-Chiari malformation. **Radiology 101:** 613-615, 1971

CHAPTER 7

THE CHIARI III AND IV MALFORMATIONS

RICHARD BROWNLEE, MD, S. TERRANCE MYLES, MD, FRCS(C), AND
MARK G. HAMILTON, MDCM, FRCS(C)

In papers published in 1891 and 1896, Hans Chiari described his autopsy findings in a series of patients with cerebellar abnormalities. He defined four distinct groups of abnormalities which have been designated Chiari malformations types I through IV.[5,6,23] Types I and II are well recognized clinical entities and are discussed in detail in other chapters of this book. Chiari III and IV malformations are uncommon and their existence as distinct entities has been questioned. This chapter reviews the diagnostic features, pathogenesis, natural history, radiological assessment, and treatment of Chiari III and IV malformations.

CHIARI III MALFORMATION

The Chiari III malformation is, in all likelihood, a real but very rare pathological entity. Chiari's original description was based on his observations in a single patient.[6] A translation of Chiari's original description was presented by Wilkins and Brody in 1971.[23] A truncated version of this translation is as follows:

> . . . of the third type changes in the cerebellum caused by chronic congenital hydrocephalus . . . the greatest degree of displacement of the cerebellum, out of the cranial cavity through the foramen magnum into the vertebral canal . . . involving deposition of nearly the entire cerebellum, which was

itself hydrocephalic, into a cervical spina bifida.

The child was a 5 month old girl admitted for operation on a spina bifida. The child had a large head and convergent strabismus. On her neck was a fluctuant, tender, and easily compressible tumor about the size of a hen's egg, extending from the occiput to the seventh cervical vertebra. It was covered with skin and was considered to be a cervical hydromyelocele, at the base of which a wide cleft in the upper vertebrae could be palpated . . . at operation the lesion was cut around its base, and a finger-sized central stalk was ligated and detached.

Postoperatively, the child developed a cerebrospinal fluid [CSF] leak and subsequently died of meningitis. The surgical specimen contained skin, dura, arachnoid and a 1-mm thick vesicle of sclerotic cerebellum.

At autopsy . . . the vesicle removed at operation had belonged to the cerebellum. . . . The lateral and third ventricles appeared greatly expanded. . . . The tentorium cerebelli was absent . . . and in place of the cerebellum there was only a walnut sized knobby body, resting on the doral surface of the pons and medulla. . . . This residue of the cerebellum lay inside the widened foramen magnum. . . . The arches of the upper three vertebrae were split and widely separated. . . . The inferior margin of the ventral surface of the pons was located at the level of the tip of the odontoid process, and the medullar oblongata lay completely within the vertebral canal. . . .

Cross section through the pons and medulla showed them to be flattened. The Sylvian aqueduct and fourth ventricle had undergone marked dilatation. The remains of the cerebellum consisted of a vesicle opened at the amputation site, with walls about 1 mm thick, and knobby widenings up to 5 mm thick. The spinal cord was very hydromyelic.

... we are dealing with a cervical cerebellar hydroencephalocele. Occipital encephaloceles often include cerebellum ... but what is noteworthy in the present case is the exit of the cerebellum from the cranial cavity ... through the foramen magnum into a cervical spina bifida. ... This extrusion of the cerebellum ... was probably the result of the hydrocephalic enlargement of the cerebrum ... and from this I believe I have the right to offer this case as representative of the third type of the sequential changes of the cerebellum that are due to cerebral hydrocephalus.

From this description it is apparent that Chiari considered the entity distinctly different from a cervical meningomyelocele or an occipital encephalocele. The key feature which Chiari identified as distinguishing the Chiari III malformation was displacement of the cerebellum below the foramen magnum into a cervical encephalocele. The medulla was also completely displaced out of the cranial cavity into the vertebral canal.

Since the original description, the Chiari III malformation has been described in various ways by different authors. Some adhere to the original definition of cerebellar displacement into a high cervical encephalocele and downward displacement of the medulla.[2,16-19] Others describe it as a displacement of the medulla, fourth ventricle, and all of the cerebellum into an occipital and high cervical encephalomeningocele.[10,21] Raimondi[20] stated that, by definition, the Chiari III malformation is a cervical encephalocele, but occipital and occipitocervical encephaloceles are commonly considered to be included in this group. Recent reports have tended to agree with Raimondi and include occipital and occipitocervical encephaloceles associated with caudal displacement of the cerebellum and medulla as part of the Chiari III group of malformations.[3,9]

The recognition of the Chiari III malformation as a distinct entity has been challenged. Bell and McCormick[1] suggested that this type of malformation is better considered as a form of rostral neural tube defect. Others have suggested that it be grouped among the occipital meningoencephaloceles.[8] Chapman et al[4] re-

ported that the degree and quality of brain morphology, as well as malformations of the meninges and skull associated with occipital encephaloceles, are remarkably variable. The encephalocele may contain variable amounts of cerebellum, occipital lobes, brain stem, fourth ventricle, or lateral ventricles. These abnormalities are frequently associated with anomalies of posterior fossa structures, including kinking of the brain stem. Despite the anatomical diversity of such lesions, certain anatomic, features can regularly be identified: 1) whenever a hindbrain anomaly is present, herniation occurs below the level of the torcula, regardless of the extent of supratentorial structures involved; 2) variable degrees of cerebellar and tectal dysplasia are present; and 3) the fluid-filled sac communicates with the fourth ventricle as a ventriculocele. Diebler and Dulac[9] presented a series of patients with occipital encephaloceles, four of whom can be considered to have Chiari III malformations. In these four patients, the cerebellum, and particularly the cerebellar vermis, was displaced caudally, although herniation of the cerebellar tissue into the encephalocele remained minimal. The fourth ventricle was displaced caudally, with the medulla and pons vertically oriented and reduction of the pontine plicature. McLaurin[13] reported that the most frequent cerebral abnormality associated with occipital encephaloceles is hydrocephalus, which is due either to aqueductal stenosis or a Chiari III malformation. Naidich et al[15] suggested that occipital and parietal encephaloceles may be related to neural tube defects and are associated with Chiari II malformations in 7% to 33% of cases. However, these authors did not comment on Chiari III malformations, suggesting that they did not recognize it as distinct entity. Cohen and Lemire[7] summarized all recognized syndromes associated with encephaloceles, listing Chiari and Dandy-Walker malformations as being associated with occipital and parietal encephaloceles but not identifying the Chiari III malformation as a distinct entity.

It is apparent that while there is considerable controversy about the exact features and even the existence of this malformation, the authors suggest that the Chiari III malformation should continue to be recognized as a distinct entity and that the distinguishing features should include a high cervical spina bifida and/or defect in the occipital squama. At least part of the cerebellum and medulla must be displaced into the spinal canal with cerebellum protruding into the encephalocele. Occipital encephalocele should only be considered as a Chiari III malformation if part of the cerebellum and medulla is displaced below the level of the foramen magnum.

Pathogenesis

The Chiari III malformation is very rare and its pathogenesis is not yet clearly understood. Chiari believed that all of the cerebellar abnormalities found in type I through III malformations resulted from congenital hydrocephalus which pushed the cerebellum and brain stem down into the vertebral canal. However, the Chiari III malformation can occur without associated hydrocephalus.[3,8,9]

Diebler and Dulac[9] suggested that defective closure of the roof plate of the rhombencephalon may be the primary cause of the Chiari III malformation. Fixation of the defective roof plate by fibrovascular adhesions, during the fourth or fifth week of embryonic development, prevents inward rotation of the membranous caudal velum, inferior vermis, and choroid plexus. The brain stem becomes elongated and kinked by traction that occurs during further development of the brain. Herniation of the membranous caudal velum and the formation of an occipitocervical hernia may be induced by the intraventricular pressure, with the bony defect occurring secondary to the hindbrain malformation.

Marin-Padilla[11,12] suggested that occipital encephaloceles result from a primary defect in the rate and degree of growth of the skull base, especially the basioccipital component of the sphenoid bone (clivus). This results in a mismatch between the growth of the skull base, which is reduced, and the posterior fossa neural structures. As a result, the neural structures are displaced. If this displacement is primarily upward against the occipital squamae, which is still at a membranous stage of development, an encephalocele may result. This hypothesis is supported by animal experiments in which the defect is induced by administering a teratogen such as vitamin A, clofibrate, or sodium arsenate.[11,12] A similar process in which the neural structures are displaced caudally could result in a Chiari III malformation.

Castillo et al[3] suggested that the pathogenesis of Chiari III malformations is similar to that which McLone and Knepper[14] have recently reported for Chiari II malformation. Accordingly, the constant escape of CSF during intrauterine life leads to failure of distention of the primitive ventricles, with the resultant development of a small skull. Displacement of the cerebellum and medulla subsequently occurs as the brain attempts to grow within this reduced space.

Radiographic Features

Computed tomography (CT) and magnetic resonance (MR) imaging can provide valuable information, although with some limitations, about the contents of the encephalocele and any associated abnormalities. Castillo et al[3] described the imaging features in nine patients with Chiari III malformations. The encephalocele contained cerebellum, occipital lobes, brain stem, fourth ventricle, lateral ventricles, and cisterns in variable amounts. All of the encephaloceles contained cerebellar tissue. However, the authors did not further differentiate the contents in relation to the site of origin and the encephalocele. Presumably, an occipital encephalocele contains herniated occipital lobe and lateral ventricle more frequently than a cervical or an occipitocervical encephalocele. Associated abnormalities which were variably present included petrous and clivus scalloping, midbrain deformity, dysgenesis of the corpus callosum, hydrocephalus (two of nine patients), and spinal cord syrinx (two patients). Of interest, they noted cerebellar tonsillar herniation in only three patients. None of their patients had isolated cervical encephaloceles and in only five of the nine were they occipitocervical in origin. A detailed description of each patient was not provided and caudal displacement of cerebellum and medulla below the foramen magnum was not specifically reported, thus raising the issue as to whether all nine patients represented true Chiari III malformations or whether some had isolated occipital encephaloceles.

Hydrocephalus is not invariably associated with the Chiari III malformation but occurs in up to 75% of cases. Hydrocephalus was present in three of four patients reported by Diebler and Dulac[9] but in only two of nine patients in the series reported by Castillo et al.[3] It is not uncommon for aqueductal stenosis to be the cause of hydrocephalus in patients with Chiari III malformations. Furthermore, hydrocephalus may be present at birth or may develop at variable times afterward.[20]

Pathological examination of the tissue resected in four patients reported by Castillo et al[3] revealed abnormalities (necrosis, gliosis, heterotopias, and meningeal fibrosis) which were not recognized on the preoperative CT or MR imaging. Aberrant deep draining veins and ectopic venous sinuses, which were encountered at surgery, were also not identified on these imaging studies. The pons and medulla, which were contained within the encephalocele in one patient, were well demonstrated on preoperative MR imaging and were preserved at surgery. None of the patients in the Castillo et al study underwent preoperative angiography.

Raimondi[20] described the angiographic appearance in a number of patients with Chiari III malformations. The site of origin of the encephalocele determined which arteries exhibited an aberrant course. Cervical encephaloceles contained cerebellar tissue which derived its vascular supply from the vertebrobasilar system, specifically branches of the posterior inferior cerebellar artery (PICA). Occipital and occipitocervical encephaloceles always contained cerebellar tissue and frequently contained portions of the occipital lobes. In these cases, the displaced cerebellum received its vascular supply from either the anterior inferior cerebellar arteries, superior cerebellar arteries, or posterior cerebral arteries which took an aberrant course into the encephalocele. The calcarine and cuneate branches of the occipital artery from the internal carotid artery supplied the occipital cortex which was within the encephalocele. The PICA was displaced downward into the spinal canal for varying distances independent of the site of origin of the encephalocele. Branches of the external carotid artery supplied the parenchymal portion of the encephalocele. The venous drainage from functioning tissue within the encephalocele was via innominate veins and not through named sinuses. The major venous return generally passed into the cervical veins surrounding the vertebral spine or entered the jugular venous system.

Natural History and Treatment

Because the Chiari III malformation is so rare, it is difficult to find adequate descriptions concerning its natural history. Pitman[19] stated that this malformation is usually incompatible with life. Castillo et al[3] suggested that the prognosis for patients with Chiari III malformations was poor. Of the nine patients in their series, four underwent surgical resection of the encephalocele: two died postoperatively and one was severely developmentally delayed. One of the patient deaths occurred postoperatively from diffuse cerebral edema thought to be due to thrombosis of the superior sagittal sinus. The remainder of their patients were lost to follow-up. Raimondi[20] stated that while mixed occipital and cervical encephaloceles represent a truly severe dysplasia of mesenchymal and neural tissue, they are not to be considered fatal lesions nor is severe neurological deficit invariable. Occipitocervical encephaloceles may be completely repaired and the child may go on to lead a normal life. In patients with occipital encephaloceles, the prognosis for survival and neurological function is thought to be related to the presence of cerebral tissue within the encephalocele, presence of hydrocephalus, and to any additional cerebral malformations.[9] Chapman et al[4] suggested that the single best prognostic indicator for survival and neurological function is the amount and type of neural tissue within the encephalocele.

Adequate surgical treatment of Chiari III malformations, like encephaloceles in general, is predicated upon a detailed understanding of the anatomy of the defect. This includes identification of the neural structures contained within the encephalocele, its vascular supply, and the presence of such associated conditions as hydrocephalus, tentorial aplasia, foraminal impaction, or a Dandy-Walker cyst. Clinical examination may fail to distinguish between a cervical, a cervico-occipital, and an occipital encephalocele.[20] Radiographic investigations including CT

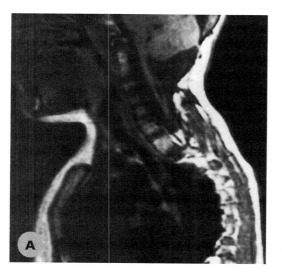 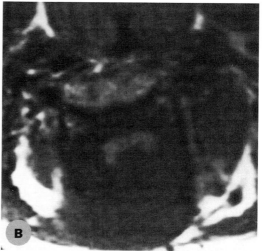

Figure 1: A) Sagittal T1-weighted MR image of a child with Chiari III malformation. Note the encephalocele with displacement of the cerebellum and brain stem into the spinal canal. **B)** Axial T1-weighted image of the same child through the posterior fossa/encephalocele region.

scanning and MR imaging (Figure 1) are valuable tools for preoperative assessment, although as discussed above, they may not reveal the full extent of the abnormality. Cerebral angiography, although not routinely utilized, demonstrates the vascularization of the herniated tissue and the locations of the venous sinuses, which may not be fully appreciated from MR images alone. The use of MR angiography to visualize venous sinus and arterial anatomy in patients with Chiari III malformations has not yet been reported, but is potentially promising when one extrapolates from other clinical experience.[22]

The timing of surgical treatment is principally determined by the competence of the encephalocele covering. If a CSF leak is present or neural tissue is exposed, early repair is advocated to prevent infection. The guiding principle in treatment should be to resect nonviable tissue and preserve all viable neural tissue. No attempt should be made to reduce the herniated occipital lobes or cerebellar hemispheres into the cranial compartment. If viable neural tissue remains outside the cranium, the bony defect should be enlarged to ensure that there is no mechanical compromise of blood vessels or neural tissue. The dura and skin should be

closed over these structures.[13,20] The closure of these latter layers may be straightforward or may require the neurosurgeon to be innovative, utilizing rotational flaps, dural grafts, or even split-thickness skin grafts as a temporary skin coverage while tissue expanders prepare the surrounding skin to provide a more permanent closure at a later time. When present, hydrocephalus should be treated with a shunting procedure. Hydrocephalus may not develop until after the encephalocele has been repaired. If present initially, treatment may be directed according to guidelines currently accepted for patients with Chiari II malformation: 1) immediate shunting; or 2) temporary ventriculostomy followed by permanent shunting. A shunting procedure may help reduce the posterior fossa contents prior to definitive repair of the encephalocele, although this is rarely of significant benefit.

Summary

The Chiari III malformation is considered to be a distinct clinical entity consisting of a cervical, occipitocervical, or occipital encephalocele associated with caudal displacement of cerebellar tissue and the medulla into the vertebral canal. It is rare and may be associated with a poor patient prognosis, depending on the extent of associated neurological abnormalities. With a good understanding of the anatomical features of the malformation, the encephalocele may be completely repaired and the child may go on to lead a normal life.

CHIARI IV MALFORMATION

In Chiari's second paper on cerebellar malformations, he described two patients with cerebellar hypoplasia, an abnormality which was later designated the Chiari IV malformation.[5] The features of this type of malformation are quite distinct from the other three types of cerebellar malformations and its existence as a distinct clinical entity is very controversial.

The morphological features described for the Chiari IV malformation include: 1) aplasia or severe hypoplasia of the cerebellar hemispheres with a funnel-shaped posterior fossa, but without displacement of cerebellar tissue out of the posterior fossa; 2) an atrophic pons with a characteristic "pigeon breast" shape; and 3) marked dilatation of the fourth ventricle and cisterna magna without enlargement of the third and lateral ventricles.[20,21] The Chiari IV malformation is at best an extremely uncommon or rare entity with few reports in the literature. Some authors, therefore, do not believe that it should be included in the category of Chiari malformations.[10,21] Bell and McCormick[1] stated that one of the cases described by Chiari would now be classified as a Dandy-Walker malformation. For these reasons, it is not possible to provide definitive information concerning the natural history or pathogenesis of the abnormality that has been defined as the Chiari IV malformation, unless extrapolations are taken from patients with Dandy-Walker malformation.

Raimondi[20] presented three patients with presumed Chiari IV malformation and described the pneumoencephalographic and angiographic features. All three children had bilateral vocal cord paralysis and none had "clinical hydrocephalus," although hydrocephalus has been reported to occur in 25% of patients. Pneumoencephalography revealed extreme di-

latation of the fourth ventricle, pontine and interpeduncular cisterns, and the cisterna magna without any expansion of the lateral ventricles or any obvious pressure effect. The dilated basal cisterns outline the pigeon-breasted deformity of the brain stem. The third and lateral ventricles are not usually enlarged. Raimondi[20] stated that it is the distinctive angiographic features that distinguish the Chiari IV malformation from those of an arachnoid cyst of the cisterna magna or a Dandy-Walker cyst. Vertebral angiography reveals a rather sharp angulation of the basilar artery which points anteriorly to form a "pigeon-breasted deformity." The main trunks of the vertebral arteries curve slightly posteriorly and then angle sharply anteriorly to join each other inferior to the angular, pigeon-breasted deformity of the basilar artery. The PICAs are completely unfolded and extend posteriorly in a gentle curve with the convexity pointing inferiorly. There is no identifiable choroidal point and the distinction between tonsillar and vermian branches is not apparent. This characteristic deformity of PICAs is the result of hypoplasia of the cerebellar hemispheres and dilatation of the fourth ventricle. The superior cerebellar arteries run almost directly posterior along a horizontal course.

The authors could find no recent reports of patients with Chiari IV malformations in the literature. However, Yuh et al[24] presented a patient with what they described as a Chiari II malformation with dysgenesis of the cerebellum and brain stem. This patient had several features of the Chiari IV malformation: a 7-year-old, mentally retarded girl with a lumbar meningomyelocele and presumptive hydrocephalus had repair of the myelomeningocele at one day of age and underwent shunting on the ninth day of life (the reason for and location of the shunt were not specified). MR imaging revealed a severely hypoplastic cerebellum and brain stem and merging of the midbrain with the pons, which lacked its normal protuberant belly. A flat band of tectum with no discrete colliculi was noted behind the aqueduct. The patient did not have an enlarged fourth ventricle, possibly because of her previous shunting procedure. The occipital lobes were unusually low, but the position of the tentorium was not identified. It is possible that the posterior fossa was small and

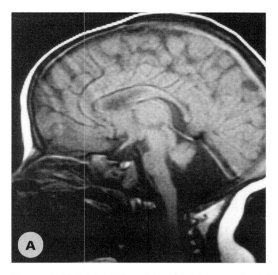
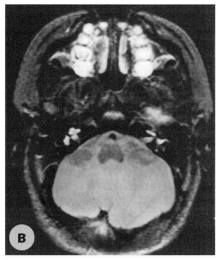

Figure 2: A) Sagittal T1-weighted MR image of a child with a Dandy-Walker malformation. **B)** Axial T2-weighted image of the same child through the posterior fossa region. This child shares many of the anatomical features that have been described for patients with Chiari IV malformations.

funnel shaped as in the Chiari IV malformation. This description suggests a malformation with several features consistent with a Chiari IV malformation.

Whether or not the Chiari IV malformation should be considered as a distinct clinical entity is still open to debate. However, it is clearly distinct from the other types of Chiari malformations. The type IV malformation may more appropriately be classified as a variant of the Dandy-Walker malformation or as a type of cerebellar hypoplasia (Figure 2).

REFERENCES

1. Bell WE, McCormick WF: **Increased Intracranial Pressure in Children: Diagnosis and Treatment.** 2nd ed. Philadelphia, Pa: WB Saunders, 1978
2. Boulter TR: The dysraphic states. **Surg Gynecol Obstet 124:**1091-1100, 1967
3. Castillo M, Quencer RM, Dominguez R: Chiari III malformation: imaging features. **AJNR 13:**107-113, 1992
4. Chapman PH, Swearingen B, Caviness VS: Subtorcular occipital encephaloceles. Anatomical considerations relevant to operative management. **J Neurosurg 71:**375-381, 1989
5. Chiari H: Über Veränderungen des Kleinhirns des Pons und der Medulla Oblongata in Folge von Congenitaler Hydrocephalie des Grosshirns. **Denkschr Akad Wiss Wien 63:**71-116, 1895
6. Chiari H: Über Veränderungen des Kleinhirns in Folge von Hydrocephalie des Grosshirns. **Dtsch Med Wochenschr 27:**1172-1175, 1891
7. Cohen MM Jr, Lemire RJ: Syndromes with cephaloceles. **Teratology 25:**161-172, 1982
8. de Reuck J, Thienpont L: Fetal Chiari's type III malformation. **Childs Brain 2:**85-91, 1982
9. Diebler C, Dulac O: Cephaloceles: clinical and neuroradiological appearance. Associated cerebral malformations. **Neuroradiology 25:**199-216, 1983
10. Harwood-Nash DC, Fitz CR: **Neuroradiology in Infants and Children.** St Louis, Mo: CV Mosby, 1976, pp 998-1019
11. Marin-Padilla M: Morphogenesis of experimental encephalocele (cranioschisis occulta). **J Neurol Sci 46:**83-99, 1980
12. Marin-Padilla M: Study of the skull in human cranioschisis. **Acta Anat 62:**1-20, 1965
13. McLaurin RL: Encephalocele and related anomalies, in Hoffman HJ, Epstein F (eds): **Disorders of the Developing Nervous System: Diagnosis and Treatment.** Boston, Mass: Blackwell Scientific, 1986, pp 153-447
14. McLone DG, Knepper PA: The cause of Chiari II malformation: a unified theory. **Pediatr Neurosci 15:**1-2, 1989
15. Naidich TP, Altman NR, Braffman BH, et al: Cephaloceles and related malformations. **AJNR 13:**655-690, 1992
16. Peach B: Arnold-Chiari malformation. Anatomic

features of 20 cases. **Arch Neurol 12:**613-621, 1965

17. Peach B: Arnold-Chiari malformation. Morphogenesis. **Arch Neurol 12:**527-535, 1965

18. Peach B: Arnold-Chiari malformation with normal spine. **Arch Neurol 10:**497-501, 1964

19. Pitman HW: The Chiari crisis. **BNI Quart 6:**10-16, 1990

20. Raimondi AJ: **Pediatric Neuroradiology.** Philadelphia: WB Saunders, 1972, pp 275-343

21. Ramsey RG: **Neuroradiology.** 2nd ed. Philadelphia: WB Saunders, 1987, pp 440-441

22. Ruggieri PM, Masaryk TJ, Ross JS: Magnetic resonance angiography. Cerebrovascular applications. **Stroke 23:**774-780, 1992

23. Wilkins RH, Brody IA: The Arnold-Chiari malformation. **Arch Neurol 25:**376-379, 1971

24. Yuh WTC, Segall HD, Senac MO, et al: MR imaging of Chiari II malformation associated with dysgenesis of cerebellum and brain stem. **J Comput Assist Tomogr 11:**188-191, 1987

Chapter 8

The Relationship Between Syringomyelia and the Chiari Malformations

John G. Piper, MD, and Arnold H. Menezes, MD

In 1891, Chiari first described a group of hindbrain malformations and proposed a classification system for these abnormalities, that continues to be used to this day with little modification.[2,28,34,64,78] The Chiari malformations are often associated with numerous congenital and developmental anomalies.[32,64,78] Of these disorders, syringohydromyelia is by far the most frequently encountered.[28,64,68,72,93] First described by Ollivier d'Angers in 1824, the pathophysiology of syringohydromyelia remains elusive and controversial.[64] This chapter will examine several major theories of syringohydromyelia formation in association with hindbrain malformations. Numerous modifications of these theories have been proposed and will also be discussed. Specific aspects of the pathophysiology of syringohydromyelia in association with hindbrain malformations have great importance in evaluating the various surgical interventions that have been proposed for these problems. An understanding of these complex pathophysiological events allows for a thoughtful and organized approach to the management of these complex disorders (Figure 1).

Characteristics of Hindbrain Malformations and Associated Anomalies

Prior to discussion of the pathogenesis of syringomyelia, a brief review of hindbrain malformations is needed. The Chiari malformations involve caudal descent of posterior fossa structures into the upper cervical canal resulting in impaction at the foramen magnum (Figures 2, 3, and 4).[2,6,8,10,17,28,53,92,97] Chiari I malformations exhibit tonsillar herniation and, if long-standing, the tonsils develop characteristic pathological changes.[2,24] The typical pattern of folia present on the surface of the tonsils is lost and the tonsils become pale and atrophic from gliotic changes and compression. In addition, dense adhesions between the tonsils, the arachnoid, and the dura can form.[10,64] If severe, a large mat of scar tissue may be present. This scarring may involve the foramen of Magendie, and possibly the foramen of Monro, compromising outflow of cerebrospinal fluid (CSF) from the fourth ventricles.[6,64] In addition, a veil of arachnoid has been described which can cover the obex or the foramina, further contributing to impediment of CSF outflow from the fourth ventricle.[6,29,34,87] The neurodysgenesis which typifies the Chiari malformations is also accompanied by numerous changes involving bony and ligamentous structures of the spine and craniovertebral junction.[3,6,28,49] Scoliosis is often identified.[25,42,49,57,68,72,73] The posterior fossa is shallow with concomitant flattening of the squamous-occipital bones.[17,28,105] With chronic tonsillar herniation, the foramen magnum may become enlarged.[64] More extensive involvement of the skull base may also include platybasia and/or basilar invagination with severe ventral cervicomedullary junction compression (Figure

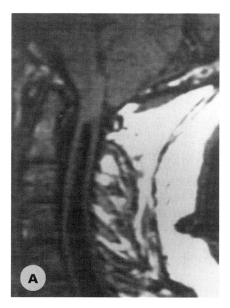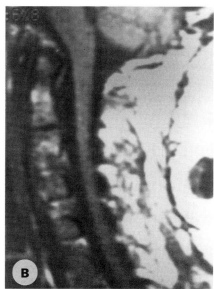

Figure 1: T-1 weighted MR imaging in the midsagittal plane documenting resolution of syringohydromyelia following posterior fossa decompression. **A)** Preoperative image demonstrating tonsillar herniation with foramen magnum impaction and midcervical syrinx. **B)** Postoperative image obtained 6 weeks following posterior fossa decompression demonstrating nearly complete resolution of syringohydromyelia following posterior fossa decompression. Note establishment of CSF pathways at the cervicomedullary junction.

3).[3,6,16,19,20,28,33,65,90] Chiari I malformations are frequently associated with Klippel-Feil syndrome, atlas assimilation, and occasionally hydrocephalus; medullary kinking may also occur.[6,25,28,33,64,92]

The other hindbrain malformations are more severe. Chiari II malformations involve caudal descent of the medulla and the pons in addition to cerebellar tonsil and vermian herniation (Figure 3).[2,28,64,93,97] Brain stem involvement includes hypoplasia of cranial nerve nuclei, a typical medullary kink, and beaking of the collicular plate.[13,17,28] The massa intermedia may also be enlarged. The vast majority of Chiari II malformations are associated with myelodysplasia. Additional findings include scalloping of the clivus and petrous-temporal bones.[63,105] The foramen magnum may also be enlarged, and other cranial anomalies include a shallow posterior fossa and cranial lacunae.[17,65] Spinal involvement is common, most often taking the form of scoliosis.[25,42] By definition, all Chiari III malformations are associated with myelodysplasia with herniation of posterior

fossa structures in a high cervical meningocele.[64]

CHARACTERISTICS OF SYRINGOHYDROMYELIA

Syringohydromyelia is a term which refers to the presence of cystic cavities within some portion of the spinal cord (Figures 1 and 2).[11,14,54,96] The most common cause of cystic cavities in the spinal cord is hindbrain anomalies, but numerous other etiologies also exist, including trauma and tumors.[14,54] Cystic cavities can be divided into several types. Hydromyelia refers to dilatation of the primitive central canal of the spinal cord and is therefore characterized by partial or complete ependymal lining of the cavity.[54] Syringomyelia pertains to cavities which lie outside the central canal and therefore lack an ependymal lining.[54] Syringomyelic cavities may or may not have a connection with the central canal. At times, a syringohydromyelic cavity may extend into or arise only within the brain

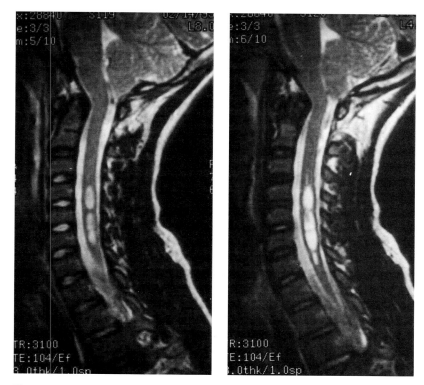

Figure 2: T-2 weighted MR imaging in the midsagittal plane documenting many of the features found in association with syringohydromyelia. In addition to the midcervical syrinx, a Chiari I malformation is demonstrated with tonsillar herniation through the level of the foramen magnum. Note obliteration of CSF at the cervicomedullary junction. Also present is mild basilar invagination and medullary kinking. Additional abnormalities include a low confluence of the sinuses.

stem, a condition called syringobulbia.[10,51] This type of cavity is thought to form in the plane which separates the primitive alar and basal plates.[64] Typically, these cavities extend no higher than the midbrain; however, a syrinx has been described within the cerebrum.[51] Under rare circumstances, hemorrhage may occur within a cystic cavity of the spinal cord or brain stem resulting in hematomyelia and hematobulbia, respectively.[63,80]

Syringohydromyelia has been subclassified as "communicating" and "noncommunicating."[2,79] Communicating syringomyelia refers to cavities which are in direct communication with the fourth ventricle through the obex.[79] This type of syringohydromyelia is strongly associated with hindbrain malformations. Noncommunicating syringomyelia refers to syringes which show no direct communication with the fourth ventricle.

While noncommunicating syringomyelia may occur in association with hindbrain malformations, they are also the type of cavities which occur in association with trauma or tumors of the spinal cord. This distinction becomes important during discussion of pathogenesis of syringohydromyelia, since the mechanisms involved in syrinx formation may differ substantially between these two subtypes of syringohydromyelia.

Histological examination of sequentially sectioned spinal cords provides insight into the development, extent, and appearance of syringohydromyelic cavities. Age-dependent stenosis of the central canal has been described with stenotic segments most commonly located in the thoracic region.[15,52,67] Histological features include ependymal injury and scarring leading to formation of ependymal rosettes, microcanals, subependymal gliovascular buds, gliosis, as

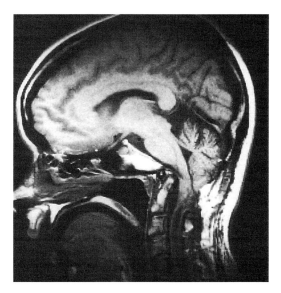

Figure 3: Syringohydromyelia is strongly associated with numerous other central nervous system anomalies. Midsagittal MR image of the brain and cervicomedullary junction revealing medullary descent with medullary kinking associated with tonsillar herniation. Also noted is mild basilar invagination and a low set confluence of the sinuses.

well as disorganization of the ependyma.[15, 67,96] Age-related changes in the histology of the ependymal lining have also been described with central canal lining being predominantly pseudostratified ciliated epithelium in the first decade of life, with a shift toward columnar and cuboidal epithelium in the second decade of life.[52] By 20 years of age, proliferation of the astrocytes and ependyma has led to central canal closure.[52]

These histological findings have a profound influence on the clinical appearance of a syringohydromyelia. Holochord syringohydromyelia is more common in young patients, with older patients typically demonstrating lower cervical and upper thoracic spinal cord cavities.[84,89] These observations correlate well with the previously mentioned studies which reveal age-dependent stenosis most commonly located in the thoracic region. Furthermore, both gross pathological and magnetic resonance imaging studies of the spinal cord often reveal a septated nature to the syringohydromyelic cavity.[55] Partial or complete stenosis of the central canal may be an underlying explanation for these septations.

PATHOGENESIS OF SYRINGOHYDROMYELIA

The pathogenesis of syringohydromyelia in association with hindbrain malformations remains quite controversial. Over the past 40 years, two dominant hypotheses and numerous minor theories have emerged in an attempt to explain the formation of the various Chiari malformations and the development of syringohydromyelia. While each hypothesis can help explain certain facets of Chiari malformations with syringohydromyelia, no one single theory succeeds in explaining all aspects of this disease state. In all likelihood, factors from each of these theories contribute to spinal cord cavity formation. The extent of contribution from each theory, though, may vary greatly in individual cases. An understanding of the pathophysiology of syringohydromyelia is imperative for successful surgical management. These major theories will be reviewed in detail and significant modifications addressed where appropriate.

The Hydrodynamic Theory

Gardner was the first to propose a unifying theory which related the development of syringohydromyelia in the presence of hindbrain malformations.[34-39] This theory, known as the hydrodynamic theory, traces the origin of the Chiari malformations and syringohydromyelia to a developmental disorder.[15,34-39] Ordinarily, a balance exists between the pulsatile pressures generated in the CSF by the choroid plexus within the lateral ventricles and the fourth ventricle. This theory proposes that an imbalance exists between these CSF pulsations, with those in the lateral ventricle exceeding those of the fourth ventricle, resulting in a small posterior fossa and herniation of the cerebellar tonsils. Also, the theory proposes that the outlets of the fourth ventricle fail to develop in the rhomboid roof, resulting in obstruction of the outlet of the fourth ventricles.[15,34-39]

The intracranial CSF arterial pulsations subsequently are directed down the central canal of the spinal cord resulting in formation and propagation of syringohydromyelia.[15,34-39] Gardner called the arterial CSF pulsations directed down the central canal the "water-hammer" effect.[34-39]

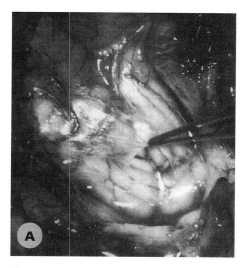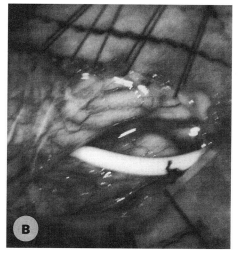

Figure 4: Intraoperative photographs of posterior fossa decompression. **A)** Dense adhesions engulf cerebellar tonsils which are being dissected free. **B)** Fourth ventricle to subarachnoid shunt is being placed to improve outflow from the ventricular system.

Once syringohydromyelia began to form, the hydrocephalus which is produced by obstruction of the outlets of the fourth ventricle was believed to become compensated by distention of the central canal. If the hydrocephalus remained severe, hydromyelia was believed to lead to neural tube rupture resulting in a meningomyelocele defect. In addition, once syringohydromyelia was initiated, its propagation was thought to become easier as the cavity enlarges. This phenomenon is analogous to blowing up a balloon, which initially is quite difficult; however, it becomes easier as the balloon is inflated more.

In support of Gardner's theory are numerous clinical and experimental observations confirming an association between obstructed fourth ventricular outflow and the development of syringohydromyelia.[2] Conway[12] examined 12 cases of syringomyelia and described partial or complete obstruction of the outlets of the fourth ventricle associated with communication between the fourth ventricle and the syrinx cavity. In a series of human and animal studies performed by Hall et al,[40-44] numerous components of the hydrodynamic theory were confirmed. Intracisternal administration of kaolin in 10 mongrel dogs resulted in hydrocephalus and syringohydromyelia via distention and subsequent rupture of the central canal of the spinal

cord.[43] Furthermore, using a similar canine model of kaolin-induced hydrocephalus and hydrosyringomyelia, radioisotope ventriculography was performed demonstrating a connection between the syrinx and the fourth ventricle.[2,41] Further studies revealed the presence of a partial one-way valve effect whereby increased ventricular pressure was transmitted to the syringohydromyelic cavity, but aspiration of the same ventricular fluid failed to lower the syrinx pressure acutely.[44] Furthermore, Hall et al[44] proposed that transmission of intra-abdominal or intra-thoracic pressures via epidural veins to the spinal subarachnoid space may lead to syrinx compression and subsequent enlargement. Finally, they performed clinical studies in 16 myelodysplastic patients demonstrating a similar relationship between hydromyelia and altered ventricular hydrodynamics using radioisotope ventriculography.[40]

A modification of Gardner's original theory was proposed by du Boulay and coworkers[23] to explain observations that patent communication may exist between the fourth ventricle and the basal cisterns in some patients with hydromyelia and Chiari malformations. These investigators observed greater displacement of CSF from the basilar cisterns during systole compared with the fourth ventricle. In the presence of a hindbrain malformation with obstruction at the foramen magnum, CSF dynamics are altered. These investigators proposed that CSF may be transmitted from the basilar cisterns into the fourth ventricle and subsequently down this central canal of the spinal cord resulting in syringohydromyelia formation. Once fluid entered the syrinx, it was prevented from escaping via a one-way valve mechanism created by posterior fossa impaction resulting in progressive enlargement of the syrinx cavity. Coughing and straining was believed to lead to further syrinx progression (see the Craniospinal Pressure Dissociation Theory).[10,27]

Not all observations are supportive of Gardner's original theory or subsequent modifications. There may not always be an observed connection between the fourth ventricle and the syringohydromyelic cavity.[54,75] Furthermore, syringohydromyelia progression has also been reported in posttraumatic syringohydromyelia or in association with neoplastic cysts which clearly are not in communication with the fourth ventricle. Therefore, it becomes difficult to explain all aspects of spinal cord cavitation by Gardner's theory alone. One potential explanation for those cavities associated with hindbrain malformations may be that a communication exists between the fourth ventricle and the syringohydromyelic cavity at the time of initiation of the syrinx but that this communication later becomes blocked off. While this is a possibility, other mechanisms are likely at work.

Craniospinal Pressure Dissociation Theory

Bernard Williams[99-103] critically examined the available data on the pathogenesis of syringohydromyelia and identified several areas which were incompatible with Gardner's theory. Williams[99-102] pointed out that the syringohydromyelic cavities are not often in communication with the fourth ventricle, at least at the time of presentation. Gardner's[74] theory failed to explain why syringohydromyelic cavities are more common in the lower cervical and upper thoracic spine rather than beginning in the upper cervical spine. Furthermore, Gardner's[74] reliance on cord dilatation resulting from the pres-

ence of mild hydrocephalus is not convincing. Typically, atresia of the foramina of Magendie and Luschka should produce hydrocephalus, rather than "mild hydrocephalus" and central canal distention.[74,100]

In order to more fully elucidate mechanisms contributing to formation of hindbrain malformations and syringohydromyelia, Williams[101] performed simultaneous ventricular and lumbar subarachnoid CSF pressure measurements in 37 patients with syringohydromyelia related to hindbrain anomalies. Pressure differential tracings often indicated an initial upward pressure deflection followed by a prolonged negative deflection during such maneuvers as coughing or blowing. Such a dissociation in the craniospinal pressure was identified in 24 of the 37 patients studied. Williams proposed that this pressure differential was caused by the hindbrain herniation which acted as a one-way valve, allowing fluid to enter the intracranial cavity from the lumbar subarachnoid space but prevented its egress. At times, the observed craniospinal pressure dissociation would exceed 100 mm Hg. With elevation of the intracranial spinal fluid pressure and a relative negative intraspinal pressure, it was proposed that spinal fluid was "sucked" into the central canal leading to syrinx formation.[101] Further support for the craniospinal pressure dissociation theory comes from observations that there is a higher incidence of syringohydromyelia in patients with Chiari malformations and concurrent subarachnoid hemorrhage from traumatic delivery. Hemorrhage was felt to cause adhesions at the cervicomedullary junction preventing CSF pressure equilibrium between the cranial and spinal fluid pressures.[10,69] On the other hand, syringohydromyelia was not identified in patients with Chiari malformations who did not have a traumatic delivery with associated subarachnoid hemorrhage.[69]

While the "sucking" mechanism helps to explain the development of syringohydromyelia, Williams[101] also proposed a further mechanism for progression of syringohydromyelia. He believed that arterial pulsations within the subarachnoid space could be transmitted to fluid within a spinal cord cavity producing fluid waves within the syrinx. Furthermore, coughing or the Valsalva maneuver could cause an elevation in the venous pressure in epidural veins which in turn could compress the thecal sac and cause further caudad fluid shifts and progression of syringohydromyelia.[10,27] Williams[101] referred to this mechanism as the "sloshing" mechanism. In addition to explaining progression of syringohydromyelia in association with hindbrain malformations, this sloshing mechanism may also explain progression of spinal cord cavities in association with trauma.

Additional support for the craniospinal pressure dissociation theory came from numerous observations which showed that Chiari malformations may be acquired, often following placement of lumboperitoneal or similar shunts.[30,47,77,98] The lumboperitoneal shunt would lead to dissociation between the cranial and spinal fluid pressures, promoting impaction of the cerebellar tonsils in the foramen magnum. Once impaction has occurred, disequilibrium between the cranial and spinal pressures becomes exacerbated. A similar mechanism has been proposed for the formation of Chiari II malformations since spinal fluid leak through an open meningomyelocele defect which leads to a similar craniospinal pressure dissociation. We have also recently seen patients with concomitant basilar invagination and Chiari malformations in whom syringohydromyelia resolved following transoral decompression of the ventral cervicomedullary junction compression. Resection of the abnormal odontoid appears to have relieved the abnormal craniospinal pressure dissociation that had caused syrinx formation.

Other Theories

Aboulker[1] advanced a theory which is now becoming, in part, more widely accepted. He believed that syringohydromyelia cavities developed within the spinal cord parenchyma itself and were not associated with the central canal except in very young children with hydrocephalus and meningomyeloceles. He proposed that stenosis of the subarachnoid space at the level of the foramen magnum from a Chiari malformation or other pathological process such as tumors or arachnoiditis was central to the pathogenesis of syringohydromyelia. Since approximately 30% of CSF is produced within the spinal subarachnoid space, stenosis at the cervicomedullary junction would prevent fluid ascent and absorption. He proposed that the excess CSF in the spinal subarachnoid space leads to spinal cord edema, cavitation, and ultimately syringohydromyelia. While the mechanism by which spinal fluid entered the cord remained vague, it was proposed that CSF filtration through the parenchyma itself or via pathways near the dorsal nerve roots were the most likely etiological factors.[1]

Ball and Dayan[5] gave further credence to Aboulker's observations. Histological sections at autopsy in a patient with syringohydromyelia revealed widened channels in the perivascular space consistent with enlargement of the Virchow-Robin band spaces. This observation was also confirmed by Brierley.[5] Furthermore, numerous clinical observations of water soluble myelographic contrast material entering syringohydromyelic cavities in a delayed fashion appeared to favor such transneural migration via the Virchow-Robin band spaces.[4,22,31,48,58,85,104]

Recent developments in magnetic resonance (MR) imaging software have contributed to the formulation of new theories regarding the pathogenesis of syringohydromyelia.[55,70,71,88,91] MR imaging is capable of detecting pulsatile motion and velocity of fluids.[55,70,71,88,91] This technology initially gave rise to the technique of MR angiography; however, another extension was the examination of CSF dynamics both in normal individuals and in patients with certain pathological conditions. Further refinement has included gating of the image acquisition to the cardiac cycle, which allows determinations of CSF flow during pulsations generated during the cardiac cycle.[70,71] In addition, intraoperative ultrasound techniques have also allowed *in situ* examination of central nervous system compression and examination of the returned pulsatility in central nervous system structures before and after decompression.[21,50] These techniques provide important information for studying the pathogenesis of abnormal CSF flow in such conditions as the Chiari malformation and syringohydromyelia. Preoperative, intraoperative, and postoperative examinations of CSF flow and can easily document changes that occur with certain types of operative intervention.

These technical advances have allowed extension of previous theories regarding the pathogenesis of syringohydromyelia in association with Chiari I malformations. Utilizing these advances in phase-contrast cine MR imaging and intraoperative ultrasonography, a recent study examined seven patients prior to, during, and following decompressive procedures for Chiari malformations.[74] Prior to the operation, occlusion of the subarachnoid space at the level of foramen magnum was identified posteriorly by impaction of the cerebellar tonsils. Tonsillar impaction also caused ventral displacement of the cervicomedullary junction with occlusion occurring anteriorly. Cervicothoracic syringohydromyelia was identified in all patients; however, no communication between the fourth ventricle and the syrinx could be identified. Foramen magnum impaction prevented normal movement of CSF across the foramen magnum. During the cardiac cycle, the arterial pulsations produced downward displacement of the cerebellar tonsils leading to a spinal subarachnoid pressure wave and constriction of the spinal cord syrinx. Furthermore, the spinal cord syrinx configuration and tonsillar movement did not vary during Valsalva maneuver or with the respiratory cycle.

From these observations, new aspects of syringohydromyelia formation were proposed by Oldfield et al.[74] Normally, the cardiac cycle produces biphasic motion of CSF within the basilar cisterns which allows CSF movement downward during systole and upward during diastole; that in turn allows accommodation of the systolic expansion of the brain. With foramen magnum impaction from ectopic cerebellar tonsils, the normal accommodative CSF movement is impeded. Systolic pressure waves result in downward displacement of the cerebellar tonsils leading to a series of pronounced systolic spinal subarachnoid pressure waves, which relentlessly over time exert adverse effects on the spinal cord ultimately leading to syrinx formation. In addition, a spinal subarachnoid pressure wave may be generated by jet-like movement of spinal fluid from the fourth ventricle into the spinal subarachnoid space via an inferiorly displaced foramen of Magendie. The mechanism by which a syrinx forms is explained by the previous observations of an extensive perivascular network (Virchow-Robin spaces) which communicates between the syrinx and the subarachnoid space.[4,5,22,31,48] Syringohydromyelia progression can also be explained, in that once a syrinx has been established the spinal subarachnoid pressure waves cause repetitive compression of the syrinx. This compression leads to downward flow of the syrinx fluid with progressive syrinx enlargement.

These observations help explain several aspects of syringohydromyelia formation that were insufficiently answered by the hydrodynamic and craniospinal pressure dissociation theories.[74] This theory is not reliant upon a patent communication between the fourth ventricle and the syrinx cavity. Furthermore, this theory would explain the relative low incidence of hydrocephalus in patients with Chiari I malformations. The hydrodynamic theory requires that the outlet of the fourth ventricle is severely compromised leading to syrinx formation. Obstruction of the outlets of the fourth ventricle should also contribute to a high incidence of hydrocephalus, which is not observed. These recent observations do not necessarily require that the outlets of the fourth ventricle be severely compromised.[75] This theory can also explain the common clinical observation that neurological deterioration occurs during episodes of sneezing or coughing. With compromise of the subarachnoid space at the level of the foramen magnum, normal cephalad movement of CSF generated by elevations in the spinal subarachnoid pressure during coughing or straining may also produce external compression of the spinal cord cavity with propagation of the syrinx.

PATHOLOGICAL OVERVIEW

No single theory adequately explains all of the complicated facets contributing to the development of syringohydromyelia in association with hindbrain malformations. When taken together, however, these theories begin to demonstrate a clear picture of the significant pathophysiological processes which need to be understood to formulate a successful operative approach to these difficult problems. Central to all three theories is the importance of abnormal

CSF dynamics at the cervicomedullary junction to the pathogenesis of syringohydromyelia. The impact that this alteration in CSF dynamics has on syrinx formation varies in each patient depending on the precise cervicomedullary pathology.

Impediment of outflow of spinal fluid from the fourth ventricle explains those cases in which hydrocephalus is present and those cases of hydrosyringomyelia in which patency exists between the fourth ventricle and the syrinx via the central canal of the spinal cord. Impaction of the cerebellar tonsils with subsequent ventral displacement of the brain stem may also lead to obstruction of the CSF pathways at the cervicomedullary junction. Williams' experimental observations clearly suggest a craniospinal pressure dissociation which may develop in relationship to maneuvers that increase intraabdominal or intrathoracic pressure and cause compression of the thecal sac via the epidural veins. It is possible that a one-way valve mechanism at the cervicomedullary junction exists and if communication is present between the syrinx and the fourth ventricle a "suck" phenomenon could occur as described by Williams.[101] In those cases where no communication between the fourth ventricle and the syrinx exists, repetitive systolic spinal subarachnoid pressure waves generated by inferior displacement of the tonsils may come into play in the formation of syringohydromyelia. The mechanism by which a syrinx can form under these circumstances was clearly demonstrated in the numerous studies that had previously shown communication between the spinal subarachnoid space and the syrinx cavity via the perivascular Virchow-Robin band spaces.[4,5,22,31,48,104] It is feasible that external compression of the spinal cord may also contribute to syrinx propagation via the "sloshing" mechanism first proposed by Williams.[101]

Clearly, the pathogenesis of syringohydromyelia is complex, but when taken together, all of these theories help explain various facets of syringohydromyelia formation and propagation. The cardiac cycle generates systolic pressure waves which may be transmitted to the spinal and intracranial CSF. In addition, straining actions such as the Valsalva maneuver or coughing produce epidural venous engorge-ment resulting in elevation and the spinal subarachnoid pressures. Under ordinary circumstances, these pressures are accommodated by the subarachnoid space but the ability to accommodate becomes compromised in the presence of foramen magnum impaction from hindbrain malformations.

IMPLICATIONS FOR SURGICAL INTERVENTION

A clear understanding of the pathogenesis of syringohydromyelia in association with hindbrain malformations is needed to formulate a thoughtful and organized approach toward the management of these complex disorders. Specific technical aspects of the operations proposed for treatment of these disorders are reviewed in later chapters and will not be addressed here in detail.

However, a brief discussion of the validity of operative interventions needs to be addressed in light of improvements in our understanding of the pathogenesis of syringohydromyelia. It is only with a thorough understanding and application of these principles that successful operative intervention can be undertaken.

THE ROLE OF POSTERIOR FOSSA DECOMPRESSION

All major theories seeking to explain the formation of syringohydromyelia share alterations in CSF dynamics at the cervicomedullary junction as the major underlying cause. These changes occur as a result of foramen magnum impaction from the Chiari malformation and fourth ventricular outflow obstruction. Therefore, to have any hopes of success, the surgical intervention needs to address these pathological features. Posterior fossa decompression has been developed as the major technique to relieve impaction created by tonsillar herniation and cause regression of symptoms.[2,26] However, components of the posterior fossa decompression vary greatly in the literature and it is often difficult to determine which interventions are necessary in a given patient.

In its simplest form, posterior fossa decompression involves bony foramen magnum decompression and cervical laminectomy to a level below the herniated tonsils.[9,12,13,15,18,24-26,33,46,87,94] Typically, this involves the C1 level and at times the C2 level, but may occasionally include laminectomy at more caudad levels.[25,26,50,59,60,72,76] In conjunction with the bony decompression, numerous intraoperative observations report the presence of a constrictive dural band near the posterior lip of the foramen magnum which prevents expansion of the thecal sac even after adequate bony decompression.[26,64] Intraoperative ultrasound has confirmed persistence of compression despite removal of bony structures.[50] Therefore, a duraplasty is absolutely an essential component to the operation in order to relieve the alterations in CSF flow at the cervicomedullary junction which leads to syrinx formation.[9,24,25,59,64,76] Typically, the patient's own fascia or dura may be used for this procedure.[64] In the past, Silastic sheets have been used for duraplasty; however, on occasion these may be associated with delayed hemorrhage near the graft with subsequent neurological deterioration. Some believe that craniectomy/laminectomy with extra-arachnoid duraplasty provides adequate treatment.[74] This approach should be viewed with caution given the lack of long-term follow-up of patients treated in this fashion and the known observation that deterioration may take years to appear.[29]

Because intraoperative observations may reveal severe arachnoid adhesions near the tonsils and outlets of the fourth ventricle which may impede CSF flow, numerous authors have recommended lysis of adhesions as an integral component to the operation (Figure 4A).[2,9,33,82] At times these adhesions can be so severe that a mass of scar tissue becomes densely adherent to the tonsils.[26,87] Microdissection with care to avoid injury to the posterior inferior cerebellar arteries can serve to open the outlet of the fourth ventricle (Figure 5).[2,9,32,61,76,86] Because of the theories proposed by Gardner, which highlighted the central importance of obstruction of fourth ventricular outflow, operative approaches have also employed fourth ventricle to subarachnoid space shunts in patients with syringohydromyelia to ensure adequate outflow (Figure 4B).[12,25,26,72,76] The need for such a procedure has become quite controversial, with more recent studies

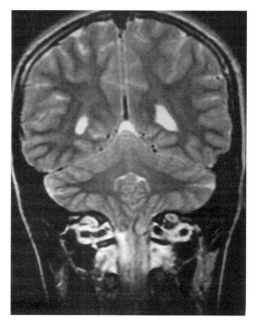

Figure 5: Coronal MR imaging of the brain and cervicomedullary junction fortuitously showing tonsillar herniation through the foramen magnum and a flow void from the posterior inferior cerebellar artery as it accompanies the tonsils, which descend through the level of the foramen magnum.

suggesting that communication between the fourth ventricle and the syrinx may be an uncommon ocurrence.[54,75] The precise role for fourth ventricle to subarachnoid shunting has not been fully elucidated.[72,76] We currently employ the shunt technique in all patients with syringohydromyelia in association with a Chiari malformation unless this intervention is not technically feasible. However, it should be recognized that this procedure is not without risk since insertion of the shunt may produce deficits in extraocular motility due to irritation of the collicular plate.[66] Typically these deficits are transient, but under rare circumstances may be permanent.[66] Insertion of a shunt is also associated in some instances with nausea and vomiting, presumably from irritation of the area postrema.[66]

Gardner's theory also places a central role in the genesis of syringohydromyelia on communication between the fourth ventricle and the syrinx cavity. In cases where a communication exists, various authors have debated whether placement of a muscle plug into the central canal at the level of the obex aids in obliteration of the communication between these two structures.[12,26,29,33,56,82] Subsequent studies have failed to demonstrate added patient benefit from such a maneuver.[59,72,83] This technique is also associated with nausea and vomiting in the postoperative period from irritation to the area postrema, which is directly adjacent to the obex in which the muscle plug is placed.[66] Because of these observations, we no longer employ muscle plug occlusion of the central canal at the level of the obex.

If posterior fossa impaction and impaired fourth ventricular outflow is severe, hydrocephalus may also develop.[26,49] It is imperative to identify hydrocephalus prior to any further surgical intervention, since the patient may have complete resolution of symptoms and/or signs following ventriculoperitoneal shunting procedures alone. This procedure may alleviate the need for more extensive procedures.[26,49] Also, posterior fossa decompression in the face of active untreated hydrocephalus may precipitate further tonsillar herniation with neurological deterioration.

As previously mentioned, there is a rare association between the development of basilar invagination and Chiari malformations.[3,6,16,19,20] It is not infrequent that syringohydromyelia develops in these patients as well. Ventral cervicomedullary junction compression from basilar invagination may be sufficient in and of itself to cause syrinx formation by alteration of normal CSF flow through the foramen magnum. Therefore, successful treatment of the Chiari malformation and syringohydromyelia requires the ventral cervicomedullary junction pathology to be addressed initially. Indeed, we have witnessed resolution of syringohydromyelia in association with Chiari malformations after transoral decompression alone without posterior fossa decompression.

THE ROLE OF SYRINGOSUBARACHNOID SHUNTING PROCEDURES

Syringosubarachnoid and syringoperitoneal shunt procedures were developed early in the treatment of Chiari malformations with syringohydromyelia.[7,18,28,45,49,81,95] These procedures typically involve placement of a Silastic tube through the dorsal root entry zone or the thinnest area of the cord to aid in drainage of CSF from within the syrinx to the subarachnoid space.[7,28,45,81] Alternatively, some authors have recommended performing a myelotomy or stent placement as equivalent treatment.[6] A terminal syringostomy has also been described where the syrinx is opened at the base of the spinal cord.[49,103] Others even combine this procedure with posterior fossa decompression, where the syrinx is approached through the upper cervical laminectomy.[53,60,62,86] While syrinx shunting is clearly beneficial in cystic cavities associated with trauma and tumors, its role in the treatment of syringohydromyelia associated with hindbrain malformations remains quite controversial.[7,45,49,53,63,95] Recent studies examining the efficacy of syringosubarachnoid shunting have called this procedure into question.[83] Certain theories of syrinx formation can help explain the pathophysiology behind the failure of the syringosubarachnoid shunts. The systolic subarachnoid pressure wave generated by downward displacement of the tonsils is proposed to cause syringohydromyelia formation via entrance of CSF through perivascular Virchow-Robin band spaces leading to fluid accumulation within the cord. The presence of a syringosubarachnoid shunt would merely result in facilitation of CSF entering into the syrinx cavity and, thus, is not an effective treatment for syringohydromyelia. In addition, syringosubarachnoid shunts performed without addressing the foramen magnum compression would also ignore the central pathology identified in all major theories of syringohydromyelia formation and therefore should be avoided.

CONCLUSION

Hindbrain malformations are frequently associated with the development of syringohydromyelia. Several major theories have been proposed to explain development of these spinal cord cysts. While no one theory explains all facets of syringohydromyelia with hindbrain malformations, a combination of these theories provides an excellent understanding of the mechanisms that may be at work in a given patient. Successful treatment of Chiari malformations and syringohydromyelia is dependent on a thorough understanding of these complex pathophysiological steps. Central to the pathogenesis of syringohydromyelia in all theories is disruption of normal CSF dynamics at the craniovertebral junction. When present, concomitant hydrocephalus and basilar invagination should be addressed prior to undertaking any intervention. Subsequently, the posterior fossa decompression procedure is the operation of choice since it addresses all major pathophysiological events that have been highlighted in the major theories of syringohydromyelia formation. This procedure should include lysis of adhesions in the region of the foramen magnum. Fourth ventricular-to-subarachnoid space shunting is also recommended in Chiari malformation patients with syringohydromyelia until clinical assessment of its necessity has been fully assessed. Muscle plug occlusion of the central canal at the level of the obex does not appear to augment results of the standard posterior fossa decompression and therefore is not necessary. While initial results with limited bony decompression and extra-arachnoid duraplasty appear encouraging, long-term follow-up is required before this treatment can be recommended. Finally, syringosubarachnoid shunting fails to address the significant pathophysiological mechanisms of syringohydromyelia formation and should be avoided except after failure of an adequate posterior fossa decompression.

REFERENCES

1. Aboulker J: La syringomyelie et les liquides intra-rachidiens. **Neurochirurgie 25 (Suppl 1)**:1-144, 1979
2. Appleby A, Foster JB, Hankinson J, et al: The diagnosis and management of the Chiari anomalies in adult life. **Brain 91**:131-139, 1968
3. Aubin ML, Vignaud J, Iba-Zizen MT, et al: NMR imaging of the cranio-cervical junction and cervical spine. Normal and pathological features. **J Neuroradiol 11**:229-237, 1984
4. Aubin ML, Vignaud J, Jardin C, et al: Computed tomography in 75 clinical cases of syringomyelia. **AJNR 2**:199-204, 1981
5. Ball MJ, Dayan AD: Pathogenesis of syringomyelia. **Lancet 2**:799-801, 1972
6. Banerji NK, Millar JHD: Chiari malformation presenting in adult life. Its relationship to syringomyelia. **Brain 97**:157-168, 1974
7. Barbaro NM, Wilson CB, Gutin PH, et al: Surgical treatment of syringomyelia. Favorable results with syringoperitoneal shunting. **J Neurosurg 61**:531-538, 1984
8. Barkovich AJ, Wippold FJ, Sherman JL, et al: Significance of cerebellar tonsillar position on MR. **AJNR 7**:795-799, 1986
9. Batzdorf U: Chiari I malformation with syringomyelia. Evaluation of surgical therapy by magnetic resonance imaging. **J Neurosurg 68**:726-730, 1988
10. Bertrand G: Dynamic factors in the evolution of syringomyelia and syringobulbia. **Clin Neurosurg 20**:322-333, 1973
11. Boman K, Iivanainen M: Prognosis of syringomyelia. **Acta Neurol Scand 43**:61-68, 1967
12. Cahan LD, Bentson JR: Considerations in the diagnosis and treatment of syringomyelia and the Chiari malformation. **J Neurosurg 57**:24-31, 1982
13. Carmel P, Bello JA: Resolution of anatomical abnormalities following posterior fossa decompression for Chiari I malformation. **J Neurosurg 80**:389A-390A, 1994 (Abstract)
14. Chandler WF, Johnson JH Jr: Syringomyelia presenting as a mass lesion of the conus medullaris. **Surg Neurol 12**:385-388, 1979
15. Conway LW: Hydrodynamic studies in syringomyelia. **J Neurosurg 27**:501-514, 1967
16. Corbett JJ, Butler AB, Kaufman B: 'Sneeze syncope,' basilar invagination and Arnold-Chiari type I malformation. **J Neurol Neurosurg Psychiatry 39**:381-384, 1976
17. Daniel PM, Strich SJ: Some observations of the congenital deformity of the central nervous system known as the Arnold-Chiari malformation. **J Neuropathol Exp Neurol 17**:255-266, 1958
18. Dauser RC, DiPietro MA, Venes JL: Symptomatic Chiari I malformation in childhood: a report of 7 cases. **Pediatr Neurosci 14**:184-190, 1988
19. de Barros M, Farias W, Ataíde L, et al: Basilar impression and Arnold-Chiari malformation. A study of 66 cases. **J Neurol Neurosurg Psychiatry 31**:596-605, 1968
20. de Barros M, Farias da Silva W, de Azevedo Filho HC, et al: Disturbances of sexual potency in patients with basilar impression and Arnold-Chiari malformation. **J Neurol Neurosurg Psychiatry 38**:598-600, 1975
21. Dohrmann GJ, Rubin JM: Intraoperative ultrasound imaging of the spinal cord: syringomyelia, cysts and tumors—a preliminary report. **Surg Neurol 18**:395-399, 1982
22. Dubois PJ, Drayer BP, Sage M, et al: Intramedullary penetrance of metrizamide in the dog spinal cord. **AJNR 2**:313-317, 1981
23. du Boulay G, Shah SH, Currie JC, et al: The mechanism of hydromyelia in Chiari type I malformations. **Br J Radiol 47**:579-587, 1974
24. Dure LS, Percy AK, Cheek WR, et al: Chiari type I malformation in children. **J Pediatr 115**:573-576, 1989
25. Dyste GN, Menezes AH: Presentation and management of pediatric Chiari malformations without myelodysplasia. **Neurosurgery 23**:589-597, 1988
26. Dyste GN, Menezes AH, VanGilder JC: Symptomatic Chiari malformations: an analysis of presentation, management, and long-term outcome. **J Neurosurg**

71:159-168, 1989

27. Ellertsson AB, Greitz T: The distending force in the production of communicating syringomyelia. **Lancet** 1:1234, 1970

28. Elster AD, Chen MYM: Chiari I malformations: clinical and radiologic reappraisal. **Radiology 183:** 347-353, 1992

29. Faulhauer K, Loew K: The surgical treatment of syringomyelia. Long-term results. **Acta Neurochir 44:** 215-222, 1978

30. Fischer EG, Welch K, Shillito J Jr: Syringomyelia following lumboureteral shunting for communicating hydrocephalus. Report of three cases. **J Neurosurg 47:** 96-100, 1977

31. Forbes WSC, Isherwood I: Computed tomography in syringomyelia and the associated Arnold-Chiari type I malformation. **Neuroradiology 15:**73-78, 1978

32. Gabrielsen TO, Seeger JF, Amundsen P: Some new angiographic observations in patients with Chiari type I and II malformations. **Radiology 115:**627-634, 1975

33. Garcìa-Uria J, Leunda G, Carrillo R, et al: Syringomyelia: long-term results after posterior fossa decompression. **J Neurosurg 54:**380-383, 1981

34. Gardner WJ: Anatomic anomalies common to myelomeningocele of infancy and syringomyelia of adulthood suggest a common origin. **Cleve Clin Q** 26:118-133, 1959

35. Gardner WJ: Anatomic features common to the Arnold-Chiari and the Dandy-Walker malformations suggest a common origin. **Cleve Clin Q 26:**206-222, 1959

36. Gardner WJ: Hydrodynamic mechanism of syringomyelia: its relationship to myelocele. **J Neurol Neurosurg Psychiatry 28:**247-259, 1965

37. Gardner WJ, Angel J: The cause of syringomyelia and its surgical treatment. **Cleve Clin Q 25:**4-8, 1958

38. Gardner WJ, Bell HS, Poolos PN, et al: Terminal ventriculostomy for syringomyelia. **J Neurosurg 46:** 609-617, 1977

39. Gardner WJ, Goodall RJ: The surgical treatment of Arnold-Chiari malformation in adults. An explanation of its mechanism and importance of encephalography in diagnosis. **J Neurosurg 7:**199-206, 1950

40. Hall PV, Kalsbeck JE, Wellman HN, et al: Clinical radioisotope investigations in hydrosyringomyelia and myelodysplasia. **J Neurosurg 45:**188-194, 1976

41. Hall PV, Kalsbeck JE, Wellman HN, et al: Radioisotope evaluation of experimental hydrosyringomyelia. **J Neurosurg 45:**181-187, 1976

42. Hall PV, Lindseth RE, Campbell RL, et al: Myelodysplasia and developmental scoliosis. A manifestation of syringomyelia. **Spine l:**48-56, 1976

43. Hall PV, Muller J, Campbell RL: Experimental hydrosyringomyelia, ischemic myelopathy, and syringomyelia. **J Neurosurg 43:**464-470, 1975

44. Hall P, Turner M, Archinger S, et al: Experimental syringomyelia. The relationship between intraventricular and intrasyrinx pressures. **J Neurosurg 52:** 812-817, 1980

45. Hida K, Iwasaki Y, Imamura H, et al: Surgical indication for and results of foramen magnum decompression versus syringosubarachnoid shunt for syringomyelia associated with Chiari malformation. **J Neurosurg 78:**351A, 1993 (Abstract)

46. Hochman MS, Kobetz SA, Sneider SE, et al: Adult Arnold-Chiari malformation type I demonstrated by CT metrizamide myelography. **Surg Neurol 16:** 467-468, 1981

47. Huang PP, Constantini S: "Acquired" Chiari I malformation. Case report. **J Neurosurg 80:**1099-1102, 1994

48. Hutchings M, Weller RO: Anatomical relationships of the pia mater to cerebral blood vessels in man. **J Neurosurg 65:**316-325, 1986

49. Isu T, Iwasaki Y, Akino M, et al: Hydrosyringomyelia associated with a Chiari I malformation in children and adolescents. **Neurosurgery 26:**591-596, 1990

50. Isu T, Sasaki H, Takamura H, et al: Foramen magnum decompression with removal of the outer layer of the dura as treatment for syringomyelia occurring with Chiari I malformation. **Neurosurgery 33:** 845-850, 1993

51. Kanev PM, Getch CC, Jallo J, et al: Cerebral syrinx with Chiari I malformation. **Pediatr Neurosurg 20:** 214-216, 1994

52. Kasantikul V, Netsky MG, James AE Jr: Relation of age and cerebral ventricle size to central canal in man. Morphological analysis. **J Neurosurg 51:**85-93, 1979

53. Kokmen E, Marsh WR, Baker HL Jr: Magnetic resonance imaging in syringomyelia. **Neurosurgery 17:** 267-270, 1985

54. Lee BCP, Zimmerman RB, Manning JJ, et al: MR imaging of syringomyelia and hydromyelia. **AJNR 6:** 221-228, 1985

55. Levy LM, Di Chiro G: MR phase imaging and cerebrospinal fluid flow in the head and spine. **Neuroradiology 32:**399-406, 1990

56. Levy WJ, Mason L, Hahn JF: Chiari malformation presenting in adults: a surgical experience in 127 cases. **Neurosurgery 12:**377-390, 1983

57. Lewonowski K, King JD, Nelson MD: Routine use of magnetic resonance imaging in idiopathic scoliosis patients less than eleven years of age. **Spine 17 (Suppl 6):**S109-S116, 1992

58. Li KC, Chui MC: Conventional and CT metrizamide myelography in Arnold-Chiari I malformation and syringomyelia. **AJNR 8:**11-17, 1987

59. Logue V, Edwards MR: Syringomyelia and its surgical treatment—an analysis of 75 patients. **J Neurol Neurosurg Psychiatry 44:**273-284, 1981

60. Love JG, Olafson RA: Syringomyelia: a look at surgical therapy. **J Neurosurg 24:**714-718, 1966

61. Margolis MT, Newton TH: Angiographic sign of cerebellar tonsillar herniation. **Neuroradiology 2:**3-8, 1971

62. Matsumoto T, Symon L: Surgical management of syringomyelia—current results. **Surg Neurol 32:** 258-265, 1989

63. McLean DR, Miller JDR, Allen PBR, et al: Posttraumatic syringomyelia. **J Neurosurg 39:**485-492, 1973

64. Menezes AH, Dyste GN, Smoker WRK: Syringomyelia, Chiari malformations and hydromyelia, in Youmans J (ed): **Neurological Surgery.** 3rd ed. Philadelphia, Pa: WB Saunders, 1990, Vol 2, pp 1421-1459

65. Menezes AH, VanGilder JC: Anomalies of the craniovertebral junction, in Youmans J (ed): **Neurological Surgery.** 3rd ed. Philadelphia, Pa: WB Saunders, 1990, Vol. 2, pp 1359-1420

66. Menezes AH: Chiari I malformations and hydromyelia—complications. **Pediatr Neurosurg 17:**146-154, 1991/1992

67. Milhorat TH, Kotzen RM, Anzil AP: Stenosis of central canal of spinal cord in man: incidence and pathological findings in 232 autopsy cases. **J Neurosurg 80:**716-722, 1994

68. Muhonen MG, Menezes AH, Sawin PD, et al: Scoliosis in pediatric Chiari malformations without myelodysplasia. **J Neurosurg 77:**69-77, 1992

69. Newman PK, Terenty TR, Foster JB: Some observations on the pathogenesis of syringomyelia. **J Neurol Neurosurg Psychiatry 44:**964-969, 1981

70. Nitz WR, Bradley WG Jr, Watanabe AS, et al: Flow dynamics of cerebrospinal fluid: assessment with phase-contrast velocity MR imaging performed with retrospective cardiac gating. **Radiology 183:**395-405, 1992

71. Njemanze PC, Beck OJ: MR-gated intracranial CSF dynamics: evaluation of CSF pulsatile flow. **AJNR 10:**77-80, 1989

72. Nohria V, Oakes WJ: Chiari I malformation: a review of 43 patients. **Pediatr Neurosurg 16:**222-227, 1990-1991

73. Nokes SR, Murtagh FR, Jones JD III, et al: Childhood scoliosis: MR imaging. **Radiology 164:**791-797, 1987

74. Oldfield EH, Muraszko K, Shawker TH, et al: Pathophysiology of syringomyelia associated with Chiari I malformation of the cerebellar tonsils. Implications for diagnosis and treatment. **J Neurosurg 80:**3-15, 1994

75. Park TS, Cail WS, Broaddus WC, et al: Lumboperitoneal shunt combined with myelotomy for treatment of syringohydromyelia. **J Neurosurg 70:**721-727, 1989

76. Paul KS, Lye RH, Strang FA, et al: Arnold-Chiari malformation. Review of 71 cases. **J Neurosurg 58:**183-187, 1983

77. Payner TD, Prenger E, Berger TS, et al: Acquired Chiari malformations: incidence, diagnosis, and management. **Neurosurgery 34:**429-434, 1994

78. Peach B: Arnold-Chiari malformation. Anatomic features of 20 cases. **Arch Neurol 12:**613-621, 1965

79. Peerless SJ, Durward QJ: Management of syringomyelia: a pathophysiological approach. **Clin Neurosurg 30:**531-576, 1983

80. Perot P, Feindel W, Lloyd-Smith D: Hematomyelia as a complication of syringomyelia: Gowers' syringal hemorrhage. Case report. **J Neurosurg 25:**447-451, 1966

81. Phillips TW, Kindt GW: Syringoperitoneal shunt for syringomyelia: a preliminary report. **Surg Neurol 16:**462-466, 1981

82. Pillay PK, Awad IA, Little JR, et al: Symptomatic Chiari malformation in adults: a new classification based on magnetic resonance imaging with clinical and prognostic significance. **Neurosurgery 28:**639-645, 1991

83. Piper JG, Muhonen MG, Sawin P, et al: Chiari malformation database report: long-term follow-up review of surgical treatment modalities. **J Neurosurg 80:**383A, 1994 (Abstract)

84. Pojunas K, Williams AL, Daniels DL, et al: Syringomyelia and hydromyelia: magnetic resonance evaluation. **Radiology 153:**679-683, 1984

85. Resjö IM, Harwood-Nash DC, Fitz CR, et al: Computed tomographic metrizamide myelography in syringohydromyelia. **Radiology 131:**405-407, 1979

86. Rhoton AL Jr: Microsurgery of Arnold-Chiari malformation in adults with and without hydromyelia. **J Neurosurg 45:**473-483, 1976

87. Saez RJ, Onofrio BM, Yanagihara T: Experience with Arnold-Chiari malformation, 1960 to 1970. **J Neurosurg 45:**416-422, 1976

88. Schellinger D, LeBihan D, Rajan SS, et al: MR of slow CSF flow in the spine. **AJNR 13:**1393-1403, 1992

89. Scotti G, Scialfa G, Landoni L, et al: Nuclear magnetic resonance in the diagnosis of syringomyelia. **J Neuroradiol 11:**239-248, 1984

90. Senelick RC: Total alleviation of downbeat nystagmus in basilar impression by transoral removal of the odontoid process. **J Clinical Neurophysiol 1:**265-267, 1981

91. Sherman JL, Citrin CM, Gangarosa RE, et al: The MR appearance of CSF pulsations in the spinal canal. **AJNR 7:**879-884, 1986

92. Spinos E, Laster DW, Moody DM, et al: MR evaluation of Chiari I malformations at 0.15 T. **AJR 144:**1143-1148, 1985

93. Stovner LJ, Rinch P: Syringomyelia in Chiari malformation: relation to extent of cerebellar tissue herniation. **Neurosurgery 31:**913-917, 1992

94. Tachibana S, Iida H, Yada K: Significance of positive Queckenstedt test in patients with syringomyelia associated with Arnold-Chiari malformations. **J Neurosurg 76:**67-71, 1992

95. Tator CH, Meguro K, Rowed DW: Favorable results with syringosubarachnoid shunts for treatment of syringomyelia. **J Neurosurg 56:**517-523, 1982

96. Taylor J, Greenfield JG, Martin JP: Two cases of syringomyelia and syringobulbia, observed clinically over many years, and examined pathologically. **Brain 45:**323-356, 1922

97. Teng P, Papatheodorou C: Arnold-Chiari malformation with normal spine and cranium. **Arch Neurol 12:**622-624, 1965

98. Welch K, Shillito J, Strand R, et al: Chiari I "malformation"—an acquired disorder? **J Neurosurg 55:**604-609, 1981

99. Williams B: A critical appraisal of posterior fossa surgery for communicating syringomyelia. **Brain 101:**223-250, 1978

100. Williams B: The distending force in the production of "communicating syringomyelia." **Lancet 2:**189-193, 1969

101. Williams B: On the pathogenesis of syringomyelia: a review. **J R Soc Med 73:**798-806, 1980

102. Williams B: Orthopaedic features in the presentation of syringomyelia. **J Bone Joint Surg (Br) 61:**314-323, 1979

103. Williams B, Fahy G: A critical appraisal of "terminal ventriculostomy" for the treatment of syringomyelia. **J Neurosurg 58:**188-197, 1983

104. Woosley RE, Whaley RA: Use of metrizamide in computerized tomography to diagnose the Chiari I malformation. **J Neurosurg 56:**373-376, 1982

105. Yu HC, Deck MDF: The clivus deformity of the Arnold-Chiari malformation. **Radiology 101:**613-615, 1971

POSTTRAUMATIC SYRINGOMYELIA

NEVAN G. BALDWIN, MD, AND DAVID G. MALONE, MD

Cavitation of the spinal cord is an entity frequently encountered in patients with spinal injury. There is some disagreement regarding the use of the terms "syringomyelia," "hydromyelia," and "syringohydromyelia" for such lesions. Hydromyelia is an expansion of the central canal of the spinal cord. Syringomyelia is an expansion beyond the central canal to involve the gray matter of the cord.[23,38] Some authors prefer the term syringohydromyelia to avoid the need for distinguishing the two entities.

Due to the mechanisms of formation, posttraumatic cavitation of the spinal cord is thought to arise most commonly from within the gray matter. Although there is usually communication with the central canal, it is frequently difficult or impossible to discern this fact with certainty. For the sake of simplicity, in this chapter the term "posttraumatic syringomyelia" refers to all posttraumatic spinal cord cavities, with or without central canal communication.

Syringomyelia is frequently classified as either communicating or noncommunicating. This terminology refers to whether or not there is direct communication between the fourth ventricle and the spinal cord dilatation.[23] In the patient with posttraumatic syringomyelia, there is usually no direct communication with the posterior fossa and, therefore, the posttraumatic variety is most commonly the noncommunicating type.[23]

The reported incidence of posttraumatic syrinx ranges from 1% to 4.5% and is higher after a complete cord injury as compared with an incomplete injury.[29] However, the actual incidence of the disease may be considerably higher than this, because diagnostic imaging is usually performed only for patients with symptoms. In a recent study of magnetic resonance imaging (MRI) scans from patients admitted to a spinal cord injury unit, none of whom demonstrated findings of ascending myelopathy, the incidence of "cysts" of the spinal cord was observed to be 51%.[5]

PATHOGENESIS

The majority of theories on formation of syringes relate to those in patients with Chiari malformations and communicating syringomyelia. These theories, generally speaking, do not pertain to the pathogenesis of the posttraumatic variety of syrinx. The theories relating mainly to the Chiari-associated types are reviewed extensively elsewhere.[21,40,41,43,48,57,65]

Blockage of cerebrospinal fluid (CSF) flow due to positional factors (i.e., neck extension) has been observed as a possible mechanism in patients with Chiari malformation.[57] This may be a factor in the posttraumatic syrinx as well, particularly if spinal instability is also present.

NONCOMMUNICATING SYRINGOMYELIA

The precise etiology of the posttraumatic syrinx has not been defined, but experimental evidence and clinical studies suggest that a number of factors are probably involved. Perhaps the most commonly cited initiating lesion is a hematoma of the cord, properly termed hematomyelia. As the hematoma resolves, a necrotic cavity and surrounding area of myelomalacia forms. Factors driving this process may include ischemia, the action of destructive enzymes or free radical products, or other toxic agents released in response to the trauma.[17,23,54] Freeman[18,19] demonstrated in the 1950s that after experimental cord trauma in animals, myelotomy at the injury level allowed the egress of necrotic material from the cord and reduced the likelihood of syrinx formation. Because of the observed role of inflammatory mechanisms in posttraumatic syrinx formation, it might be viewed essentially as an abortive attempt at healing and regeneration.[53]

Studies in rats using a photochemically induced vascular thrombosis model of spinal cord injury have shown that the histological and ultrastructural changes arising from vascular spinal cord injury are very similar to those observed with compression or contusion models.[13] In this rat model, cavitation of the spinal cord occurred in a predictable sequence of events. This may argue for the presence of a vascular component in the pathogenesis of posttraumatic syrinx formation. There has been extensive study of this subject in other animal models as well. These other models also support the finding that vascular mechanisms are a key component in the occurrence of "secondary" spinal cord injury.[58]

THE ROLE OF ARACHNOIDITIS

Arachnoiditis can lead to adhesions which alter the dynamics of CSF flow and lead to syrinx formation.[8,9] Generally found in the thoracic region, these syringes are distinguished from the more common cervical variety.[56] It is possible that persistent spinal cord compression after injury can also lead to syrinx formation. This may be due to ischemia of the cord with resulting secondary changes in the gray matter. This can occur with intra- or extradural compression, or with abnormalities of the skull base.[25,33,59] Alternatively, damage to the glial elements of the spinal cord with resulting enlargement of the Virchow-Robin spaces may provide an abnormal entry pathway for the accumulation of CSF in the spinal cord.[14] Arachnoid adhesions may also play a role by forming a one-way valve mechanism, trapping CSF from the subarachnoid space and allowing the CSF pulsations to then force fluid into the cord parenchyma.[15,23]

It is interesting to note that in a rabbit model, syrinx formation was observed in up to 55% of subjects following spinal cord trauma and chemical induction of arachnoiditis, while arachnoiditis alone produced no syrinx formation. Trauma alone, without induction of arachnoiditis, led to syrinx formation in only 12% of subjects.[15] Arachnoiditis may therefore be a factor both in the formation and the enlargement of spinal cord cavities.

Barnett and colleagues[7] described a series of patients with progressive myelopathy after spinal trauma and suggested that these may be related to cystic change in the cord. Tension, torsion, and cord distortion related to neck movement with resulting continued spinal trauma were believed to be possible factors leading to progression. Tethering of the spinal cord, usually due to changes associated with arachnoiditis in the region of the conus medullaris, may also lead to these same tension-related effects.[4,61]

Clinicopathological studies have led to the concept of a spectrum of posttraumatic spinal cord pathology. This spectrum courses from arachnoiditis to microcystic degeneration to syringohydromyelia.[27,34,54,67] A continuum of noncystic to cystic myelopathy to syrinx is therefore believed to represent the series of changes occurring over highly variable time periods after injury.[27]

ANATOMY AND CLINICAL PRESENTATION

Patients with posttraumatic syringomyelia often present with clinical findings identical to those with syringes of other etiologies. The disruption of sensory fibers for pain and temperature as they cross the anterior commissure of the spinal cord causes loss of sensation resulting in burns or other injuries to the hands or arms that are painless. Atrophy or pain in the neck, arms, or hands is also common. Examination of the patient may reveal the typical capelike distribution of loss of pain and temperature sensation. Touch, pressure, position sense, and vibratory sensation are usually unaffected. The loss of pain and temperature with preservation of these other modalities is referred to as dissociated sensory loss. A number of unusual symptoms may also be seen in syringomyelia, particularly if the cavity is ascending in the cervical region. Reported presenting symptoms include segmental hyperhidrosis, episodic unconsciousness, hiccups, trigeminal paresthesias, and tinnitus.[31,36,37,55]

In patients with spinal cord injuries and preexisting neurological deficits, documentation of neurological deterioration can be more difficult. Often it is simply a feeling by the patient that his level of sensory loss is ascending or a similar complaint that leads to medical attention. In the spinal cord injured patient who complains of worsening neurological deficits, syringomyelia should be high on the list of conditions to be ruled out.

Posttraumatic syrinx formation can occur following any degree of trauma to the spinal cord.[46,60] Four types of spinal trauma are recognized in association with syringomyelia: severe single trauma, trauma followed by arachnoiditis, repeated microtrauma, and single minor trauma. Single minor trauma is an extremely rare cause of syringomyelia, but the others clearly have a common association.[12,61] Posttraumatic syringes are seen in all age groups and the condition has even been reported in a neonate following birth injury.[39] The time course from injury to presentation is extremely variable. Cases of posttraumatic syringomyelia have been cited occurring from 2 weeks to 41 years after spinal cord injury.[5,12,36,60] However, in only one patient has time from injury to syrinx formation been reported to be less than 2 months. It is possible that this case represented a pre-existing lesion and not a true posttraumatic syrinx.

Clinical progression is highly variable in syringomyelia. Permanent physical disability usually does not occur until many years after the onset of symptoms. However, in 5% to 10% of the patients suffering from this condition, severe disability occurs within 2 to 5 years after the onset of symptoms.[28,50,53]

Evoked potentials have demonstrated that alterations of posterior column function do occur in association with syringomyelia.[38] However, this was demonstrated in patients with Chiari malformations and the changes in posterior column function might therefore be related to hindbrain malformation, having little to do with the syrinx itself. Posterior column dysfunction, and subsequently the value of evoked potential use, has not been well evaluated in patients in whom the syrinx was posttraumatic in nature. Since patients with posttraumatic syringomyelia most commonly have complete spinal cord injuries, evoked potentials are of questionable utility. They might, however, be used to demonstrate worsening function as a syrinx ascends above the level of injury.

Scoliosis may be the first presenting symptom of syringomyelia. The possibility of a syrinx should be included in the differential diagnosis of any abnormal spinal curve.[46] Many patients in whom scoliosis is considered to be idiopathic probably have a neurogenic etiology relating to the presence of a syrinx.[51] In a series of more than 1,000 patients with scoliosis, syrinx was observed in 18% of the male patients and 3% of females.[3] A cervical curve, high thoracic double curve, or a painful curve should elicit suspicion of possible syringomyelia.[51] In a patient with Charcot's neuropathic arthropathy, a syrinx should be considered a likely diagnostic possibility.[22,32] Neuropathic joints are found in 25% to 32% of patients with syringomyelia.[16,22,24,32]

DIAGNOSTIC EVALUATION

The evaluation of a patient with a suspected syrinx or follow-up for a known syrinx should include MRI. This is widely regarded as the modality of choice for imaging both the syrinx and any associated spinal cord abnormality.[20,23,27,44,49,56] Although no longer the primary technique for evaluation of syringes, the myelogram and postmyelography computed tomography (CT) scan are of considerable value in selected instances.[10,26,28,46] This is especially true in the posttraumatic type because myelography will reveal arachnoiditis and will delineate complete canal blockage more definitively than MRI. Knowledge of whether the subarachnoid space is patent for the flow of CSF may be an important factor in the selection of an appropriate surgical treatment. Delayed CT scanning at 3 and 6 hours after the myelogram will often show that passage of contrast into the syrinx has occurred, thereby confirming communication of the cavity with the subarachnoid space.

Following surgery, the use of radioisotopes is a valuable technique in syrinx patients if shunt malfunction is suspected. Historically, radioiodinated serum albumin (^{131}I RISA) was injected into the intrathecal space, and the abdomen (or whichever body cavity the shunt was directed toward) was then monitored for radioactivity. The albumin component, however, was found to cause arachnoiditis in some cases and newer isotopes were developed. Currently, the two isotopes used for this purpose are ^{111}In diamine triamine penta-acetic acid (DTPA) and ^{99m}Tc DTPA. The advantages of the indium compound include a 3-day half-life, which allows long study periods, and it is approved for intrathecal use. However, since this compound is not routinely used in most nuclear medicine departments and has a very short shelf life, it is not usually found in stock and must be ordered, thereby creating a one day delay.

The technetium compound (^{99m}Tc DTPA) has not been fully approved for intrathecal use, although it is very commonly utilized for this "off-label" purpose. The advantages of this compound include excellent photon flux, which improves image quality, and it is stocked in any nuclear medicine department, so availability is usually immediate. If the shunt to be tested has a reservoir, a known volume of ^{99m}Tc DTPA can be injected (or this can be placed in the thecal space) and the rate of shunt flow can be calculated with reasonable precision using the measured decay rates. Because this compound has a half-life of only 6 hours, studies are limited to no more than 24 hours after injection.

If the patency of a shunt system is in question, those devices having a reservoir can be tapped percutaneously. Evaluation of flow can be done by simple manometer testing or by injecting a small amount of a myelographic contrast agent into the shunt and evaluating flow with plain radiography or CT.

In the patient whose symptoms may not be related to the syrinx, for example a patient with headache only, percutaneous drainage of the syrinx may be of diagnostic value.[29] If the symptoms respond to drainage, then surgical intervention may be warranted.

Although the larger syringes are often the most symptomatic, it should be borne in mind that small cavities can result in dramatic symptoms and disability. The following case vignette demonstrates this fact.

A 52-year-old male patient was evaluated for progressive lower-extremity spasticity which had resulted in the loss of ambulation. He had suffered a cervical fracture dislocation more than 20 years earlier, following which he was mildly quadriparetic. Mild gait spasticity had been present but he was able to ambulate and remain working as a rancher.

Approximately one year prior to evaluation, he began to notice bilateral hand pain and numbness. His gait became more spastic in the ensuing months, and he sought evaluation when he had become unable to ambulate without assistive devices. An MRI scan revealed a small syrinx at the cervicothoracic junction, and no other significant cord abnormalities were seen (Figure 1A). A syringosubarachnoid shunt was placed and postoperative imaging demonstrated collapse of the syrinx (Figure 1B). The patient's pain resolved completely and his gait returned to baseline by 3 weeks postoperatively. The sensory loss was unchanged.

At surgery, it is often difficult to define the extent of a syrinx simply by the appearance of the cord. Intraoperative endomyelography (direct instillation of contrast medium into the

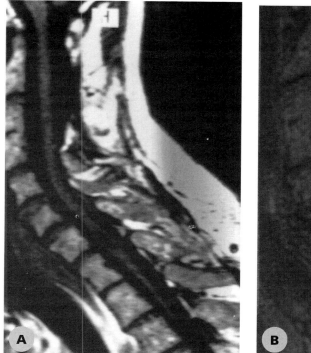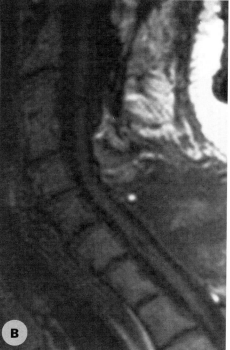

Figure 1: A) T1-weighted MRI demonstrating a small cervicothoracic syrinx in a 52-year-old patient whose symptoms worsened more than 20 years after he suffered a spinal cord injury. The lesion did not enhance when contrast medium was administered. **B)** A study obtained 3 weeks postoperatively demonstrating reduction in the size of the syrinx. The patient made a substantial neurological recovery.

syrinx) can be used if questions exist about possible septations or double cavities.[49] The presence of septations is not a contraindication to the placement of a single catheter into one region of the syrinx. The cavities most often communicate either directly or via the central canal.[2,61] Ultrasound is frequently employed for intraoperative guidance and can be especially helpful to localize small cavities. However, the use of this modality is limited to the extent of the laminectomies.[49]

Surgical Treatment

It is difficult to clearly define the indications for surgical intervention in posttraumatic syrinx patients, since the natural history of the problem varies from spontaneous and complete resolution to devastating neurological defi-

cits.[11,35,52] Surgical treatment is indicated for the patient with documented progression of neurological deficits.[23] Mariani and colleagues[35] reported that a more nearly normal cord size was associated with a benign clinical course in their series of patients treated conservatively. However, if significant cord dilatation was seen, symptoms tended to progress. Therefore, it is probably reasonable to consider surgical intervention in those patients noted to have clear radiographic progression of their syringes even in the absence of symptom progression.

The first reported surgical treatment of syringomyelia involved a syringostomy performed by Abbe and Coley in 1892.[1] Since that time, a host of surgical treatments have been developed. Despite the newer methods and microsurgical techniques, comparison of historical results with those of the microsurgical era shows that success rates are essentially the same.[4] The simplest of the surgical treatments remains the syringostomy. Lysis of dural adhesions can be performed simultaneously and, to ensure free communication of CSF flow, the dura can be left open to create an artificial meningocele. Using syringostomy, Shannon et al[53] noted marked improvement of patients whose predominant symptom was pain. Patients with sensory symptoms were not improved with syringostomy. Problems with the syringostomy method include locating the optimal site for the myelotomy and difficulty keeping the stoma open.[4]

The most commonly used methods at present for posttraumatic syrinx treatment are shunting techniques to drain the syrinx fluid into the subarachnoid space, pleural space, or the peritoneum. The simplest of these methods is syringosubarachnoid shunt placement. In theory, implantation of the shunt catheter helps to prevent closure of the myelotomy. Some authors, however, report less favorable results with this technique than with shunting to other body cavities.[6,42,61]

Since the role of arachnoiditis in the propagation of syrinx cavities is believed to relate to the differentials in CSF pressure created by the adhesions, the broad opening of the dura and creation of a pseudomeningocele has been advocated as a treatment for posttraumatic syringomyelia.[66] This can be done alone or in combination with the placement of a syringopleural shunt. In patients with complete myelopathy, transection of the spinal cord at the distal terminus of the cavity can also be performed, provided, of course, that this is below the level of cord injury.[66]

Perhaps the most popular method for treatment of posttraumatic syrinx at present is the syringoperitoneal shunt. Using this technique, Lesoin et al[28] demonstrated neurological improvement in seven of eight patients with syringes of mixed etiologies. Other authors have likewise reported favorable results with this method, but its complication rate may be higher than for other techniques.[6,42,61] In patients with syringes in the thoracic region, it may be easier to shunt to the thoracic cavity due to the proximity of the pleural space.[47] Syringopleural shunting can be performed with minimal paraspinous muscle dissection and little risk of pneumothorax.[45,47]

The use of thecoperitoneal (lumboperitoneal) shunting has recently been touted as an effective treatment for syringes. However, most of the reported cases of this method involve patients with Chiari malformation and the reported experience in patients with posttraumatic syringes is limited.[62-64] Progressive enlargement of a posttraumatic syrinx after lumboperitoneal shunting has also been reported.[61]

Recent advances in neuroendoscopy have created another attractive alternative for the treatment of syringomyelia. Endoscopic release of arachnoid adhesions, syringotomy, and intrasyringeal septotomy are procedures that may soon allow surgical management of syringomyelia with far less invasive strategies.[4,30]

RESULTS

The combined results of all surgical therapies for syringomyelia demonstrate that improvement can be expected in about 50% of patients and stabilization of progression is seen in an additional 20% to 30%.[4] Patients receiving a syringosubarachnoid shunt may have a somewhat lower rate of deterioration.[4] Reduction in the size of the syrinx appears to be a key factor in neurological improvement.[20,35] Improvement in pain and motor symptoms is common after surgical intervention but sensory improvement is uncommon.[60]

COMPLICATIONS

The complications seen after surgical intervention for posttraumatic syringomyelia are generally straightforward and their management is a matter of routine. Infection, worsening neurological condition, and leakage of CSF are among the common complications. Failure to improve due to myelotomy closure or malfunction of shunt devices may be observed. Other complications of shunts, such as low pressure headaches or formation of subdural fluid collections, may also occur.

REFERENCES

1. Abbe R, Coley WB: Syringomyelia, operation—exploration of cord—withdrawal of fluid—exhibition of patient. **J Nerv Ment Dis 19:**512-520, 1892

2. Adams RD, Salam-Adams M: Chronic nontraumatic diseases of the spinal cord. **Neurol Clin 9:**605-623, 1991

3. Arai S, Ohtsuka Y, Moriya H, et al: Scoliosis associated with syringomyelia. **Spine 18:**1591-1592, 1993

4. Aschoff A, Kunze S: 100 years of syrinx-surgery—a review. **Acta Neurochir 123:**157-159, 1993

5. Backe HA, Betz RR, Mesgarzadeh M, et al: Post-traumatic spinal cord cysts evaluated by magnetic resonance imaging. **Paraplegia 29:**607-612, 1991

6. Barbaro NM, Wilson CB, Gutin PH, et al: Surgical treatment of syringomyelia. Favorable results with syringoperitoneal shunting. **J Neurosurg 61:**531-538, 1984

7. Barnett HJM: The pathogenesis of syringomyelic cavitation associated with arachnoiditis localized to the spinal canal, in Barnett HJM, Foster JB, Hudgson P: **Syringomyelia.** London: WB Saunders, 1973, pp 220-243

8. Barnett HJM: Syringomyelia associated with spinal arachnoiditis, in Barnett HJM, Foster JB, Hudgson P: **Syringomyelia.** London: WB Saunders, 1973, pp 245-259

9. Barnett HJM, Botterell EH, Jousse AT, et al: Progressive myelopathy as a sequel to traumatic paraplegia. **Brain 89:**159-174, 1965

10. Barnett HJM, Fox A, Vinuela F, et al: Delayed metrizamide CT observations in syringomyelia. **Ann Neurol 8:**116, 1980 (Abstract)

11. Birbamer G, Buchberger W, Felber S, et al: Spontaneous collapse of posttraumatic syringomyelia: serial magnetic resonance imaging. **Eur Neurol 33:**378-381, 1993

12. Bleasel A, Clouston P, Dorsch N: Post-traumatic syringomyelia following uncomplicated spinal fracture. **J Neurol Neurosurg Psychiatry 54:**551-553, 1991

13. Bunge MB, Holets VR, Bates ML, et al: Characterization of photochemically induced spinal cord injury in the rat by light and electron microscopy. **Exp Neurol 127:**76-93, 1994

14. Castillo M, Quencer RM, Green BA, et al: Syringomyelia as a consequence of compressive extramedullary lesions: postoperative clinical and radiological manifestations. **AJR 150:**391-396, 1988

15. Cho KH, Iwasaki Y, Imamura H, et al: Experimental model of posttraumatic syringomyelia: the role of adhesive arachnoiditis in syrinx formation. **J Neurosurg 80:**133-139, 1994

16. Cleveland M, Wilson HJ Jr: Charcot disease of the spine. A report of two cases treated by spine fusion. **J Bone Joint Surg (Am) 41:**336-340, 1959

17. Fox JL, Wener L, Drennan DC, et al: Central spinal cord injury: magnetic resonance imaging confirmation and operative considerations. **Neurosurgery 22:**340-347, 1988

18. Freeman LW: Ascending spinal paralysis. Case presentation. **J Neurosurg 16:**120-122, 1959

19. Freeman LW, Wright TW: Experimental observations of concussion and contusion of the spinal cord. **Ann Surg 137:**433-443, 1953

20. Fujii K, Natori Y, Nakagaki H, et al: Management of syringomyelia associated with Chiari malformation: comparative study of syrinx size and symptoms by magnetic resonance imaging. **Surg Neurol 36:**281-285, 1991

21. Gardner WJ, Angel J: The cause of syringomyelia and its surgical treatment. **Cleve Clin Q 25:**4-8, 1958

22. Harrison MJ, Sacher M, Rosenblum BR, et al: Spinal Charcot arthropathy. **Neurosurgery 28:**273-277, 1991

23. Jack CR Jr, Kokmen E, Onofrio BM: Spontaneous decompression of syringomyelia: magnetic resonance imaging findings. Case report. **J Neurosurg 74:**283-286, 1991

24. Johnson JTH: Neuropathic fractures and joint injuries. Pathogenesis and rationale of prevention and treatment. **J Bone Joint Surg (Am) 49:**1-30, 1967

25. Kaden B, Cedzich C, Schultheiss R, et al: Disappearance of syringomyelia following resection of extramedullary lesion. A contribution to the aetiological enigma of syringomyelia. **Acta Neurochir 123:**211-213, 1993

26. Kan S, Fox AJ, Viñuela F: Delayed metrizamide CT enhancement of syringomyelia: postoperative observations. **AJNR 6:**613-616, 1985

27. Kerslake RW, Jaspan T, Worthington BS: Magnetic resonance imaging of spinal trauma. **Br J Radiol 64:**386-402, 1991

28. Lesoin F, Petit H, Thomas CE III, et al: Use of the syringoperitoneal shunt in the treatment of syringomyelia. **Surg Neurol 25:**131-136, 1986

29. Levy R, Rosenblatt S, Russell E: Percutaneous drainage and serial magnetic resonance imaging in the diagnosis of symptomatic posttraumatic syringomyelia: case report and review of the literature. **Neurosurgery 29:**429-33, 1991

30. Lewis AI, Crone KR: Advances in neuroendoscopy. **Contemp Neurosurg 16:**1-6, 1994

31. Loft LM, Ward RF: Hiccups. A case presentation and etiologic review. **Arch Otolaryngol Head Neck Surg 118:**1115-1119, 1992

32. Louthrenoo W, Ostrov BE, Park YS, et al: Pseudoseptic arthritis: an unusual presentation of neuropathic arthropathy. **Ann Rheum Dis 50:**717-721, 1991

33. Lovely TJ, Buchheit WA: Syringomyelia as a postoperative sequela of the resection of a chordoma of the clivus: case report. **Neurosurgery 28:**431-433, 1991

34. Macdonald RL, Findlay JM, Tator CH: Microcystic spinal cord degeneration causing posttraumatic myelopathy. Report of two cases. **J Neurosurg 68:**466-471, 1988

35. Mariani C, Cislaghi MG, Barbieri S, et al: The natural history and results of surgery in 50 cases of syringomyelia. **J Neurol 238:**433-438, 1991

36. McComas CF, Frost JL, Schochet SS Jr: Posttraumatic syringomyelia with paroxysmal episodes of unconsciousness. **Arch Neurol 40:**322-324, 1983

37. Morgan D, Williams B: Syringobulbia: a surgical appraisal. **J Neurol Neurosurg Psychiatry 55:**1132-1141, 1992

38. Morioka T, Kurita-Tashima S, Fujii K, et al: Somatosensory and spinal evoked potentials in patients with cervical syringomyelia. **Neurosurgery 30:**218-222,

1992

39. Morota N, Sakamoto K, Kobayashi N: Traumatic cervical syringomyelia related to birth injury. **Childs Nerv Syst 8**:234-236, 1992

40. Oldfield EH, Muraszko K, Shawker TH, et al: Pathophysiology of syringomyelia associated with Chiari I malformation of the cerebellar tonsils. Implications for diagnosis and treatment. **J Neurosurg 80**:3-15, 1994

41. Olivero WC, Dinh DH: Chiari I malformation with traumatic syringomyelia and spontaneous resolution: case report and literature review. **Neurosurgery 30**:758-760, 1992

42. Phillips TW, Kindt GW: Syringoperitoneal shunt for syringomyelia: a preliminary report. **Surg Neurol 16**: 462-466, 1981

43. Pillay PK, Awad IA, Hahn JF: Gardner's hydrodynamic theory of syringomyelia revisited. **Cleve Clin J Med 59**:373-380, 1992

44. Pillay PK, Awad IA, Little JR, et al: Symptomatic Chiari malformation in adults: a new classification based on magnetic resonance imaging with clinical and prognostic significance. **Neurosurgery 28**: 639-645, 1991

45. Pitts LH: Technique for syringopleural shunting for the treatment of syringomyelia. **Spine 15**:985, 1990 (Letter)

46. Pravda J, Ghelman B, Levine DB: Syringomyelia associated with congenital scoliosis. A case report. **Spine 17**:372-374, 1992

47. Ram Z, Findler G, Tadmor R, et al: Syringopleural shunt for the treatment of syringomyelia. Technical note. **Spine 15**:231-233, 1990

48. Rice-Edwards M: Syringomyelia and the Chiari malformation, in Dudley H, Carter D, Russell RCG, et al (eds): **Rob and Smith's Operative Surgery**. London: Butterworths, 1989, pp 135-145

49. Robertson DP, Narayan RK: Intraoperative endomyelography during syrinx drainage: technical note. **Neurosurgery 30**:246-249, 1992

50. Rossier AB, Werner A, Wildi E, et al: Contribution to the study of late cervical syringomyelia syndromes after dorsal or lumbar traumatic paraplegia. **J Neurol Neurosurg Psychiatry 31**:99-105, 1968

51. Samuelsson L, Lindell D, Kogler H: Spinal cord and brain stem anomalies in scoliosis. MR screening of 26 cases. **Acta Orthop Scand 62**:403-406, 1991

52. Santoro A, Delfini R, Innocenzi G, et al: Spontaneous drainage of syringomyelia. Report of two cases. **J Neurosurg 79**:132-134, 1993

53. Shannon N, Symon L, Logue V, et al: Clinical features, investigation and treatment of post-traumatic syringomyelia. **J Neurol Neurosurg Psychiatry 44**: 35-42, 1981

54. Stevens JM, Olney JS, Kendall BE: Post-traumatic cystic and non-cystic myelopathy. **Neuroradiology 27**:48-56, 1985

55. Sudou K, Tashiro K: Segmental hyperhidrosis in syringomyelia with Chiari malformation. **J Neurol 240**: 75-78, 1993

56. Sze G: MR imaging of the spinal cord: current status and future advances. **AJR 159**:149-159, 1992

57. Tachibana S, Iida H, Yada K: Significance of positive Queckenstedt test in patients with syringomyelia associated with Arnold-Chiari malformations. **J Neurosurg 76**:67-71, 1992

58. Tator CH, Fehlings MG: Review of the secondary injury theory of acute spinal cord trauma with emphasis on vascular mechanisms. **J Neurosurg 75**:15-26, 1991

59. Tumiati B, Casoli P: Syringomyelia in a patient with rheumatoid subluxation of the cervical spine. **J Rheumatol 18**:1403-1405, 1991

60. Umbach I, Heilporn A: Review article: post-spinal cord injury syringomyelia. **Paraplegia 29**:219-221, 1991

61. Van den Bergh R: Pathogenesis and treatment of delayed post-traumatic syringomyelia. **Acta Neurochir 110**:82-86, 1991

62. Vassilouthis J, Papandreou A, Anagnostaras S: Thecoperitoneal shunt for post-traumatic syringomyelia. **J Neurol Neurosurg Psychiatry 57**:755-756, 1994

63. Vassilouthis J, Papandreou A, Anagnostaras S, et al: Thecoperitoneal shunt for syringomyelia: report of three cases. **Neurosurgery 33**:324-327, 1993

64. Vengsarkar US, Panchal VG, Tripathi PD, et al: Percutaneous thecoperitoneal shunt for syringomyelia. Report of three cases. **J Neurosurg 74**:827-831, 1991

65. Williams B: Pathogenesis of syringomyelia. **Acta Neurochir 123**:159-165, 1993

66. Williams B: Post-traumatic syringomyelia: an update. **Paraplegia 28**:296-313, 1990

67. Yamashita Y, Takahashi M, Matsuno Y, et al: Chronic injuries of the spinal cord: assessment with MR imaging. **Radiology 175**:849-854, 1990

CHAPTER 10

Syringomyelia Associated With Intraspinal Neoplasms

Seth M. Zeidman, MD, Paul McCormick, MD, and Richard G. Ellenbogen, MD

In syringomyelia, a longitudinal cavity extends over several levels within the spinal cord. The most common cause of syringomyelia is a structural lesion at the foramen magnum, such as a hindbrain malformation (Chiari I or II). The association of syringomyelia and spinal cord tumors is well established. More accurately, these fluid collections should be termed "tumor-associated cysts" because they lack a true ependymal lining. These terms are used interchangeably in the present discussion. In many cases, patients with intramedullary spinal cord tumors will also present with syringomyelia; only rarely do those with extramedullary spinal cord tumors present with syringomyelia. Additionally, postoperative or postirradiation syringomyelia has been reported in patients with spinal cord tumors. Each of these entities, along with their history, clinical presentation, pathophysiology, and the results of therapy, are discussed.

Posttraumatic syringomyelia was first described by Henry C. Bastian in 1867, and later elaborated upon by Struempel in 1880. Simon, in 1875, was the first to recognize the association of syringomyelia and spinal cord tumors. He speculated that the syrinx was formed by the softening of a glioma. Other authors reported patients with syringomyelia and a simultaneous spinal tumor.[42]

Recently, Samii and Klekamp[41] reviewed 100 intramedullary tumors operated on in 94 patients between 1977 and 1992. Of these, 45% presented with associated syringomyelia. The tumors most often noted in connection with syringomyelia are glial in origin.[5] Ependymoma and hemangioblastoma are more commonly associated with syringomyelia than is astrocytoma.[41] However, syringomyelia can occur with virtually any type of neoplasm.[20] Additionally, there is no apparent difference in histology between spinal cord tumors associated with syringomyelia and those that are not.[5]

Intramedullary spinal cord tumors have an incidence of associated syringomyelia between 25% and 58%.[5] Postmortem studies on patients with syringomyelia show an associated spinal cord neoplasm in 8% to 16% of patients.[5]

The syrinx is more likely to be located above (49%) than below (11%) the tumor level. In 40%, the syrinx extended both above and below the level of the tumor. Regardless of histology, the higher the spinal level, the more likely a syrinx will be encountered.[41]

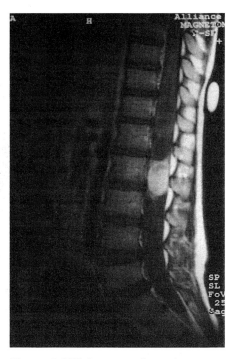

Figure 1: MRI demonstrating syringomyelia in association with an intramedullary ependymoma of the spinal cord.

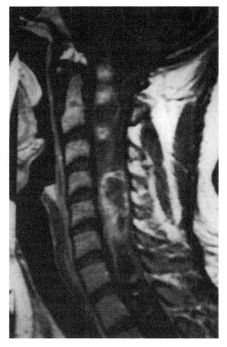

Figure 2: T1-1 weighted gadolinium-enhanced MRI demonstrating syringomyelia found in association with an intramedullary subependymoma. This cyst extended up into the medulla. Intratumoral cysts are present along with a large syrinx (syringobulbia).

PRESENTATION

The presentation in patients with syringomyelia associated with a spinal cord tumor can take many forms and is not unlike that observed with idiopathic or posttraumatic syringomyelia. Two somewhat unusual clinical presentations that should alert the examiner to the possibility of tumor-associated syringomyelia are torticollis and scoliosis.

There are multiple causes of acquired torticollis. It is important to exclude an intramedullary spinal cord tumor with associated syringomyelia in the differential diagnosis of patients with acquired torticollis. Kiwak et al[21] presented three children with syringomyelia and spinal cord tumor in whom torticollis was an early finding.

Scoliosis is another common presentation for patients with spinal cord tumors. Nokes et al[29] examined the spinal cords of 28 scoliosis patients who underwent magnetic resonance imaging (MRI). In 15 patients (54%), neuropathological abnormalities demonstrated by MRI, including spinal cord tumors, significantly affected their clinical course. The advantages of MRI in the evaluation of the scoliotic spine in children include a high sensitivity for the occult conditions associated with scoliosis, good anatomical demonstration of the cord, and an absence of bone artifacts.

GLIAL TUMORS

Low-grade glial tumors frequently have a cystic component (Figures 1 and 2). Despite advances in our understanding of syringomyelia, the pathogenesis of syringomyelia in conjunction with intramedullary tumors remains poorly defined. Multiple pathophysiological mechanisms for the creation of syringes associated with neoplasms have been proposed. Edema,[12] blockage of the perivascular spaces with resultant tissue fluid stasis,[24] cavitation secondary to disordered spinal cord circulation,[39] and spontaneous intratumoral hemorrhage or autolysis have all been postulated as the causal or sustaining entity in syrinx formation.

Numerous authors have documented the association of intramedullary spinal cord tumors and syringomyelia, and all favor classification of the latter lesion as a true neoplastic growth.[5,14,32,34,46] Tumor-associated syringes often contain a yellow, extremely proteinaceous, turbid fluid which likely represents a "neoplastic cyst." In order to more precisely define the mechanism of formation of the tumor-associated syringomyelia, Lohle et al[25] intraoperatively obtained syrinx fluid associated with an intramedullary ependymoma and measured the concentrations of several proteins in the syrinx fluid, the cerebrospinal fluid (CSF), and the blood serum. Protein analysis revealed an exudative character of the fluid.

Those cavities with CSF-like fluid may represent true syringomyelic cavities. An alternative mechanism of formation of the latter may be obstruction of CSF flow created by a mechanism similiar to that observed with obstructive arachnoiditis. This may be the mechanism of syrinx formation observed with extramedullary neoplasms.[50]

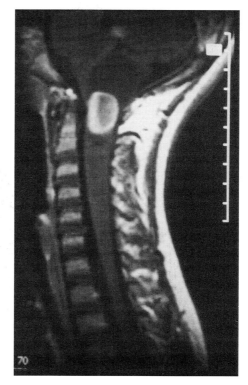

Figure 3: MRI demonstrating syringomyelia in association with a hemangioblastoma of the spinal cord and medulla (syringobulbia). Resection of the tumor resulted in complete resolution of the syrinx.

HEMANGIOBLASTOMA

Hemangioblastomas are the third most common type of intramedullary spinal cord tumor and comprise approximately 3% of primary spinal cord tumors. They occur most often in the cervical or thoracic region and are intramedullary in 60% of cases. Intradural extramedullary and extradural lesions have also been reported. Spinal cord hemangioblastomas usually present as a discrete mass involving the dorsal spinal cord and dorsal roots.

Spinal hemangioblastomas most commonly present as solitary lesions (79%). However, approximately 30% of patients with spinal hemangioblastomas have von Hippel-Lindau syndrome. This syndrome is an autosomal dominant disorder characterized by an inherited susceptibility to various forms of cancer, including hemangioblastomas of the central nervous system and retina, pheochromocytomas, pancreatic tumors, and renal cell carcinoma. More than two-thirds of patients with intramedullary hemangioblastoma have an associated syrinx (Figure 3).

The formation of a syringomyelic cavity or a syrinx with a wall consisting of a fibrillary gliotic layer is thought to occur without dilatation of the central canal or in relation to an ependymal cell lining. Fifty percent of spinal hemangioblastomas are accompanied by cysts near the tumor. Many explanations have been offered for the relationship between these cysts and syringomyelic cavities. One theory hypothesizes that syringomyelic cavities are formed by softening of the spinal cord resulting from damage to the spinal cord or the intramedullary vessels by the tumor. Another theory attaches importance to the secretion or transudation of fluid from the tumor vessels. This latter theory appears to be the most likely, given the high amounts of vascular endothelial growth factor found in the syrinx fluid (Zeidman, unpublished data).

Spinal cord hemangioblastoma is associated with extensive syringomyelia, which can be evaluated by myelography, postmyelographic computed tomography (CT), MRI, and angiography.[18]

Until recently, clinical and conventional radiological techniques were often unable to detect tumor niduses in the wall of a syrinx. During surgical exploration, the tumor was frequently missed, leading to misinterpretation of the pathological entity as syringomyelia, spinal gliosis, or low-grade spinal astrocytoma. Postoperative clinical deterioration was common due to persistent tumor and spinal cord edema. MRI allows the exact preoperative localization of the intramedullary lesion distinct from the accompanying cysts.[49]

MRI can differentiate the various components of these tumors, including the tumor nodule, edema, cysts, and syringomyelia. The tumor nodule is identified as an isointense area surrounded by edema, a cyst, or syringomyelia, or as an area adjacent to a signal void (which represents feeding and draining vessels). Tumor nodules demonstrate intense enhancement following gadolinium administration. Edema appears as an ill-defined region of moderately low signal intensity in T1-weighted images and moderately high signal intensity in T2-weighted images. Cysts and syringes appear as well-defined regions of low signal intensity on T1-weighted images and high signal intensity on T2-weighted images.[16]

Particularly in hemangioblastoma, resection of the tumor nidus results in obliteration of the syrinx without the necessity for additional shunting procedures. Mock et al[28] reported a 2-year-old child with an acute inability to bear weight. Radiological investigation revealed a large cervicothoracolumbar syrinx without apparent etiology. At surgery, a small thoracic spinal cord hemangioblastoma was discovered and excised. Complete recovery with syrinx collapse followed. Wong et al[54] presented a patient

with sleep apnea and a cervicomedullary hemangioblastoma. Syringomyelia resolved following tumor nidus excision.

SYRINGOMYELIA WITH INTRAMEDULLARY METASTASIS

A number of patients with syringomyelia associated with spinal cord tumors have intramedullary metastasis from systemic tumors.[15,23,51] Foster et al[15] reported two cases of syringomyelia associated with intramedullary metastasis. The first case presented with hyperesthesia in the right arm and bilateral pyramidal leg weakness; the second case presented with a partial right-sided Brown-Séquard syndrome with a sensory level at T6. Landan et al[23] reported a patient with syringomyelia involving the entire spinal cord secondary to a spinal intramedullary tumor. CSF cytology and microscopic evaluation of gross necropsy specimens revealed a primary large cell lymphoma.

CAUDA EQUINA LESIONS

Cauda equina tumors rarely produce syringomyelia. When it occurs, it is typically by means of tumor extension to the conus medullaris,[1,8] but occasional cases of noncontiguous lesions have been reported.[47] Chee et al[8] presented a patient with syringomyelia secondary to a cauda equina meningioma involving the conus medullaris. Removal of the tumor with decompression of an adjacent cyst and syrinx resulted in resolution of the symptoms and radiological appearance. Aoki[1] reported an infant with lumbosacral lipoma and a syrinx arising just above the lipoma. Progression of the syrinx was observed in conjunction with rapid growth of the lipoma. Radical excision of the lipoma yielded definite shrinkage of the syrinx. Aoki postulated that syrinx formation resulted from compression by the extramedullary lipoma. Steel et al[47] presented a patient with cauda equina paraganglioma in association with cervicothoracic syringomyelia. Surgical resection of the tumor and syringostomy eradicated the patients' symptoms without residual pathology.

SYRINGOMYELIA WITH A POSTERIOR FOSSA TUMOR

Formation of a syrinx may also occur with posterior fossa tumors (e.g., cerebellar astrocytoma). The mechanism of formation may be comparable to that proposed for communicating syringomyelia. That is, it may result from a displacement of structures in the region of the posterior fossa, with resultant perturbation of CSF dynamics. Resulting syringomyelia is not distinct from typical communicating syringomyelia, but is important to consider because it affects overall prognosis, and overlooking posterior fossa lesion-producing syringomyelia is possible.

In the Midland Centre for Neurosurgery and Neurology database of 545 cases of syringomyelia and related disorders, there were four patients with syringomyelia and hindbrain herniation secondary to posterior fossa tumors. All of these were intrinsic tumors (midbrain gliomas),[53] although the association with meningiomas of the posterior fossa and even supratentorial meningiomas has been reported.[22]

SYRINGOMYELIA WITH A SUPRATENTORIAL LESION

The simultaneous occurrence of syringomyelia and an intracranial tumor has been documented in several studies.[22,53] In the rare case, in which a syrinx exists in the presence of a supratentorial neoplasm, the combined occurrence of these lesions should be considered coincidental.

EXTRAMEDULLARY LESIONS

The association between syringomyelia and extramedullary spinal cord tumors only rarely occurs (Figure 4). Blaylock[6] and Quencer et al[36] have reported cases of the simultaneous presentation of syringomyelia with extramedullary tumors. Barnett and Rewcastle[5] tabulated the published series of extramedullary tumors associated with syringomyelia and identified only seven cases. They suggested that these tumors may have interfered with the blood supply or venous drainage to or from the syringomyelic cavity. Rhyner et al[37] presented a patient with this association documented by MRI. Puca et al[35] reported a patient with an extramedullary spinal neurenteric cyst in association with Klippel-Feil deformity, spinal lipoma, and syringomyelia documented on MRI and myelography.

POSTOPERATIVE AND POSTIRRADIATION SYRINGOMYELIA

Late neurological deterioration after spinal cord surgery mandates evaluation to exclude syrinx formation and/or tumor recurrence. The pathogenesis of spinal cord cavitation after tumor removal and the relationship with therapeutic intervention are poorly defined. Castillo et al[7] reported five cases where postoperative development of syringomyelia was documented after excision of an extramedullary tumor. The effects of chronic spinal cord compression may be accelerated by stresses on the spinal cord and/or spinal cord tethering. Therapeutic techniques include lysis of adhesions and/or shunting procedures. These are most efficacious when performed at or rostral to the level of original tumor removal.[9]

Avrahami and colleagues[3,4] reported the results of MRI in 31 patients with insidious progressive myelopathy 2 to 8 years after cervical spine surgery. Syringomyelia and cystic lesions of the spinal cord were noted in 15 patients operated on for vascular malformations or intramedullary tumors. Seven patients had recurrent tumor and spinal atrophy. Cusick and Bernardi[9] reported two patients with symptomatic noncommunicating syringomyelia after the excision of benign intradural extramedullary neoplasms. Takayasu et al[48] reported a patient presenting with syringomyelia 20 years after surgery for a foramen magnum meningioma.

Although primary intramedullary tumors of the spinal cord with syrinx formation are well documented, there have been few reports of extensive syrinx formation or cystic degeneration due to radiation injury. Saltuari et al[40] reported a young woman with a retroperitoneal neuroblastoma and secondary syringomyelia. The etiology of the syringomyelia was unclear

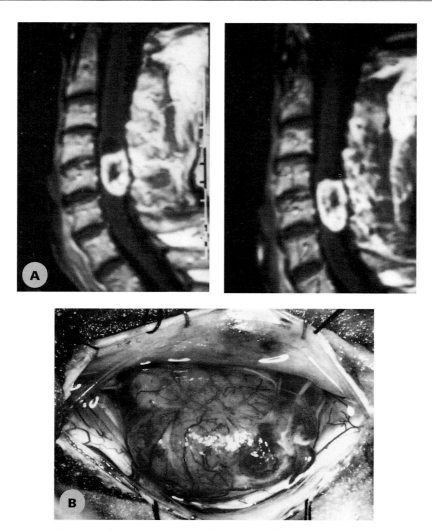

Figure 4: Examples of intradural extramedullary schwannoma in the cervical region. **A)** T1-weighted gadolinium-enhanced sagittal MRI scans of the tumor with syrinx in the suprajacent spinal cord. **B)** Intraoperative photograph of the tumor demonstrating its extramedullary nature. At surgery, an extramedullary tumor (nerve sheath tumor) was identified and completely resected. This demonstrates the occasional occurrence of a tumor arising from an extramedullary tumor.

given the distance between the tumor and the spinal cord. The most likely explanation is that the syringomyelia resulted from arachnoiditis due to postoperative irradiation. Phuphanich et al[33] reported a 49-year-old woman with a 5-year history of astrocytoma grade II of the cervical cord, who developed radiation necrosis and

syrinx formation after surgery and irradiation which progressed to quadriparesis. MRI of the cervical and thoracic spine demonstrated an enlarged cervical cord with diffuse increased signal and gadolinium-enhancing mass, as well as a syrinx from T4 to T10. Autopsy revealed a residual glioma in the upper cervical areas, but the diffuse parenchymal abnormality observed on MRI was radiation necrosis with cyst formation.

IMAGING

There has been a rapid evolution in spinal cord imaging within the past 20 years. The development of such diverse imaging modalities as CT myelography, intraoperative ultrasound, and MRI has dramatically improved the diagnosis and management of syringomyelia associated with neoplasms.

Kan et al[19] examined six patients with syringomyelia associated with intramedullary tumor using myelography and delayed CT. All cases showed syrinx opacification 7 to 24 hours following myelography. Metrizamide passes from the subarachnoid space into the syrinx cavity, emphasizing the role of transneural fluid passage in the origin of such cavities.

Dynamic intraoperative imaging of the spinal cord, using real-time ultrasound, has gained widespread application in the evaluation of tumor-associated syringomyelia. Delineation of the intradural space and spinal cord, including the central canal and the dentate ligaments, is possible prior to dural opening. Anterior and posterior spinal arteries can often be seen. Cavities may be visualized and drained or shunted. Spinal cord cysts or cystic components of tumors can be precisely identified. Intramedullary tumors can be demonstrated sonographically, as can the location and extent of intradural extramedullary tumors and tumors that have both extradural and intradural components.[11]

Intraoperative imaging in patients with syringohydromyelia reveals a smooth, regular, cystic space located symmetrically in the spinal cord. Tumor appears as an echogenic, hypoechoic, or cystic expansile lesion that both narrows the subarachnoid space and obliterates the spinal canal.[17] Guidance for placement of syringosubarachnoid shunts reduces the amount of surgical manipulation.[31] Completeness of tumor removal can be determined, precise locations for biopsy of intramedullary lesions made, periodic motion of the spinal cord detected. This motion is produced by transmitted pulsations from the anterior spinal artery and is most pronounced when the artery is compressed between a mass and the spinal cord. This contradicts the commonly held notion that spinal cord motion implies cord freedom within the thecal sac.[38]

Percutaneous puncture is a relatively safe and efficacious technique for differentiating cystic neoplasms from syringomyelia. Percutaneous puncture permits accurate lesion delineation as well as histological, biochemical, and cytological analyses of the aspirated cystic fluid. This permits improved surgical planning by elucidating tumor location and syrinx dynamics. Additionally, aspiration of cystic tumors decompresses the spinal cord and often brings symptomatic relief to the patient, albeit temporary. Dietemann et al[10] reported four patients who underwent percutaneous aspiration of intramedullary cystic lesions. Mirfakhraee et al[27] modified this technique, incorporating CT myelography.

For demonstrating and delineating the extent of syringomyelia, MRI is superior to CT and myelography. In the detection of intramedullary tumors, MRI is more sensitive than CT and myelography and provides additional information on the extent of the tumor.[13]

To determine the MRI criteria effective for differentiating intramedullary neoplasms from syringo- or hydromyelia, Williams et al[52] reviewed MRI of 33 patients with surgically confirmed cord abnormalities, including nine intramedullary neoplasms and 20 cysts (syringo- or hydromyelia). The combination of distinct margins and uniform signal intensity equal to that of CSF correlated consistently (88%) with spinal cord cysts. Other combinations were less reliable for diagnosing a cyst or tumor.[52]

Slasky et al[45] used gadolinium-enhanced MRI to differentiate between syringomyelia, syringomyelia in association with tumor, and cystic tumor in the spinal cord. Enhancement occurred in all 12 histologically proven cases of tumor and enabled clear demarcation of neoplastic tissue from syrinx or cyst. Eleven of the 12 tumors observed in association with spinal cord cavitation were malignant; all tumors except one (a schwannoma) were intramedullary in location. Enhanced scans were more helpful than unenhanced scans in diagnosing and defining the extent of tumors associated with a syrinx or cyst.[45]

Gadolinium-diethylenetriamine pentacetic acid (Gd-DTPA) improves MRI sensitivity and specificity in the evaluation of spinal lesions. Forty-eight Gd-DTPA-enhanced MRI examinations of the spine were performed in 40 patients referred for imaging because of clinically suspected spinal tumor or for further evaluation of an expanded spinal cord. The study group consisted of 32 patients with spinal tumors (seven ependymomas; seven astrocytomas; four hemangioblastomas; four meningiomas; two arteriovenous malformations; two unidentified intramedullary neoplasms; and single cases of metastatic breast carcinoma, cavernous hemangioma with associated hematomyelia, neurinoma, angiolipoma, drop metastasis from medulloblastoma, and epidermoid with diastematomyelia). In the remaining eight patients, other diagnoses were established: syringomyelia secondary to arachnoiditis (four), thoracic disc herniation (two patients), lumbosacral meningocele (one), and expanded cord secondary to gliotic tissue (one). All but two diagnoses were proved histologically by biopsy, surgery, or autopsy; in the two patients with arteriovenous malformations, the definitive diagnosis was made by spinal angiography. Contrast enhancement occurred in 30 of the 32 spinal tumors, and Gd-DTPA-enhanced T1-weighted images proved helpful to define and outline intra- and extramedullary spinal neoplasms. In all cases, ependymomas and astrocytomas (including low-grade astrocytomas) enhanced. In meningiomas, an immediate and uniform contrast uptake was demonstrated. Gadolinium-enhanced MRI permits differentiation of solid tumor components versus syrinx or cyst or pseudotumoral areas of cord expansion, and the differentiation of residual or recurrent tumor from scar tissue in postoperative patients.[30]

Fifty-eight patients with spinal cord cavities were studied with MRI. Patients were separated into four groups, and the appearance of the cavities were compared. There were 24 patients (41.4%) with communicating syringomyelia (associated with the Chiari I malformation). Sixteen patients (27.6%) had posttraumatic syringomyelia, nine patients (15.5%) had associated tumors, and nine patients (15.5%) had idiopathic syringomyelia. There is a striking similarity in the appearance of many syrinx cavities, regardless of the cause. Characteristics that were found in some patients in every group included areas of increased intensity on T2-weighted images, the presence of CSF flow void in the syrinx cavity, eccentric cavities, beaded cavities, and cord enlargement. Tonsillar ectopia alone does not indicate that a syrinx is of the communicating type, because it was present in two (13%) of 16 patients with trauma and in two (40%) of five patients with tumors. T1-weighted images were most useful in evaluating the anatomical characteristics of the syrinx and the cerebellar tonsils. Most syrinx cavities involved the cervicothoracic junction. The average length was between five and nine vertebral segments but ranged from one to 20 segments. T2-weighted images revealed areas of increased intensity in the spinal cord in 13 patients without tumors. Two of these cases had gliosis on histopathological review. CSF flow voids were present in the syrinx cavities of 23 patients (40%), probably reflecting pulsatile movements of the syrinx fluid.[44]

Schubeus et al[43] reviewed the MRI examinations of 30 patients with idiopathic syringomyelia and 10 patients with cavities associated with intramedullary neoplasms to determine MRI features typical to both groups. All tumor-associated cases resembled idiopathic syringomyelia in some portions of the cavity. At the tumor site, however, tumor-associated cases demonstrated typical findings: the cavities showed abrupt changes in diameter (10/10) and position (8/10), and the surrounding spinal cord demonstrated an uneven thickness (10/10), an increased signal intensity on T2-weighted images (10/10), and pathological contrast enhancement (7/7). Displacement of cerebellar tonsils below the level of the foramen magnum (21/30) and enlargement of the spinal canal (7/29) were characteristic features of idiopathic cases.

Another technique for differentiating syringomyelia from tumor-associated cyst is the application of non-motion compensated imaging. Syrinx cavities of significance show fluid motion and signal loss on the second echo of the T2-weighted image. Tumor cysts do not demonstrate this type of fluid motion. Additionally, tumor-associated cysts often have high signal intensity without motion in contrast to syringomyelic fluid, which exhibits low signal intensity on T2-weighted images with motion.[2]

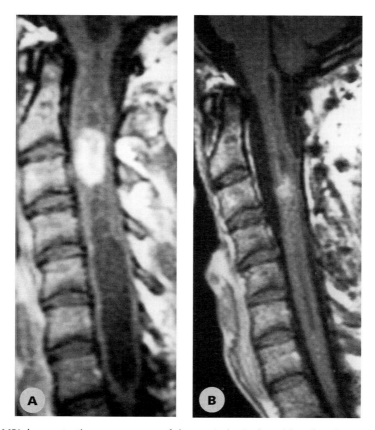

Figure 5: MRI demonstrating astrocytoma of the cervical spinal cord (C2-3) with a tumor-associated syrinx extending into the medulla. **A)** Preoperative scan. There is also an inferior syrinx which extended caudally. There is not an obvious connection between the superior syrinx and the top of the tumor. The tumor can occur at a significant distance from the syrinx. **B)** Sagittal gadolinium-enhanced MRI obtained three years after surgery. Resection of the tumor resulted in complete obliteration of the syrinx without an additional shunting procedure. There is still some residual tumor. This patient did not receive any postoperative radiation therapy and is being followed clinically.

SURGICAL TREATMENT AND RESULTS

Available treatment methods are not consistently successful in alleviating or reversing the clinical symptoms produced by syringomyelia.[55] An incomplete understanding of the underlying patholophysiology has prevented the development of consistently effective treatment methods.[26]

In general, the presence of an associated syrinx favors the resectability of the tumor, because it indicates a displacing rather than an infiltration by tumor. Patients with syringo-myelia and intramedullary spinal cord tumors recovered from surgery sooner than those without associated syringomyelia. However, surgical results and long-term prognosis are not significantly influenced by an associated syrinx. The most important factor determining long-term outcome was the preoperative neurological function.[41]

Often, the use of the syrinx cavity to gain access to the tumor and to facilitate surgical resection is helpful. Removal of the tumor generally results in obliteration of the syrinx without a need for additional shunting procedures (Figure 5). Discovery of a syrinx, particularly in

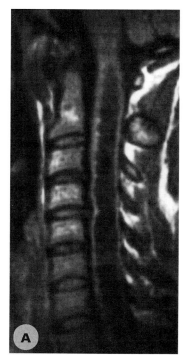
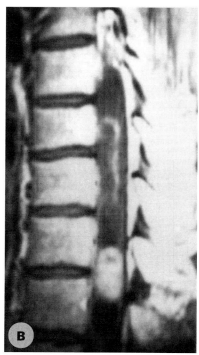

Figure 6: A) T-1-weighted sagittal MRI demonstrating a large syrinx extending throughout the cervical and thoracic spinal cord. There is no obvious hindbrain malformation. Opening into the syrinx revealed yellow proteinaceous fluid. **B)** Subsequent gadolinium-enhanced MRI revealing an intramedullary tumor in the lower thoracic spine. Discovery of a syrinx in the absence of a hindbrain malformation should prompt an aggressive search for an underlying neoplasm.

the absence of a hindbrain anomaly, should prompt a concerted search to exclude a tumor as the etiology (Figure 6).

SUMMARY

Cavitary lesions of the spinal cord have been recognized for centuries; however, only recently have effective, noninvasive imaging techniques allowed antemortem diagnosis. Optimal management of syringomyelia associated with intramedullary and extramedullary spinal cord tumors requires an understanding of the pathogenesis and natural history of these lesions. Improved diagnostic modalities, including MRI and detailed physiological investigations, are helping to elucidate the pathophysiology of syringomyelia. New surgical techniques that directly address the underlying pathophysiological

perturbation are improving management. However, resection of the underlying tumor will typically result in collapse of the syrinx, often without the need for additional shunting procedures.

REFERENCES

1. Aoki N: Syringomyelia secondary to congenital intraspinal lipoma. **Surg Neurol 35:**360-365, 1991
2. Armonda R, Citrin CM, Foley KT, et al: Quantitative cine-mode magnetic resonance imaging of Chiari I malformations: an analysis of cerebrospinal fluid dynamics. **Neurosurgery 35:**214-224, 1994
3. Avrahami E, Herskovitz PI, Cohn DF: Magnetic resonance imaging of syringomelia occurring after operation on spinal intramedullary tumours by Cavitron ultrasonic aspirator. **Br J Radiol 60:**701-702, 1987
4. Avrahami E, Tadmor R, Cohn DF: Magnetic resonance imaging in patients with progressive myelopathy following spinal surgery. **J Neurol Neurosurg Psychiatry 52:**176-181, 1989
3. Barnett HJM, Rewcastle NB: Syringomyelia and tumors of the nervous system, in Barnett HJM, Fos-

ter JB, Hudgson P (eds): **Syringomyelia.** London: WB Saunders, 1973, pp 261-301

6. Blaylock RL: Hydrosyringomyelia of the conus medullaris associated with a thoracic meningioma. Case report. **J Neurosurg** 54:833-835, 1981

7. Castillo M, Quencer RM, Green BA, et al: Syringomyelia as a consequence of compressive extramedullary lesions: postoperative clinical and radiological manifestations. **AJR** 150:391-396, 1988

8. Chee CP, Tan CT, Nuruddin R: Syringomyelia associated with a cauda equina meningioma involving the conus medullaris. **Br J Neurosurg** 4:529-533, 1990

9. Cusick JF, Bernardi R: Syringomyelia after removal of benign spinal extramedullary neoplasms. **Spine** 20:1289-1294, 1995

10. Dietemann JL, Babin G, Wackenheim A, et al: Percutaneous puncture of spinal cysts in the diagnosis and therapy of syringomyelia and cystic tumors. **Neuroradiology** 24:59-63, 1982

11. Dohrmann GJ, Rubin JM: Intraoperative ultrasound imaging of the spinal cord: syringomyelia, cysts, and tumors—a preliminary report. **Surg Neurol** 18: 395-399, 1982

12. Feigin I, Ogata J, Budzilovich G: Syringomyelia: the role of edema in its pathogenesis. **J Neuropathol Exp Neurol** 30:216-232, 1971

13. Fenzl G, Heywang SH, Lissner J, et al: Magnetic resonance imaging compared with computed tomography and myelography in the diagnosis of spinal masses. **Acta Radiol Suppl** 369:257-259, 1986

14. Ferry DJ, Hardman JM, Earle KM: Syringomyelia and intramedullary neoplasms. **Med Ann DC** 38:363-365, 1969

15. Foster O, Crockard HA, Powell MP: Syrinx associated with intramedullary metastasis. **J Neurol Neurosurg Psychiatry** 50:1067-1070, 1987

16. Hoff DJ, Tampieri D, Just N: Imaging of spinal cord hemangioblastomas. **Can Assoc Radiol J** 44:377-383, 1993

17. Hutchins WW, Vogelzang RL, Neiman HL, et al: Differentiation of tumor from syringohydromyelia: intraoperative neurosonography of the spinal cord. **Radiology** 151:171-174, 1984

18. Kaffenberger DA, Shah CP, Murtagh FR, et al: MR imaging of spinal cord hemangioblastoma associated with syringomyelia. **J Comput Assist Tomogr** 12: 495-498, 1988

19. Kan S, Fox AJ, Viñuela F, et al: Delayed CT metrizamide enhancement of syringomyelia secondary to tumor. **AJNR** 4:73-78, 1983

20. Kernohan JW, Woltman HW, Adson AW: Intramedullary tumors of the spinal cord: a review of 51 cases, with an attempt at histologic classification. **Arch Neurol Psychiatry** 25:679-701, 1931

21. Kiwak KJ, Deray MJ, Shields WD: Torticollis in three children with syringomyelia and spinal cord tumor. **Neurology** 33:946-948, 1983

22. Kosary IZ, Braham J, Shaked I, et al: Cervical syringomyelia associated with occipital meningioma. **Neurology** 19:1127-1130, 1969

23. Landan I, Gilroy J, Wolfe DE: Syringomyelia affecting the entire spinal cord secondary to primary spinal intramedullary central nervous system lymphoma. **J Neurol Neurosurg Psychiatry** 50:1533-1535, 1987

24. Liber AF, Lisa JR: Rosenthal fibers in non-neoplastic syringomyelia: a note on the pathogenesis of syringomelia. **J Nerv Ment Dis** 86:549-558, 1937

25. Lohle PNM, Wurzer HAL, Hoogland PH, et al: The pathogenesis of syringomyelia in spinal cord ependymoma. **Clin Neurol Neurosurg** 96:323-326, 1994

26. Madsen PW III, Yezierski RP, Holets VR: Syringomyelia: clinical observations and experimental studies. **J Neurotrauma** 11:241-254, 1994

27. Mirfakhraee M, Benzel EC, Crofford MJ, et al: Combined CT metrizamide syringography and needle aspiration of cystic intramedullary spinal cord lesions. **Spine** 12:214-221, 1987

28. Mock A, Levi A, Drake JM: Spinal hemangioblastoma, syrinx, and hydrocephalus in a two-year-old child. **Neurosurgery** 27:799-802, 1990

29. Nokes SR, Murtagh FR, Jones JD III, et al: Childhood scoliosis: MR imaging. **Radiology** 164:791-797, 1987

30. Parizel PM, Balériaux D, Rodesch G, et al: Gd-DTPA-enhanced MR imaging of spinal tumors. **AJR** 152: 1087-1096, 1989

31. Pasto ME, Rifkin MD, Rubenstein JB, et al: Real-time ultrasonography of the spinal cord: intraoperative and postoperative imaging. **Neuroradiology** 26: 183-187, 1984

32. Peerless SJ, Durward QJ: Management of syringomyelia: a pathophysiological approach. **Clin Neurosurg** 30:531-576, 1983

33. Phuphanich S, Jacobs M, Murtagh FR, et al: MRI of spinal cord radiation necrosis simulating recurrent cervical cord astrocytoma and syringomyelia. **Surg Neurol** 45:362-365, 1996

34. Poser CM: **The Relationship Between Syringomyelia and Neoplasm.** Springfield, Ill: Charles C Thomas, 1956

35. Puca A, Cioni B, Colosimo C, et al: Spinal neurenteric cyst in association with syringomyelia: case report. **Surg Neurol** 37:202-207, 1992

36. Quencer RM, el Gammal T, Cohen G: Syringomyelia associated with intradural extramedullary masses of the spinal canal. **AJNR** 7:143-148, 1986

37. Rhyner PA, Hudgins RJ, Edwards MSB, et al: Magnetic resonance imaging of syringomyelia associated with an extramedullary spinal cord tumor: case report. **Neurosurgery** 21:233-235, 1987

38. Rubin JM, Dohrmann GJ: The spine and spinal cord during neurosurgical operations: real-time ultrasonography. **Radiology** 155:197-200, 1985

39. Russell DS: Capillary hemangioma of spinal cord associated with syringomyelia. **J Pathol Bacteriol** 35:103-112, 1932

40. Saltuari L, Formisano R, Birbamer G, et al: Association of ganglioneuroblastoma with syringomyelia. Case report. **Clin Neurol Neurosurg** 91:139-143, 1989

41. Samii M, Klekamp J: Surgical results of 100 intramedullary tumors in relation to accompanying syringomyelia. **Neurosurgery** 35:865-873, 1994

42. Schlesinger H: **Die Syringomyelie.** Leipzig: Deutiche, 1902

43. Schubeus P, Schörner W, Hosten N, et al: Spinal cord cavities: differential-diagnostic criteria in magnetic resonance imaging. **Eur J Radiol** 12:219-225, 1991

44. Sherman JL, Barkovich AJ, Citrin CM: The MR appearance of syringomyelia: new observations. **AJR** 148:381-391, 1987

45. Slasky BS, Bydder GM, Niendorf HP, et al: MR imaging with gadolinium-DTPA in the differentiation of tumor, syrinx, and cyst of the spinal cord. **J Comput**

Assist Tomogr 11:845-850, 1987

46. Slooff J, Kernohan J, MacCarty C: **Primary Intra-medullary Tumors of the Spinal Cord and Filum Terminale.** Philadelphia, Pa: WB Saunders, 1964

47. Steel TR, Botterill P, Sheehy JP: Paraganglioma of the cauda equina with associated syringomyelia: case report. **Surg Neurol 42:**489-493, 1994

48. Takayasu M, Shibuya M, Kouketsu N, et al: Rapid enlargement of a syringomyelia cavity following syringo-subarachnoid shunt: case report. **Surg Neurol 45:** 366-369, 1996

49. Trost HA, Seifert V, Stolke D: Advances in diagnosis and treatment of spinal hemangioblastomas. **Neurosurg Rev 16:**205-209, 1993

50. Vinters H: Neuropathology of syringomyelia, in Batzdorf U (ed): **Syringomyelia: Current Concepts in Diagnosis and Treatment.** Baltimore, Md:

Williams & Wilkins, 1991, pp 35-58

51. Weitzner S: Coexistent intramedullary metastasis and syringomyelia of cervical spinal cord. Report of a case. **Neurology 19:**674-678, 1969

52. Williams AL, Haughton VM, Pojunas KW, et al: Differentiation of intramedullary neoplasms and cysts by MR. **AJR 149:**159-164, 1987

53. Williams B, Timperley WR: Three cases of communicating syringomyelia secondary to midbrain gliomas. **J Neurol Neurosurg Psychiatry 40:**80-88, 1977

54. Wong CW, Wai YY, Lui TN, et al: Bilateral glossopharyngeal neuralgia after excision of a solitary cervicomedullary haemangioblastoma: case report. **Acta Neurochir 114:**64-67, 1992

55. Zeidman SM, North RB, Ducker TB: Syringomyelia, in Johnson RT, Griffs JN (eds): **Current Therapy in Neurology and Disease.** 4th ed. Philadelphia, Pa: BC Decker, 1993

CHAPTER 11

Management Schemes for Syringomyelia: Surgical Indications and Nonsurgical Management

Bernard Williams, MD, ChM, FRCS

Definitions

Syringomyelia

The term "syringomyelia" indicates the presence of longitudinally disposed tubular cavities within the spinal cord, usually of greater than two or three segments in length. The cavity contains fluid that is either cerebrospinal fluid (CSF) or indistinguishable from CSF.

Syringobulbia

Neurologists use the term "syringobulbia" to indicate bulbar features.[20,31,47,56,60] These include hindbrain hernia headache as perhaps the most significant manifestation.[47,60] Other features may be related to cranial nerves or to diffuse signs of bulbar dysfunction. Cranial nerves are not necessarily involved; related features include paralysis of eye movement, double vision, and numbness and tingling of the face. Syringobulbia may also be associated with atypical facial pain, tinnitus, deafness, palatal dysfunction, sometimes with fluid coming down the nose, swallowing difficulty, voice problems often associated with unilateral palsy of the larynx and wasting of the tongue, and disturbance of taste or anisocoria. Inequalities of the palpebral fissures are less commonly seen. Diffuse bulbar dysfunction is indicated by nystagmus, oscillop-

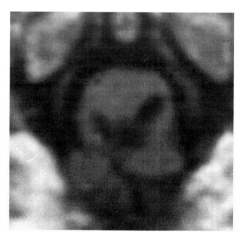

Figure 1: Syringobulbia due to clefts running out of the fourth ventricle. Patients of this class require correction of hydrocephalus as well as a careful craniovertebral decompression and opening up of the normal outflow tracks of the fourth ventricle, if possible.

sia, syncopal attacks, drop attacks, and occasionally apneic attacks, which may cause sudden death.[20]

A neuropathologist is likely to regard syringobulbia as the development of fourth ventricular clefts which run out as splits from the bottom part of the floor of the fourth ventricle (Figure 1). For either of the above definitions of

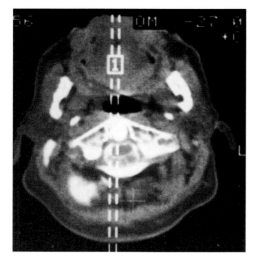
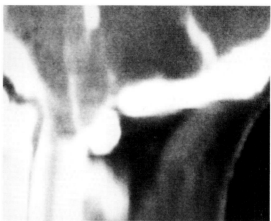

Figure 2: Postmyelography computed tomography scans of a patient with hydrocephalus and a pouch in the cerebellum. The filling mechanism of a pouch such as this is usually that CSF is forced into the pouch by upward movement and then the hindbrain closes over the mouth of the pouch. In this instance, moderate hydrocephalus was associated with this patient and, under these circumstances, a direct attack on the tonsils may correct the hydrocephalus as occurred here.

syringobulbia, syringomyelia is not necessary; they are both manifestations of hindbrain herniation.

Ascending syringomyelia is not infrequently seen, particularly when syringomyelia is not hindbrain related. If the patient has a hindbrain hernia, for example, the tonsils pressing against the upper part of the cord frequently seem to prevent the split in the cord from tracking further upward. An alternative explanation might be that the presence of the tonsillar tips there actually causes the syringomyelia to develop slightly further down. Patients with hindbrain-related syringomyelia may sometimes have the ascending form of syringobulbia. If an ascending syrinx joins clefts in the floor of the fourth ventricle, then this may be a variety of communication between the syrinx and the floor of the fourth ventricle.

Arnold-Chiari Deformity

The term "Arnold-Chiari deformity" is used by the *Index Medicus*. It is not a good description but is better than "Arnold-Chiari malformation." This deformation is not a malformation. It was not described well by Arnold nor

was it first described by Arnold, and if it is to be eponymously named, then "Cleland deformity" would have been preferable. Chiari's division into type I, which includes the herniation associated with development at birth or in later life, is relevant and his type II, which describes the prenatal deformity usually associated with spina bifida, may be justifiable.[9] They are both, however, herniations of the partially developed hindbrain and they differ only in degree; they are caused by pressure differences acting across the foramen magnum. The grotesque nature of the type II malformation is induced by low pressure in the spine, consequent upon the spina bifida, and leads to severe overfolding of the medulla and upper spinal cord, maldevelopment of the vermis, enlargement of the foramen magnum, and so on.[58] The more mature type of deformity is not as clearly distinguished from type II as is sometimes supposed; for example, medullary deformity is not uncommon. This author much prefers the term "hindbrain herniation" to describe all varieties of such deformity, and recommends retention of types I and II.

Hindbrain herniation appears to cause not only hydrocephalus and syringomyelia but also pouches containing CSF within the posterior fossa (Figures 2 and 3).

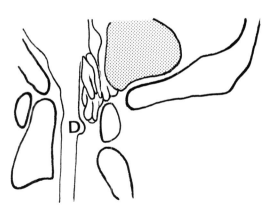

Figure 3: Drawing depicting Figure 2 *right*. The position of the pouch is marked as a speckled area. D = the deformation of the medulla.

Meningeal Fibrosis

Meningeal fibrosis, or abnormal collagenosis of the meninges, is found in many conditions. In conjunction with hindbrain-related syringomyelia, it is found around the foramen magnum and is most commonly due to birth injury.[6,57] Non-neonatal head injuries are also a known cause, as are inflammatory processes such as tuberculous meningitis.[1] Lower down the spine, meningeal fibrosis is most commonly found in relation to spinal injuries.[4,11,14,20,23,43,59,62] After this, the commonest cause is idiopathic followed by reaction to Myodil or Pantopaque, tuberculous meningitis, epidural abscess, Pott's disease, and occasionally other causes such as operation for tumor or disc disease.[4,14,23,59,62] Idiopathic meningeal fibrosis is a well-known cause of syringomyelia, but it is unclear what the mechanisms are.

The usual term used to describe collagenosis involving the dura and the arachnoid and the pia is "arachnoiditis."[1] This is an unfortunate term because more than the arachnoid is involved. Additionally, "arachnoiditis" implies an active inflammatory process, whereas what the surgeon sees is the result of tissue reaction rather than an active inflammatory process. The term "arachnoiditis" therefore has much to condemn it and should be abandoned.

CLASSIFICATION OF SYRINGOMYELIA

The major divisions of syringomyelia may be determined by the associated lesions. These are, of course, likely to be causes of the syringomyelia, but are not necessarily so. The principal separation is between "hindbrain-related" syringomyelia and what may be called either "primarily spinal" syringomyelia or "nonhindbrain-related" syringomyelia. The approximate numbers encountered in a practice expressing an interest in patients with syringomyelia are given in Table 1. Obviously, the interrelationship with some associated conditions (e.g., spina bifida) is complex.[21,22,33] Likewise, hydrocephalus may be regarded as causative of syringomyelia, particularly when there is a wide communication from the floor of the fourth ventricle linking the hydrocephalus to the inside of the syrinx, but conversely it is reasonable to regard it as additional evidence of disease of the CSF pathways. The entire symptom complex may be due to some other disorder (e.g., previous head injury or meningitis). Idiopathic syringomyelia is extremely uncommon and, when it occurs, it is not infrequently associated with idiopathic meningeal fibrosis.

Skull deformities such as may be found with rickets, Paget's disease, acro-osteolysis, or varieties of fragilitas osseum (osteogenesis imperfecta) provide management problems whether or not associated with syringomyelia.[6,7,13,21,28,32,33,40,45] In these conditions, the odontoid peg frequently becomes displaced backward, as well as basilar invagination occurring.[46]

A degree of basilar invagination may be on occasion related to birth injury.[6] Family traits are also sometimes found with basilar invagination, although the mechanisms involving genetic bone disorder are not well understood.

CLINICAL PRESENTATION

Hindbrain Herniation Alone

The assessment of patients with hindbrain-related syringomyelia involves deciding whether it is the hindbrain herniation that is symptomatic or whether it is the cord lesion. A proportion of patients with hindbrain herniation do

TABLE 1

CLASSIFICATION ACCORDING TO ASSOCIATED CONDITIONS*

Hindbrain-related syringomyelia	72%
Hindbrain herniation	
Idiopathic herniation (Chiari I)	32%
Secondary to birth injury	39%
Secondary to tumors	1-2%
Bony or meningeal tumors of the posterior fossa	<1%
Tumors forming the hindbrain hernia	<1%
Intrinsic brain tumors above the lower 4th venticle	<1%
Secondary to bony abnormality	
Basilar invagination (idiopathic or birth injury)	10%
Sclerostenosis	<1%
Rickets	<1%
Acro-osteolysis	<1%
Osteogenesis imperfecta	<1%
Associated with hydrocephalus	10%
Intracranial arachnoid pouches	2%
Dandy-Walker cysts	<1%
Early onset hydrocephalus (aqueductal stenosis)	<1%
Meningeal fibrosis of cisterna magna	
Birth-injury related	9%
Postinflammatory	<1%
Posttraumatic (postnatal)	1%
Infections	<1%
Nonhindbrain-related syringomyelia	22%
Spinal tumors	1%
Intramedullary	1%
Cysts wholly or partly within the tumor	
Cysts outside the tumor extending in the cord	
Extramedullary intradural tumors	<1%
Extradural tumors, including disc disease	<1%
Meningeal fibrosis	
Idiopathic	1%
Postinflammatory	<1%
Pyogenic meningitis	<1%
Epidural abscess	<1%
Tuberculous meningitis	<1%
Myodil (Pantopaque)	1%
Posttraumatic	13%
Secondary to spinal bony deformities	
Posttraumatic	11%
Tuberculous bone disease	<1%
Idiopathic scoliosis	<1%
Dysraphic lesions	
With hydrocephalus	2%
With hindbrain hernia	1%
With both the above	4%
With neither of the above	7%
Unknown cause (no associated conditions)	<1%

*The percentages are from a database of syringomyelia and related diseases and do not add up to 100% because of overlapping (e.g., post-traumatic syringomyelia is associated with meningeal fibrosis and bony deformity). Some factors such as head injury are difficult to interpret. Others such as hydrocephalus, spina bifida occulta, or basilar impression are matters of degree.

not have syringomyelia and this group of patients, therefore, presents with the features of syringobulbia.[31,47,49]

Hindbrain hernia headache is characteristic and should be carefully sought during the examination. Many patients do not seem to notice that they have headache in relation to straining, coughing, or sneezing and it is useful to ask them to blow into a sphygmomanometer. If patients are asked to blow to a pressure of 40 mm of mercury for five seconds, characteristic intensification of the pain may occur with symptomatic hindbrain herniation. Sometimes the pain comes on at the moment of blowing, suggesting that craniospinal pressure dissociation has its onset at that time. Rather more frequently, the pain intensifies at the end of blowing, suggesting that a post Valsalva rebound has a part to play.

It may not occur to patients to complain of some features that they do not connect with the main symptom pattern. This is particularly true of breathing difficulties while asleep. Deafness and tinnitus often have to be specifically inquired about. Audiometry commonly shows a high tone loss which, if present, is objective evidence of symptomatic hindbrain herniation but may not be reported by the patient.

Nystagmus is difficult to attribute. It is difficult to localize it anatomically, but when it has a strong vertical element, often with rotation, nystagmus is good evidence of compression of the hindbrain.[20,31] Double vision is a presentation that often does not lead to diagnosis, and some patients degenerate to severely disabled status because of failure to appreciate the clinical significance of the onset of double vision in childhood or early adult life. It is rarely due to a nerve palsy and seems, as the nystagmus is, predicated by central disorders involving structures related to the medial longitudinal bundle.

Syringomyelia Without Hindbrain Herniation

Syringomyelia without hindbrain herniation illustrates aspects which may be attributable to the cord cavity alone. This includes the characteristic sensory loss, which is usually unilateral and in the hindbrain-related varieties commonly affects one forequarter.[20] The sensory disturbances are often difficult to analyze. They vary from day to day, sometimes depending on the patient's activity. Although well known, the dissociated sensory loss (such as when a patient sustains burns) is not the only sensory change. The other modalities are commonly affected.[24]

Kyphoscoliosis, which frequently affects the vertebral column at the time of the growth spurt or even before, is often present before any other features suggest syringomyelia.[22] Kyphoscoliosis may be present without syringomyelia in the presence of hindbrain herniation but this is uncommon and it is usually the case that the cord cavity appears to be the cause of the deformity of the thoracic spine. It has to be noted that the side and the level have no correlation with the side or the level of the syrinx.

Sweating disturbance and anisocoria are both sometimes found with hindbrain-related syringomyelia, but they seem to be proportionately more common in primarily spinal syringomyelia associated with meningeal fibrosis.[59]

Motor features include, of course, the lower motor neuron involvement of the upper limbs and upper motor neuron involvement of the lower limbs. Spasticity of the arms is not infrequently found with syringomyelia, but the assumption is that this is probably due to compression of the brain stem and the long tracts at the level of the hindbrain. Spasticity of the upper limbs in someone with syringomyelia secondary to a spinal fracture is almost unknown. Under these circumstances, fasciculation, weakness, and wasting with early loss of the tendon reflexes are characteristic.[20] Spasticity of the lower limbs was the commonest neurological finding reported by Barnett, Foster, and Hudgson and the patients often have nothing more striking than a complaint of gait difficulty which, because of the diffuse motor and sensory changes, may be difficult to analyze.[20]

Clinical history suggesting the slosh mechanism is often valuable in determining when a syrinx is being symptomatic. If the patient has pain in or below the neck related to coughing or sneezing, it seems likely that this is due to surging of fluid within the syrinx cavity inflicting damage by distending the cavity. This may not only produce pain but also alteration in sensitivity and, for instance, sometimes weakness in response to exertion.

Hydrocephalus Associated With Syringomyelia

The hydrocephalus which is associated with syringomyelia may of itself be symptomatic. Headaches, therefore, may not only be related to straining through impaction of the hindbrain but may also be related to raised intracranial pressure. Likewise, bladder dysfunction may be due to cord damage or may be associated with hydrocephalus. Gait difficulty is one of the characteristic features of symptomatic hydrocephalus; given the difficulties in ascribing such gait difficulties to a cord lesion, the possibility that there may be a contribution from hydrocephalus may need to be borne in mind. Hydrocephalus does not need to be symptomatic to justify being treated first.

DETERMINING WHICH OPERATION

Concepts of pathogenesis of hindbrain herniation and syringomyelia abound[2,6,9,21,26,28-30,48,49,56,58-63] and every surgeon needs to have some sort of intellectual basis for his/her actions. In this area, however, some of the earlier concepts, notably those of Gardner,[21,28] have been useful although clearly flawed.

There are many operations available for syringomyelia and many technical variations. Overwhelmingly, the most useful operation for hindbrain-related syringomyelia and symptomatic hindbrain herniation is craniovertebral decompression.[7,8,12,13,31,33,39,42,51,52,55,56,59-63] This operation is not easy and is best done by a surgeon who has experience with the technique.

Hydrocephalus Operations

Hydrocephalus is not an "all or nothing" phenomenon; some degree of ventriculomegaly is not uncommon, and around 30% of patients with hindbrain-related syringomyelia have ventricles that a radiologist would consider to be enlarged.[54] Only about 3% of patients have severe hydrocephalus and, of this group, patients with overtly high pressure and papilledema are a tiny proportion, constituting less than 1% of patients attending the Syringomyelia Clinic. When the hydrocephalus is sizable, it is recommended that this disorder be treated first.

The author favors Medos adjustable valves for patients with severe hydrocephalus and for those in whom CSF drainage is chosen as a treatment for syringomyelia. Gross enlargement of the ventricles in adults is likely to be complicated by subdural collections, and the adjustable valve may help in dealing with this situation.

When the presence of hydrocephalus is questionable, the surgeon may perform a craniovertebral decompression procedure in the belief that correcting this aspect of the CSF pathways disorder will resolve the hydrocephalus. This may indeed occur, but it is unwise to hope for this since hydrocephalus may become exacerbated following the hindbrain hernia operation. The author tends to shunt the hydrocephalus first, even when it is not symptomatic and not especially large. There may be other indications to favor hydrocephalus operation, for example, the history of a difficult birth. Such patients are likely to be associated with hindbrain meningeal fibrosis, which makes the hindbrain operation more difficult.

Enlargement of the fourth ventricle and the presence of fourth ventricular clefts also may be a relative indication for ventricular shunting. Communication between the floor of the fourth ventricle and syringomyelia might also be thought to favor hydrocephalic shunting (Figure 4). This is common in patients with spina bifida. In patients with a previously placed shunt, possibly done many years before, and in whom it is uncertain whether this shunt is working, then a shunt revision may often produce a pleasing improvement in syringomyelia symptoms as well as helping hydrocephalic features. There is no proof that patients with communicating hydrocephalus do better following a shunt placement than others, but it seems a reasonable additional indication for favoring ventricular shunting.

Lowering pressure by shunting CSF from the spinal subarachnoid space to the peritoneum may control syringomyelia.[25,37] Lumboperitoneal shunting may, however, cause hindbrain impaction.[10,17,53] Any degree of hindbrain herniation is therefore a contraindication and any case treated in this way demands vigilance.

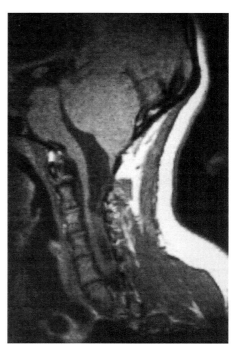

Figure 4: MRI of a patient with spina bifida with severe hydrocephalus and communicating syringomyelia. This patient did well after ventricular shunting. There is no value in operating on the hindbrain directly. In this case, the fluid is the problem, not the tissues around it. The fluid might be regarded as being internally decompressed once the overall CSF pressure has been lowered.

The idea of lowering the overall CSF pressure in the treatment of syringomyelia without hydrocephalus has a varied history.[25,26,37] It is possible to improve syringomyelia in this way. As a treatment, however, it is not universally successful and paradoxical results can sometimes occur such that a syringomyelia worsens after shunting hydrocephalus. It is, therefore, not reasonable to rely upon this method of treatment and vigilance is required, including repeat magnetic resonance imaging (MRI) scans to assess syrinx size.

Craniovertebral Decompression

Descriptions of the position, exposure, dural opening, dealing with the arachnoid, and dealing with the tonsils are dealt with elsewhere in this book.

Syrinx Drains

On seeing a lesion such as syringomyelia, it might be thought a natural temptation to a surgeon to insert a drain into it.[2,4,14,21,23,36,51] On being faced with a domestic flood, however, no neurosurgeon would send for a plumber to put a drain into his carpet. Better to find out where the water is coming from and to prevent its arrival. If this is dealt with, then the situation may be salvaged. The carpet may be somewhat damaged but it will not be as badly damaged as it would have been had a drain been added to the other problems from which it has suffered. Similarly, with the spinal cord, it is not possible to perform a myelotomy without causing some damage to the cord; in addition, the CSF will still accumulate if the factors leading to the cord's filling are undisturbed. The domestic analogy is strained because it is difficult to work out how the fluid is being forced into the spinal cord. It seems clear that it has to do with the local anatomy. In the most straightforward analysis, local anatomy is almost always an obstruction in the subarachnoid space. This is the case whether that obstruction is due to hindbrain herniation or meningeal fibrosis at the hindbrain or to a zone of meningeal fibrosis lower down the spine.

In addition to that common-sense observation for subarachnoid shunts, if the drain is inserted in relation to local anatomical features which are causing fluid to ingress, then the fluid may be able to enter the cord readily through the drain.

There are two basic forms of syrinx drainage which may be employed. One is to open the syrinx to the subarachnoid pathways; this includes the simplest kind of operation, which is a myelotomy.[2,4,14,23,36,51,61-63] The commonest modification is to put some sort of drain in the hole in the syrinx wall, or something else that will keep it open such as a wick or a nerve root. The other is to drain the syrinx to a site outside the neuraxis, such as the pleural or peritoneal cavities.[62] The pleura is, in general, a more useful cavity than the peritoneum, as it is easily opened with the patient in the same position as for an exposure of the cord. The pressure in the pleural cavity is satisfactorily low, and there is no potentially obstructing omentum in the pleural cavity

which may help to keep it patent.[4,62] The drain should not, of course, be allowed to drain all the CSF from the neuraxis. The pleura would not be able to absorb this quantity of fluid and the patient may suffer from low intracranial pressure. If the purpose of drainage is to lower overall CSF pressure, such as for example in the presence of hydrocephalus, then the peritoneum should be chosen.[4]

Syringosubarachnoid Shunting

Procedures for syringosubarachnoid shunting include the oldest operations for syringomyelia and they are still spoken of with respect by some practitioners.[2,36,63] There seems to be little doubt that they sometimes work and may continue to work for a long period. Presumably in these circumstances, they are sited at an area where the natural tendency of the fluid is to escape and by aiding this process and utilizing the natural elasticity of the walls of the cord, a period of deflation enables the cavities to heal. Under these circumstances, it may be that the filling mechanisms have previously spontaneously resolved or been disturbed by surgery. The size of the syrinx may have contributed to the obstruction. It may be that when the syrinx reaches a certain size, it is more energy efficient for the body to transmit pulsation within the syrinx rather than outside it. Under these circumstances, the second law of thermodynamics may be better satisfied, for a section of the spinal canal with syringomyelia in it, by having fluid move within the syrinx rather than on the outside. If the syrinx can be made flat and the anatomy in some other part of the spine has been dealt with, then it is possible that the drain may assist everything to resolve.

In cases where the syringomyelia goes as far as the conus, one neat variety of myelotomy is to cut off the bottom of the cord. This operation was favored by Gardner in his latter years. He claimed that syringomyelia would communicate with the conus through the central canal. MRI studies suggest that this is not the case but, nevertheless, the cavity not infrequently does go to the bottom of the cord. Under those circumstances cutting off the conus and a short length of filum, "terminal ventriculostomy" as Gardner called it, may help a syrinx to deflate.[38,61] This may equalize pressure between syringomyelia above a block and that below. It is not a physiologically appealing method of equalizing these pressures, however, because it involves using the cord as a permanent conduit for fluid, which is a function for which it was not designed and from which the surgeon should be trying to protect it.

Lapras has suggested that, in cases where the MRI scan shows a syrinx extending down to the tip of the conus, this might be a reasonable adjunct to surgery directed against the cause of the disorder.[63]

Syrinx to Extrathecal Shunting

When syrinx to extrathecal shunting is instituted, it should not be hampered by the use of a hydrocephalus shunt valve. Such a valve is designed to keep the pressure in the normal range and since the majority of syringomyelia patients have a normal overall CSF pressure, the valve may prevent the drain from working.

One objection to this form of drainage is that it is too efficient. If the drain is allowed to run freely it will produce energetic flattening of the cord. This imposes an immediate stress on the cord, as illustrated in Figures 5 and 6. It is not uncommon for neurological symptoms to first manifest at a separate level from the myelotomy, and this factor has led Lapras to suggest that syringosubarachnoid shunting may be less injurious to the cord.[57] Of greater significance is the observation that when the syrinx collapses energetically around a drain, it necessarily blocks it.[43] The glial tissues will grow into the drain wherever the fluid has been able to ingress and if the syrinx mechanisms remain intact the syrinx will then re-form and excavate its way in a new plane past the gliosis. This will form a syrinx often just as severe as the previous one, sometimes affecting the opposite side, and it leaves the drain uselessly immured in the wall of the cavity.

Having said this, the proponents of syringoperitoneal and syringopleural drains report their findings with varying degrees of enthusiasm. References dealing with the negative aspects of drains are less common.[16,51] The results of syrinx drainage have been collected and reviewed by Sgouros and Williams.[43]

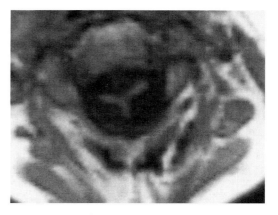

Figure 5: MRI of a patient with the slit cord syndrome. This patient underwent a regular hindbrain hernia decompression procedure but remained symptomatic with a full syrinx. After syringoperitoneal shunting, the cord is excessively flattened.

Odontoid Peg Resection

A proportion of patients with severe skull base deformities will have syringomyelia. These include dysmorphic patients such as those with genetic forms of basilar impression, hypoplasia of the condyles, os odontoideum, and hypoplasia of the dens. There are also secondary varieties of basilar invagination due to Paget's disease, rickets, achondroplasia, Morquio's syndrome, osteogenesis imperfecta, acro-osteolysis, and so on which may frequently be complicated by syringomyelia. In most of these patients the syringomyelia is relatively unimportant, but in some it constitutes the presenting symptom. The clinical considerations are often not primarily those of CSF dynamics and the first consideration is for stability of the craniocervical junction and correction of the neural compression.[7,33,46]

Often the main compression is plainly coming from ventral to the medulla, and under these circumstances transpharyngeal removal of the odontoid peg is a reasonable strategy. If the compression is equal from the front and from the back, then an approach from behind is often easier and gives a better decompression. It is also easier to provide stability with a posterior approach. The author agrees with Lapras that a Cone fusion with a block of bone placed between the superior articulation of the axis and the lateral mass of the atlas is often useful and has a particular advantage in not placing metal

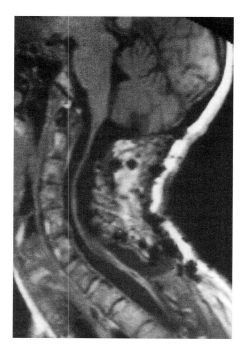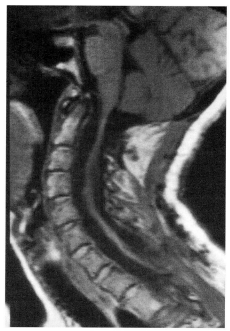

Figure 6: MRI of the same patient as Figure 5. Laminectomy of C5-7 had been performed and a drain taken to the left pleural cavity. The drain (*left*) can be seen and the severe collapse of the cord is visible (also seen in Figure 8). Observe the good hindbrain result in this case, with a generous cisterna magna rounding off of the tonsils and opening up of the outlet of the fourth ventricle. It is not clear why the syrinx did not respond. Unfortunately, this result is not rare. It is possible that either a ventriculoperitoneal shunt to lower the overall pressure or a syrinx-to-subarachnoid shunt would have helped this patient. She did not have a terminal ventriculostomy because two syringes were not in certain communication. The lower syrinx, however, went flat after the upper one was drained.

where subsequent imaging is important. Distracting the skull above the arch of C1 may also assist in lessening the odontoid pressure.

Another important consideration when approaching a patient with a moderate degree of odontoid backward displacement and either tight hindbrain herniation or syringomyelia is that the posterior approach allows a much greater decompression of the CSF spaces. Both syringomyelia and symptomatic hindbrain compression are CSF pressure-related disorders. For these reasons, the author has no experience of odontoid peg resection in cases of syringomyelia (Figures 7 to 9).

COMPLICATIONS FOLLOWING SURGERY

Persistence of the Syrinx

The most irritating complication encountered is persistence of the syrinx. Following surgery, the syrinx rarely disappears; rather, in the majority of cases, it becomes concave in some part, indicating a satisfactory collapse. The patients in whom the syrinx remains substantially full may show good clinical improvement. Under these circumstances, it would seem unwise to attempt further surgery unless there

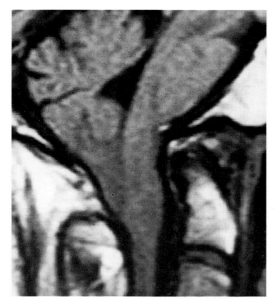

Figure 7: MRI demonstrating symptomatic hindbrain herniation with a prominent odontoid peg. The suggestion had been made that this odontoid peg should be removed, but it seems clear that greater correction of the CSF abnormality can be attained by a posterior decompression procedure.

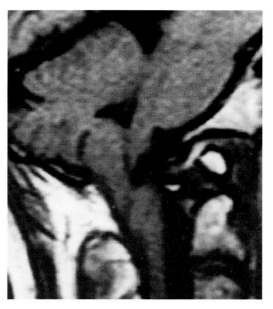

Figure 8: MRI of the same patient as Figure 7. Observe the severe impression made by the vertebral artery on a cut a little to one side of the midline. Vascular impression of this kind is not likely to be corrected by removal of the odontoid peg.

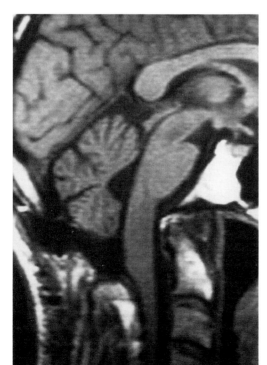

Figure 9: MRI of the same patient as Figure 7. Observe that the decompression from behind has allowed the tonsils to reshape themselves. The midline outflow track of the fourth ventricle has opened up; there is a neat artificial cisterna magna and the patient's symptoms were markedly improved. The arteries were not sutured laterally. Observe that the odontoid peg now appears relatively harmless.

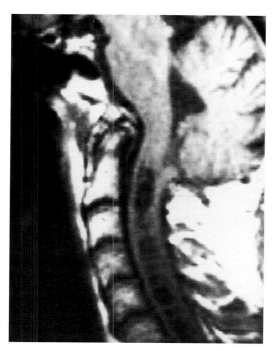

Figure 10: MRI of a patient with a prominent odontoid peg, pronounced basilar invagination, and failure to provide an artificial cisterna magna. The bottom end of the skull had been markedly inverted and it was difficult to gain a clear passageway. The cerebellum has slumped into this space. The fourth ventricle and the syrinx remain prominent and did not respond to ventricular shunting. This woman is overweight and had a complicated response to the first operation, requiring the shunt and tracheostomy. An attack upon this odontoid peg may be justifiable, but she is currently neurologically stable and is being observed with some apprehension.

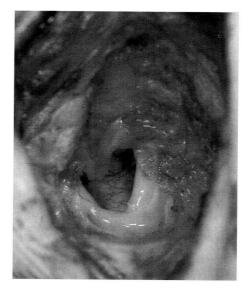

Figure 11: Operative photograph of re-exploration after inadequate craniovertebral decompression. A graft had been placed, leaving a small hole. Note the smooth surface of tissues left in contact with the CSF. A good artificial cisterna magna was present but was cut off from free access to the CSF pathways by this graft. The hole has been dissected and enlarged, turning a small flap of the graft upward.

is something that invites surgical attention, such as hydrocephalus or persistence of the central canal to the conus.

A number of patients will show no clinical improvement and a persistently full syrinx. The most frequent cause of this is the manner in which the operation was done (Figure 10). This most frequently relates to technical considerations at the time of the operation. The commonest failing is to not address the tonsils. The tonsils may at times appear as they did before operation and before the dura has been reconstituted (sometimes with a graft), with a conical firm sheath around the tonsils into which they continue to be jammed. The desired result is that the tonsils should ascend after decompres-

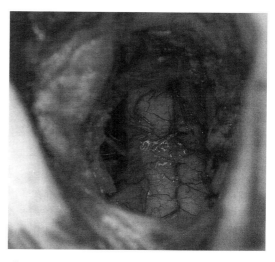

Figure 12: Operative photograph of same patient as Figure 11. There was no point in clearing the graft off the tonsils and exposing the tonsils because there was good access underneath the tonsil on either side.

sion,[3,5,12,41] even if other parts of the hindbrain may descend slightly.[12,41] The tonsils should also become rounded and not descend or slump.[5] Patients in this situation invite reoperation and an energetic attack on the tonsils (Figures 11 and 12). Reoperation may be as successful as a primary operation. The situation may be more difficult if a graft has been inserted, because a graft not only occupies space but it also promotes fibrosis. If Silastic had been used, there is likely to be a dense fibrotic sheet, which may be largely intact over the front of the graft involving the arachnoid and the pia over the tonsils and which may be adherent to the medulla. Concerns with grafts include hemorrhage[18,19] as well as fibrosis.[34,50] Under these circumstances, the operation is more difficult. Similarly, a graft of tissue such as pericranium, pericardium,[18] or fascia lata may develop vascularity and if fluid has built up behind this and pressed it forward then it will adhere to and try to gain a blood supply from the central nervous system structures (Figure 13). Under these circumstances, reoperation may be successful, but there is an increased risk of both vascular and medullary damage.

In some cases, severe meningeal fibrosis around the hindbrain has defeated the first surgical attempt. The appearances in such cases can be formidable. The likely result of such a case is that the foramen of Magendie has not been opened. Under these circumstances, there may be hydrocephalus. The hydrocephalus may be localized to the fourth ventricle and the patient's condition may deteriorate neurologically because of fourth ventricular clefts (Figure 1). Reoperation under these circumstances is difficult. It is tempting to insert a shunt from the lateral ventricle to the peritoneal cavity and wait to see the effect on the syrinx symptoms. If there is modest hydrocephalus or dilatation of the fourth ventricle, then it is reasonable to operate on the posterior fossa and to use the dilatation to gain access to the fourth ventricle. This involves a risk of medullary or cerebellar damage. Some surgeons advocate placement of drains from the fourth ventricle to the sub-arachnoid space; sometimes even drainage from the syrinx to the posterior fossa CSF has been proposed.

The author prefers not to leave drains from one part of the subarachnoid space to another

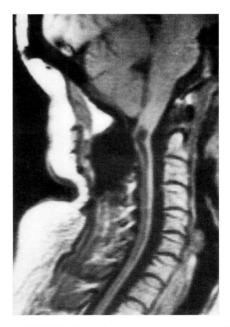

Figure 13: MRI of a patient in whom the surgical procedure was too low. The cerebellum has not been adequately decompressed. The tonsils have not been tackled; a graft was placed which continues to fill and has caused adhesion at the back of the upper cord. Nevertheless, the syrinx is substantially collapsed. The neurology is not a problem; there is no hydrocephalus and no further recommendation for surgery was made.

because such drains are rigid, may compress neural structures, and may provoke fibrosis around both ends, usually becoming walled off. Although the author devised small tapered drains with triangular cross section for the posterior fossa, these devices have not been used because of concerns about fibrosis. It is the author's view that there are few indications for the use of such devices.

Stents are rigid devices that assist in the healing of soft tissue and are then removed. The typical use for a stent in the situation where there has been a previous posterior fossa decompression is to place the tip of the stent into the fourth ventricle. This needs to be done carefully so that there is no chance that postoperative manipulations by the patient will cause impingement on the medulla. If the stent is positioned carefully, using the muscular attachments to the axis to prevent ventral displacement and bringing it out through the skin well below the axis, then this tube will not press on the medulla. The tube may be positioned inside the fourth ventricle; it can be weakened by the careful fashioning of extra holes and can lie comfortably. The tip should be within the ependymal lining of the fourth ventricle. The stent may then be removed between the third and the fifth postoperative day. Local edema around the tonsils may be less by that time and it seems probable that the communication between the ventricular system and the surgically fashioned artificial cisterna magna may persist.

The other alternative, which can be tried by inserting a tube into the fourth ventricle, is to drain the entire CSF space. This operation is reserved for cases in which there is a good artificial cisterna magna after the first procedure. The author places the proximal end of a regular valve system in the way described, that is to say using the arch and spinous process of C2 to direct the catheter tip. The lower end of the drain can be put into the skin between the clavicle and the trapezius muscle. At the end of the posterior fossa procedure, the patient can be laid supine and the bottom of the tube mobilized and attached to a valve and the lower end taken to the peritoneum. Once again, the author favors Medos adjustable valves, which can be placed to the right of the sternum just medial to the breast tissue. A straight posteroanterior radiograph allows the valve setting to be checked; a slightly oblique view helps to clear the spine off the valve. Reopening the posterior fossa in this way and lowering the overall CSF pressure at the same time has on occasion been conspicuously successful.

Hydrocephalus

When noted at the time of the initial diagnosis, hydrocephalus may improve after hindbrain operation. This is particularly the case if there is a pouch in relation to the hindbrain. Deflation of the pouch and normalization of all the tissue relationships at that site will often resolve the hydrocephalus (Figures 2 and 3). Batzdorf[7] notes that a minor degree of hydrocephalus can be ignored, although vigilance in the postoperative period is necessary. Major hydrocephalus should not be ignored.

"Slumping" of the Cerebellum

It is naturally a bad principle to treat a hernia by making the hole wider. If the cerebellum becomes jammed in an enlarged aperture in the occipital bone, then the situation can become worse, the hindbrain can move further down, and the patients may suffer increased symptomatology, particularly headache. In cases where the posterior fossa is too small for the contained cerebellum, this is a difficult situation to avoid. However, the problem is usually only seen when either the removal of the bone and dura has been excessive, so that the cerebellum slumps downward under gravity or, more commonly, the craniospinal pressure dissociation has not been corrected and the cerebellum continues to be sucked into the aperture (Figure 10). Another possibility is persisting hydrocephalus with some obstruction to the outlets of the fourth ventricle. Another cogent cause of intensified hindbrain herniation is either the presence of a thecoperitoneal shunt below the hindbrain or a syrinx drain which is overdraining and producing the same effect as lowering pressure below the hindbrain. The question of determining the size of decompression is interesting. The author has tended to make the exposures smaller over the years and to launch progressively more intense attacks upon the tonsils. This policy obviously has its limitations, and there comes a point when a proportion of cases will not be adequately decompressed because of the proximity of the bony margins. The way that the tonsils and the lower cerebellum are diminished in size will produce a complication rate proportional to the amount of aggression and the number of vessels that are sacrificed around the tonsils (Figures 14 to 16).

An interesting contrary view has come from Sahuquillo et al,[41] who noted the earlier observations by Duddy and Williams[12] that the size of the decompression as assessed on the sagittal MRI scan seemed to correlate with failure of the fourth ventricle and brain stem to descend. Sahuquillo proposed making large decompressions. His group has reported early success with this method and, provided that the cerebellum is not disrupted from its support by leaving the arachnoid intact as Sahuquillo suggests, then the size of the decompression does not matter;

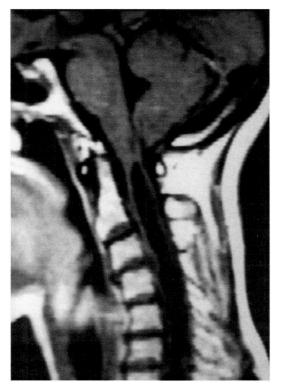

Figure 14: MRI of a patient with regular hindbrain-related syringomyelia. This was not severe hindbrain herniation, and there was no history of difficult birth or hydrocephalus.

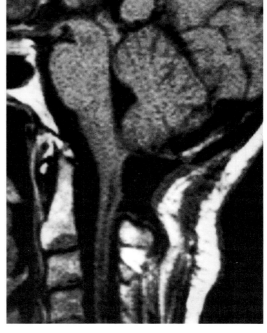

Figure 16: Postoperative MRI of the same patient as Figure 14. Note that the artificial cisterna magna is capacious but not in free communication with the fourth ventricle. The top of the cord is angulated slightly backward even though no graft was used. This patient had an excessive meningeal fibrosis. She was drowsy in the postoperative period with respiratory stridor and Cheyne-Stoke respirations. Ventricular shunting and tracheostomy were performed and resulted in immediate improvement of her level of consciousness.

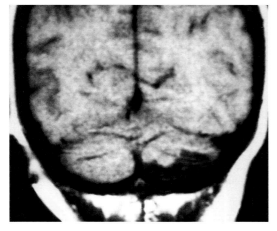

Figure 15: MRI of the same patient as Figure 14 demonstrating infarction of the lower cerebellum due to dissection of tonsils with excessive meningeal fibrosis. This degree of damage was accompanied by a slight increase in gait instability, but the patient's overall neurological picture was improved following this procedure.

what matters is the adequacy of the decompression in the zone where craniospinal pressure dissociation is engendered.

Postoperative Deterioration

Following the craniovertebral decompression procedures, there is a significant morbidity rate and occasional mortality; at times, immediate postoperative deterioration is seen. Perhaps the most dangerous condition is persistent hydrocephalus as discussed above, but the following additional factors need consideration.

Respiratory Inadequacy

Patients with kyphoscoliosis and muscular deficits are in a poor physical condition to withstand major surgery, especially in the presence of a condition which may produce distortion and dysfunction of the respiratory centers. Patients who do not breathe well after operation constitute a major problem. The phenomenon of mortality following surgery is not unknown and for any suspect cases it is recommended that an anoxia monitor or other form of respiratory monitor should be used over the first three days. If the patient has a diminished respiratory drive, it is the author's policy to opt for tracheostomy early rather than after a prolonged period of endotracheal ventilation. It is common for the patient to have difficulty in clearing secretions from the chest, and the tracheostomy helps. Also, the patient usually has a normal level of consciousness, and endotracheal intubation prevents conversation. During the phase of recovery, it is a bigger insult for the patient to have an endotracheal tube removed prematurely than it is to have a tracheostomy in place without ventilation for a while. Drowsiness and respiratory inadequacy together often raise the question of whether there is an element of hydrocephalus present. Since it is untidy to insert a shunt when a tracheostomy is in position with sometimes unpleasant flora on the patient's skin, it is the author's policy to insert a shunt and then a tracheostomy at the same operation. This combined procedure has been done three times in the past 20 years at the Syringomyelia Clinic.

Vascular Damage

The major hazard of an energetic approach to reducing the size of the tonsils is damage to the vascular supply of the cerebellum or the medulla. This hazard is greatest when there is a degree of meningeal fibrosis. If the meningeal fibrosis is Grade 4, the vasculature may be plainly abnormal, occasionally with large veins giving rise to the suspicion of an arteriovenous malformation. Usually this is due to pre-existing hydrocephalus disturbing the normal drainage pathway and causing hypertrophy of the posterior fossa veins as well as the diploic venous channels. This degree of meningeal fibrosis is almost always confined to patients with birth injury or those with spina bifida, where the problem is additionally compounded by prenatal hydrocephalus and gross hindbrain herniation. Patients with the more common type of hindbrain herniation, where the tonsils can be separated easily, are not immune to the possibility of vascular damage. In debulking the tonsils, any sizable artery should be spared and the posterior inferior cerebellar artery should be respected (Figures 14 to 16). In lifting the tonsils off the medulla, there may be small strands with vessels that apear to run from the medulla to the cerebellum. These vessels are not normally present and it is usually safe to lift up the tonsil and dissect the cerebellomedullary fissure. The rule is not to cauterize anything that could possibly be supplying the medulla but to try and extract such vessels from the cerebellar tissues. The vessels usually turn out to be loops and dissection can be carried up beyond the obex on either side. When the tonsils are evacuated and sutured, there is normally a free passageway with no likelihood of vascular damage.

Damage to the medulla can be severe. A touch by the diathermy can produce symptoms. If the syrinx comes up beneath the pia, even a covering of tissue which appears extremely thin and looks as though it could not possibly contain functional fibers should not be myelotomized or excised.

Reoperation

If the patient initially underwent a craniovertebral decompression procedure which was not successful, then reoperation by reopening the posterior fossa is difficult. Obviously, if the dura has been closed or grafted, the tonsils have not been removed and the syrinx looks the same; in this case, it is probably better to go straight into the posterior fossa once more, rather than to opt for a shunt (Figures 11 and 12). Sometimes, the situation becomes markedly worse at the posterior fossa with closure of the foramen of Magendie and hydrocephalus formation in the fourth ventricle, possibly with clefts. Once again, if the hydrocephalus has been dealt with by ventricular shunting, reintervention in the posterior fossa is possible and stenting may be successful.

NONSURGICAL MANAGEMENT OF SYRINGOMYELIA

Contraindications to Surgery

Some patients are in an extreme degree of dilapidation when encountered by the surgeon. Respiratory reserve compromised by kyphoscoliosis or severe limb deficits such that the patient cannot walk and has little function in the hands might seem to be contraindications to surgery. Nevertheless, patients in that condition who have progressive bulbar deficits may be grateful for operation; additionally, they may also achieve unexpected benefits such as recovery of sitting balance as well as preservation of swallowing and respiratory function. Too pessimistic an attitude should be avoided.

Patients in Stable Condition

Sometimes patients with severe deficit have had no progression for many years, even though the hindbrain anatomy and the syrinx cavity appear inviting for surgery. If the disease had progressed fairly rapidly in the early stage and then became stable, there is probably a good case to be made for nonsurgical treatment.

Patients With Spontaneous Cure

Sometimes patients will be seen who have a completely flat or substantially empty syrinx, which may be calcified, and the hindbrain may be disimpacted. This is uncommon, but clearly such patients do not need to undergo surgery. This phenomenon is seen in less than 1% of cases, and the idea of awaiting a spontaneous cure is not recommended.[35]

Asymptomatic Patients

In some patients, syringomyelia is accidentally discovered on an MRI scan performed for some other reason. If the patient is otherwise well, some authors recommend a waiting policy. In the majority of patients that this author has seen in whom the disorder has come on after the age of 50 years, the symptoms are difficult to ameliorate and a firm recommendation is made that asymptomatic patients should be regarded as an opportunity to prevent this disorder from

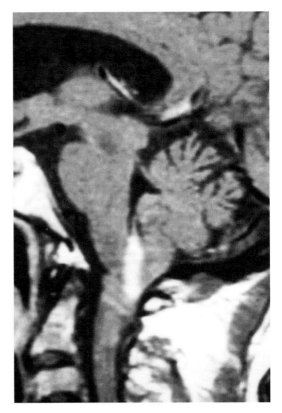

Figure 17: MRI of a patient with hindbrain herniation due to tumor blocking the outflow track of the fourth ventricle. This not only enhanced with gadolinium but was also calcified. The patient was 61 years old at the time of onset of gait disorder, swallowing, and incontinence. He had Rombergism and nystagmus and mild spasticity. The patient was not referred for surgery, provided that associated hydrocephalus was dealt with; the tumor was not likely to enlarge quickly. MRI outpatient review was recommended.

becoming symptomatic. Treatment should be proceeded with expeditiously. Such a policy must respect the patient's age (Figure 17).

When the patient has asymptomatic hindbrain herniation without syringomyelia, it is difficult to know under what circumstances the condition can be left and when it should be operated upon. One difficulty concerns patients in whom there is another pathology; examples are proven multiple sclerosis and hindbrain herniation that looks as though it might be contributing to such problems as diplopia, oscillopsia, and long tract features. If causative demyelinating lesions cannot be identified on the

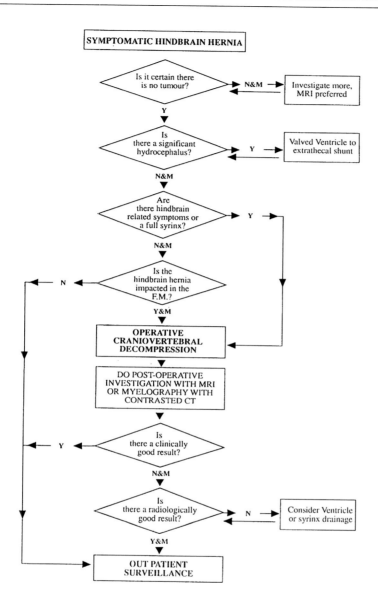

Figure 18: A decision tree for hindbrain herniation. Note that "maybe" (M) is sometimes an answer to such questions as whether hydrocephalus is significant. CT = computed tomography; Y = yes; N = no; F.M. = foramen magnum.

MRI scan, it would seem reasonable for these patients to undergo craniovertebral decompression.

The Spindle Syrinx

A spindle is a small object sharply pointed at both ends. This characteristic shape is sometimes seen in patients with syringomyelia which is usually discovered in the course of investigation for pain. Whether the syrinx is causing the pain is debatable. In the absence of webs of meningeal fibrosis (sometimes forming pouch-like diverticula), the correction of which may cure such syringes, there seems little to do. The spindle shape indicates the probability that the syrinx is not tense and not surging in response to slosh. Such syringes are commonly not circular in cross section and may have a diamond-shaped outline which is reminiscent of the stage in the development of the spinal cord before the central canal is closed. It is tempting, therefore, to suppose that this is a primary form of dysraphism. Similar lesions are sometimes seen with spina bifida manque or transitional lesions between the occult and the overt.

Magnetic Resonance Imaging Assessment

MRI has revolutionized the management of syringomyelia, not only by revealing the anatomy but also by making a start in analysis of flow.[3,5,12,15,23,27,44,49,52] It is probable that in the future, MRI scanning will be of sufficient quality to show craniospinal pressure dissociation, either by impaction of the tonsils in the rebound phase after straining or, perhaps even better, by showing an arrest of CSF pulsation past the impacted tonsils. The development of such MRI methods is obviously a much-awaited tool for the assessment of all patients of this class.

Summary

Decisions about when and how to operate on syringomyelia are not easy to make (Figure 18). Each patient should be taken into the surgeon's confidence and the difficulties not minimized. Hydrocephalus should be dealt with as a priority when dealing with hindbrain-related syringomyelia, and careful postoperative surveillance is necessary to ensure that further procedures are not required. Procedures directed against the filling mechanism are preferable to drainage operations. As with many other neurosurgical procedures, concentration of expertise is likely to be beneficial.

References

1. Appleby A, Bradley WG, Foster JB, et al: Syringomyelia due to chronic arachnoiditis at the foramen magnum. **J Neurol Sci 8:**451-464, 1969
2. Aschoff A, Kunze S: 100 Years of Syrinx-Surgery. Proceedings of a workshop, December 13–15, 1991 at Heidelberg. **Acta Neurochir 123:**157-159, 1993
3. Balagura S, Kuo DC: Spontaneous retraction of cerebellar tonsils after surgery for Arnold-Chiari malformation and posterior fossa cyst. **Surg Neurol 29:** 137-140, 1988
4. Barbaro NM: Surgery for primarily spinal syringomyelia, in Batzdorf U (ed): **Syringomyelia: Current Concepts in Diagnosis and Treatment.** Baltimore, Md: Williams & Wilkins, 1991, pp 183-198
5. Barkovitch AJ, Sherman JL, Citrin CM, et al: MR of postoperative syringomyelia. **AJNR 8:**319-327, 1987
6. Battersby RD, Williams B: Birth injury: a possible contributory factor in the aetiology of primary basilar impression. **J Neurol Neurosurg Psychiatry 45:** 879-883, 1982
7. Batzdorf U: Syringomyelia related to abnormalities at the level of the craniovertebral juntion, in Batzdorf U (ed): **Syringomyelia: Current Concepts in Diagnosis and Treatment.** Baltimore, Md: Williams & Wilkins. 1991, pp 163-182
8. Blagodatsky MD, Larionov SN, Manohin PA, et al: Surgical treatment of "hindbrain related" syringomyelia: new data for pathogenesis. **Acta Neurochir 124:** 82-85, 1993
9. Chiari H: Über die Pathogenese der Sogennanten Syringomyelie. **Z Heilkunde 9:**307-336, 1888
10. Chumas PDL, Armstrong DC, Drake JM, et al: Tonsillar herniation: the rule rather than the exception after lumboperitoneal shunting in the pediatric population. **J Neurosurg 78:**568-573, 1994
11. Di Lorenzo N, Maleci A, Williams BM: Severe exacerbation of post traumatic syringomyelia after lithotripsy. Case report. **Paraplegia 32:**694-696, 1994
12. Duddy MJ, Williams B: Hindbrain migration after decompression for hindbrain hernia: a quantitative assessment using MRI. **Br J Neurosurg 5:**141-152, 1991
13. Dyste GN, Menezes AH, VanGilder JC: Symptomatic Chiari malformations. An analysis of presentation, management, and long-term outcome. **J Neurosurg 71:**159-168, 1989
14. Edgar RE: Surgical management of spinal cord cysts. **Paraplegia 14:**21-27, 1976
15. Enzmann DR, O'Donohue J, Rubin JB, et al: CSF pulsations within nonneoplastic spinal cord cysts. **AJR 149:**149-157, 1987
16. Firsching R, Sanker P: MRI follow-up in syringomyelia. Observations from twelve cases. **Acta Neurochir 123:**206-207, 1993
17. Fischer EG, Welch K, Shillito J Jr: Syringomyelia following lumboureteral shunting for communicating hydrocephalus. Report of three cases. **J Neurosurg 47:**96-100, 1977
18. Fisher WS III, Braun D: Closure of posterior fossa dural defects using a dural substitute: technical note. **Neurosurgery 31:**155-156, 1992
19. Fontana R, Talamonti G, D'Angelo V, et al: Spontaneous haematoma as unusual complication of Silastic dural substitute. Report of 2 cases. **Acta Neurochir 115:**64-66, 1992
20. Foster JB: Neurology of syringomyelia, in Batzdorf U (ed): **Syringomyelia: Current Concepts in Diagnosis and Treatment.** Baltimore, Md: Williams & Wilkins, 1991, pp 91-115
21. Gardner WJ: **The Dysraphic States: From Syringomyelia to Anencephaly.** Amsterdam: Excerpta Medica, 1973
22. Hall PV, Lindseth RE, Campbell RL, et al: Myelodysplasia and developmental scoliosis: a manifestation of syringomyelia. **Spine 1:**48-56, 1976
23. Hida K, Iwasaki Y, Imamura H, et al: Posttraumatic syringomyelia: its characteristic magnetic resonance imaging findings and surgical management. **Neurosurgery 35:**886-891, 1994
24. Honan WP, Williams B: Sensory loss in syringomyelia: not necessarily dissociated. **J R Soc Med 86:** 519-520, 1993
25. Krayenbühl H: Evaluation of the different surgical approaches in the treatment of syringomyelia. **Clin Neurol Neurosurg 77:**111-128, 1974

26. Kruse A, Rasmussen G, Børgesen SE: CSF-dynamics in syringomyelia: intracranial pressure and resistance to outflow. **Br J Neurosurg 1**:477-484, 1987

27. Maier SE, Hardy CJ, Jolesz FA: Brain and cerebrospinal fluid motion: real time quantification with M-mode MR imaging. **Radiology 193**:477-483, 1994

28. Marín-Padilla M: Cephalic axial skeletal-neural dysraphic disorders: embryology and pathology. **Can J Neurol Sci 18**:153-169, 1991

29. Milhorat TH, Johnson WD, Miller JI: Syrinx shunt to posterior fossa cisterns (syringocisternostomy) for bypassing obstructions of upper cervical theca. **J Neurosurg 77**:871-874, 1992

30. Milhorat TH, Miller JI, Johnson WD: Anatomical basis of syringomyelia occurring with hindbrain lesions. **Neurosurgery 32**:748-754, 1993

31. Morgan D, Williams B: Syringobulbia: a surgical appraisal. **J Neurol Neurosurg Psychiatry 55:** 1132-1141, 1992

32. Murovic JA, Posnick JC, Drake JM: Hydrocephalus in Apert syndrome: a retrospective review. **Pediatr Neurosurg 19**:151-155, 1993

33. Oakes WJ, Gaskill SJ: Symptomatic Chiari malformations in childhood, in Park TS (ed): **Spinal Dysraphism**. Oxford: Blackwell Scientific, 1992, pp 104-124

34. Ohbayashi N, Inagawa T, Katoh Y, et al: Complication of Silastic dural substitute 20 years after dural plasty. **Surg Neurol 41**:338-341, 1994

35. Olivero WC, Dinh DH: Chiari I malformation with traumatic syringomyelia and spontaneous resolution: case report and literature review. **Neurosurgery 30**:758-760, 1992

36. Padovani R, Cavallo M, Gaist G: Surgical treatment of syringomyelia: favorable results with syringosubarachnoid shunting. **Surg Neurol 32**:173-180, 1989

37. Park TS, Cail WS, Broaddus WC: LP shunting in cases of Chiari malformation. **J Neurosurg 71**:953, 1989

38. Pillay PK, Awad IA, Hanh JF: Gardner's hydrodynamic theory of syringomyelia revisited. **Clev Clin J Med 59**:373-380, 1992

39. Raftopoulos C, Sanchez A, Matos C, et al: Hydrosyringomyelia—Chiari I complex. Prospective evaluation of a modified foramen magnum decompression procedure: preliminary results. **Surg Neurol 39:** 163-169, 1993

40. Ryken TC, Menezes AH: Cervicomedullary compression in achondroplasia. **J Neurosurg 81**:43-48, 1994

41. Sahuquillo J, Rubio E, Poca MA, et al: Posterior fossa reconstruction: a surgical technique for the treatment of Chiari I malformation and Chiari I/syringomyelia complex—preliminary results and magnetic resonance imaging quantitative assessment of hindbrain migration. **Neurosurgery 35**:874-885, 1994

42. Samii M, Klekamp J, Sepehrnia A, et al: Syringomyelia associated with Arnold-Chiari-I-malformation and tumours of the posterior fossa. Long-term results of syringo-subarachnoid shunting and decompression of the posteria fossa. **Acta Neurochir 123**:195, 1993

43. Sgouros S, Williams B: A critical appraisal of drainage for syringomyelia. **J Neurosurg 82**:1-10, 1995

44. Sherman JL, Barkovitch AJ, Citrin CM: The MR appearance of syringomyelia: new observations. **AJR 148**:381-391, 1987

45. Stein SA, Witkop C, Hill S, et al: Sclerostenosis: neurogenetic and pathophysiologic analysis of an American kinship. **Neurology 33**:267-277, 1983

46. Stevens JM, Chong WK, Barber C, et al: A new appraisal of abnormalities of the odontoid process associated with atlanto-axial subluxation and neurological disability. **Brain 117**:133-148, 1994

47. Stovner LJ: Headache associated with the Chiari type I malformation. **Headache 33**:175-181, 1993

48. Stovner LJ, Bergan U, Nilsen G, et al: Posterior cranial fossa dimensions in the Chiari I malformation: relation to pathogenesis and clinical presentation. **Neuroradiology 35**:113-118, 1993

49. Stovner LJ, Rinck P: Syringomyelia in Chiari malformation: relation to extent of cerebellar tissue herniation. **Neurosurgery 31**:913-917, 1992

50. Thompson DNP, Taylor WF, Hayward RD: Silastic dural substitute: experience of its use in spinal and foramen magnum surgery. **Br J Neurosurg 8:** 157-167, 1994

51. Tognetti F, Calbucci F: Syringomyelia: syringo-subarachnoid shunt versus posterior fossa decompression. **Acta Neurochir 123**:196-197, 1993

52. Vaquero J, Martínez R, Arias A: Syringomyelia-Chiari complex: magnetic resonance imaging and clinical evaluation of surgical treatment. **J Neurosurg 73:** 64-68, 1990

53. Welch K, Shillito J, Strand R, et al: Chiari I "malformation"—an acquired disorder? **J Neurosurg 55:** 604-609, 1981

54. West RJ, Williams B: Radiographic studies of the ventricles in syringomyelia. **Neuroradiology 20:** 5-16, 1980

55. Williams B: A blast against grafts—on the closing and grafting of the posterior fossa dura. **Br J Neurosurg 8**:275-278, 1994

56. Williams B: A critical appraisal of posterior fossa surgery for communicating syringomyelia. **Brain 101**:223-250, 1978

57. Williams B: Difficult labour as a cause of communicating syringomyelia. **Lancet 2**:51-53, 1977

58. Williams B: Further thoughts on the valvular action of the Arnold-Chiari malformation. **Z Kinderchir Grenzgebiete Suppl 25 (13)**:105-112, 1971

59. Williams B: Post traumatic syringomyelia, in Floman Y, Farcy JP, Argenson C (eds): **Thoraco-Lumbar Spine Fractures**. New York, NY: Raven Press, 1993, pp 429-448

60. Williams B: Surgery for hindbrain related syringomyelia. **Adv Tech Stand Neurosurg 20**:107-164, 1993

61. Williams B, Fahy G: A critical appraisal of "terminal ventriculostomy" for the treatment of syringomyelia. **J Neurosurg 58**:188-197, 1983

62. Williams B, Page N: Surgical treatment of syringomyelia with syringopleural shunting. **Br J Neurosurg 1**:63-80, 1987

63. Williams B, et al: Overview: session on hindbrain herniation, in Samii M (ed): **Skull Base Surgery**. Basel: Karger, 1994, pp 1114-1117

CHAPTER 12

SUBOCCIPITAL AND CERVICAL DECOMPRESSION

ANDREA L. HALLIDAY, MD

Several studies have enhanced our understanding of the abnormal cerebrospinal fluid (CSF) flow dynamics present in Chiari I malformations and syringomyelia. Enhanced understanding of the pathophysiology of syringomyelia has altered the surgical treatment of this malformation. There is still, however, controversy over the best initial surgical approach for syringomyelia and the Chiari malformation.

RATIONALE OF SURGICAL TREATMENT

Many of the surgical procedures used to treat Chiari malformation and associated syringomyelia were based on prevailing theories of the pathogenesis of syringomyelia developed in the era before magnetic resonance imaging (MRI).[6,11,17-19,27] Theories by Gardner[6] and Williams[27] are among the most well known of these. The hydrodynamic theory of Gardner proposed that syringomyelia resulted from the "water-hammer" transmission of pulsatile CSF pressure via a communication between the fourth ventricle and the central canal of the spinal cord through the obex.[17]

A microsurgical modification of the Gardner procedure was used to treat most cases in a series of 35 patients treated at the Cleveland Clinic.[18] This modification included suboccipital craniectomy, microsurgical lysis of adhesions, opening the fourth ventricular outlet, plugging of the obex in patients with syringomyelia, and placing a dural patch graft. Plugging of the obex and opening of the fourth ventricular outlet as treatment of syringomyelia are based on Gardner's hydrodynamic theory.

For the treatment of syringomyelia associated with the Chiari malformation, Rhoton[19] recommended a posterolateral myelotomy and placement of a Silastic wick anchored to the dura above and threaded downward into the myelotomy. Rhoton modified the Gardner procedure by placing a Silastic wick attached to the dura in the new midline opening of the fourth ventricle to maintain the opening of the outlet. To avoid the risk of damaging the hypoglossal and vagal nuclei, Rhoton did not recommend plugging of the obex with muscle.

Studies using cadavers[11,14] or MRI[13,16,17] rarely confirm the presence of a functional communication between the fourth ventricle and the syrinx in cases of syringomyelia with Chiari malformation. Therefore, plugging of the obex and exploring the fourth ventricular outlet are becoming less common. This has resulted in a reduction in complications such as bradycardia and postoperative respiratory distress following the procedure.[3,11]

In Williams' theory,[27] the syrinx develops in patients with Chiari malformation from a differential between intracranial pressure and spinal pressure caused by a valve-like action at the foramen magnum. This in turn causes partial obstruction to the downward movement but not the upward movement of CSF. This leads to intermittent abrupt pressure differences transmitted from the central venous pressure (associated with Valsalva maneuvers), leading in turn to the movement of CSF from the obex to the syrinx.[27] The surgical strategy outlined by Batzdorf is based on Williams' theory. Batzdorf[3] recommended dissecting the arachnoid off the tonsils under magnification and separating the cerebellar tonsils in the midline, lifting them away from the underlying cervicomedullary junction, as long as they are not adherent. To maintain the exposure of the fourth ventricle, bipolar coagulation, subpial dissection, and application of clips or fine Nurolon suture are used. If the tonsils cannot be mobilized, Batzdorf places a shunt from the fourth ventricle to the subarachnoid space.

An opening between the fourth ventricle and syrinx has rarely been demonstrated by MRI or cadaver studies,[10,12,13,15,16] and direct measurement of cranial and spinal CSF pressures does not support a cranial-spinal pressure dissociation with intracranial pressure greater than lumbar spinal pressure.[7,17] Additionally, dynamic MRI and intraoperative ultrasound studies are inconsistent with both Gardner's and Williams' theories of the pathogenesis of syringomyelia associated with the Chiari malformation.

Advances in MRI technology that provide dynamic imaging of CSF flow have helped to elucidate the pathophysiology of syrinx formation associated with the Chiari malformations. This enhanced understanding of the etiology of syrinx formation associated with the Chiari malformation is guiding the current thinking regarding the best approach to the surgical treatment of this malformation. Oldfield et al[16] used phase-contrast and phase-contrast cine MRI and intraoperative ultrasound to examine the flow of CSF and syrinx fluid. Their observations suppported the hypothesis that progression of syringomyelia occurs because the herniated cerebellar tonsils occlude the sub-arachnoid space at the foramen magnum, preventing rapid flow of CSF at the foramen magnum and acting as a piston during systole, pushing fluid longitudinally into the syrinx and possibly originating the syrinx by forcing CSF into the cord through the perivascular and interstitial spaces. Ball and Dayan[1] in 1972 proposed that CSF enters the cord through dilated perivascular and interstitial spaces, resulting in syringomyelia. Other studies which show the presence of fluorescein, labeled albumin, horse-radish peroxidase, and metrizimide in the syrinx after intrathecal injection support this hypothesis. Additionally, simultaneous measurements of intracranial pressure by Park et al[17] have also suggested that CSF under pressure moves into the spinal cord. The mechanism of syringomyelia formation proposed by Oldfield et al[16] supports decompression of the cerebellar tonsils alone as the first step in the surgical treatment of this disorder.

In several series, reduction or resolution of the syrinx resulted from tonsillar decompression alone by a suboccipital craniectomy and upper cervical laminectomies, leaving the arachnoid intact.[8,11,16,26,27] Leaving the arachnoid intact decreases postoperative complications such as CSF collection in the operative wound, pseudomeningocele or meningitis, and arachnoid scarring.[3,8,11] Not mobilizing the tonsils minimizes the risk of injury to the medulla and the posterior inferior cerebellar arteries.[3] The indications for surgery in patients with the Chiari I malformation are symptoms from foramen magnum compression, syringomyelia, and/or cerebellar dysfunction and include suboccipital and lower central neck pain, particularly provoked by Valsalva manuevers, capelike dissociated sensory loss, dysesthesias, gait difficulty, nystagmus, upper or lower extremity weakness, cranial nerve dysfunction, and blurred vision.[11,18] Headache, neck pain, and sensory disturbances are the most common symptoms. Progression of symptoms is usually slow; therefore, there is no indication to operate on an asymptomatic Chiari malformation. Because of this slow progression of symptoms and because patients may not improve or may be worse after surgery, some centers advocate waiting for signs of neurological deterioration before operating.[9,11] Others, however, argue that deterioration may be sudden and that surgical intervention is warranted in symptomatic Chiari malformations when the condition is diagnosed, as long as the patient is not severely disabled from the disorder and is in good medical condition.[27] Most authors argue against surgical intervention if the patient is disabled to the point of being confined to a wheelchair, as the surgery is not without risk and it is very unlikely to significantly reverse such severe neurological compromise.

SURGICAL TECHNIQUE

Patients are placed prone on chest rolls in Mayfield pin fixation with the head slightly flexed. Excessive neck motion should be avoided during intubation and positioning of the patient, as the neural elements are already compressed by the cerebellar tonsils and/or the syrinx. Marked flexion of the neck during surgery has been reported to cause postoperative neurological deficit or respiratory problems.[15] The shoulders are pulled caudally with broad tape applied to the shoulders and attached to the bottom of the table. A Foley catheter is placed in all patients. A suboccipital craniectomy is performed, using either rongeurs or the craniotome to remove the lower two-thirds of the squama of the occipital bone, and is carried out laterally with rongeurs (Figure 1). If rongeurs are used for bony removal, the high-speed drill is used to thin the bone, especially in the midline where a prominent midline keel is usually present. Care is taken to leave the dura intact during the bony removal. Batzdorf[3] argues that the posterior fossa craniectomy should not be carried too far laterally so as to prevent delayed cerebellar ptosis, which Batzdorf believes contributes to re-expansion of the syrinx cavity after posterior fossa decompression. This view, however, has recently been brought into question by Sahuquillo et al.[21] They treated 10 patients with an extensive craniectomy, a wide opening of the foramen magnum and dura while leaving the arachnoid intact, patching of the dura to allow for a spacious posterior fossa, and tenting of the dural graft. Postoperative MRI demonstrated formation of a new cisterna magna with upward migration of the cerebellum in all cases.

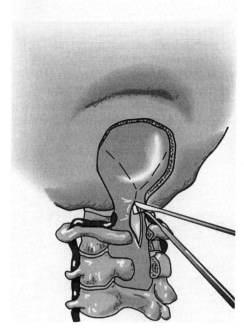

Figure 1: Illustration of a suboccipital craniectomy and cervical laminectomies demonstrating the extent of the bony removal, the position of the vertebral arteries, and the technique used for opening the dura while leaving the arachnoid intact.

The foramen magnum is exposed using curettes, dissecting instruments, and rongeurs, being careful to strip the dura and not to lever bone fragments into the cervicomedullary junction. The laminae of Cl, C2, and sometimes C3 are removed to entirely expose the herniated tonsils. Approximately 1.5 cm of the foramen magnum and the ring of Cl on either side of the midline are removed. The decompression need not be wider than the width of the spinal cord and extension farther laterally risks injury to the vertebral arteries (Figure 1). Care is taken to remove all soft tissue from the bone fragments prior to their removal so as not to lever fragments into the vertebral artery or the perivertebral venous plexus. When bleeding from the venous plexus is encountered, it is treated by packing with Surgicel or thrombin-soaked Gelfoam. Meticulous hemostasis must be achieved prior to opening of the dura.

The dura is opened in a Y-shaped fashion, being careful to keep the underlying arachnoid

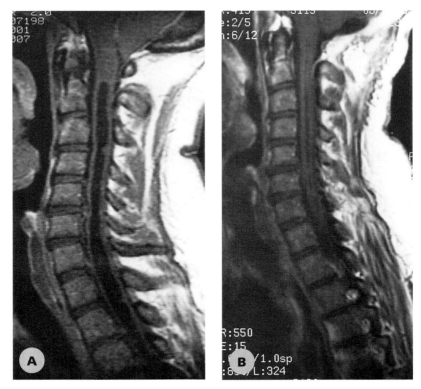

Figure 2: Preoperative **(A)** and postoperative **(B)** sagittal T1-weighted MRI demonstrating significant reduction in the size of a cervical syrinx associated with the Chiari malformation after suboccipital and cervical decompression.

intact (Figure 1). Enough dura is left between the dural and bony openings to facilitate a watertight closure. The occipital sinus is either coagulated with bipolar forceps or clipped with titanium Weck clips. The dural opening is carried inferior to the herniated tonsils. The underlying arachnoid is gently separated from the dura as the dura is held back and tacked up with stay sutures. The dura is then patched with either an autologous pericranial or fascia lata graft, lyophilized dura, or bovine pericardium. A watertight closure is performed to prevent the postoperative complications of pseudomeningocele, CSF leak, or meningitis.[8] Inadequate collapse of the syrinx postoperatively may result from the pressure effect of a pseudomeningocele. The tightness of the dural closure is tested with a Valsalva maneuver. Meticulous hemosta-sis is achieved with the bipolar forceps and bovie cautery, and the wound is closed in layers.

A recent report by Isu et al[8] advocated removing just the outer layer of dura to provide added insurance that the subarachnoid space is not entered. They found this technique to be just as effective as removing both layers of the dura when treating syringomyelia and the Chiari malformation, with reduction in the size of the syrinx on postoperative MRI as well as a wider cisterna magna on all seven patients treated thus far. Ultrasound examination of all patients was carried out intraoperatively to demonstrate that good pulsation of the cerebellar tonsils with restoration of the subarachnoid space posterior to the cerebellar tonsils was achieved with removal of the outer layer of dura alone. This approach, however, remains unproven.

RESULTS

Plugging the obex, exposing and opening the fourth ventricle, and placing a stent in the foramen of Magendie are not supported by the current theory of the pathophysiology of this disorder and have not been shown to improve the surgical results.[4,10-12,27] They can also lead to complications, including vasomotor instability and respiratory difficulty from injury to the structures on the floor of the fourth ventricle.[2,11,12,27] Most authors currently recommend bony decompression with opening and patching of the dura as the initial treatment for syringomyelia occurring with Chiari malformation. In several small series, reduction or disappearance of the syrinx has occurred in all patients.[3,10-12,16,21,26] This has been our experience as well (Figure 2). Foramen magnum decompression as the initial surgical treatment for syringomyelia associated with Chiari I malformation is in keeping with the growing body of evidence regarding the pathophysiology of syringomyelia associated with Chiari malformations and with minimizing operative risk. Shunting of the syrinx to the subarachnoid space, pleura, or peritoneum carries with it the risk of spinal cord injury accompanying myelotomy and insertion of the catheter, hemorrhage, shunt dysfunction or disconnection, infection, a shunt-related inflammatory response, or arachnoid fibrosis and postoperative dysesthetic pain.[8,16,23] Furthermore, Sgouros and Williams[24] recently examined the long-term results of treating syringomyelia with drains. Ten years after the shunting or drainage procedures, only one-half of the patients remained clinically stable and the procedures had a 15.7% complication rate. They concluded that surgical treatment of syringomyelia associated with the Chiari malformation should be directed at reconstructing normal CSF pathways.

In most cases, decompression of the foramen magnum combined with cervical laminectomies to expose the cerebellar tonsils relieves the symptoms caused by tonsillar compression.[4,10-12,20] Improvement in symptoms related to the syrinx, however, is less predictable. Cahan and Bentson[4] and Saez et al[20] reported a 70% and 80% improvement rate,

respectively, in patients with intracranial hypertension or cerebellar dysfunction. However, of patients with a central cord syndrome characterized by dysesthetic pain, dissociated sensory loss in a cape distribution, segmental weakness, and long-tract signs, only 33% improved regardless of the surgical approach. These results are in agreement with those reported by Levy et al[10] and Pillay et al.[18] Using a logistic regression analysis, Dyste et al[5] defined preoperative features associated with a poor outcome. They found that being symptomatic for over 2 years and the presence of ataxia, nystagmus, bulbar symptoms, muscle atrophy, and dorsal column dysfunction were predictive of a poor outcome. Stevens et al[25] found an association between the degree of descent of the cerebellar tonsils and outcome. They also found that the clinical features least likely to improve were bulbar symptoms, ataxia, and nystagmus. Cahan and Bentson[4] found that bulbar symptoms and pathological pain were least likely to improve. Persistent dysesthetic pain can occur despite radiographic improvement or collapse of the syrinx on the postoperative MRI.[2,18] This has also been demonstrated in case reports of spontaneous resolution of syrinxes in patients with Chiari malformations who were not treated surgically.[9,22]

CONCLUSION

The current trend in the literature regarding the surgical treatment of syringomyelia associated with Chiari I malformations is to try to restore the normal flow of CSF at the foramen magnum as the first step. Drainage of the syrinx is advocated as an adjuvant, only if the first surgery fails. Series reporting initial success with the management of this disorder are small, however, and lack long-term follow-up. Although foramen magnum decompression as the initial surgical treatment for syringomyelia associated with the Chiari malformation remains unproven, it is consistent with the most recent theory, based on advances in MRI technology, of the pathophysiology of syrinx formation in this disorder.

REFERENCES

1. Ball MJ, Dayan AD: Pathogenesis of syringomyelia. **Lancet** 2:799-801, 1972
2. Batzdorf U: Chiari I malformation with syringomyelia. Evaluation of surgical therapy by magnetic resonance imaging. **J Neurosurg** 68:726-730, 1988
3. Batzdorf U: Chiari malformation and syringomyelia, in Apuzzo MLJ (ed): **Brain Surgery: Complication Avoidance Management**. New York: Churchill Livingstone, 1993, vol 2, pp 1985-2001
4. Cahan LD, Bentson JR: Considerations in the diagnosis and treatment of syringomyelia and the Chiari malformation. **J Neurosurg** 57:24-31, 1982
5. Dyste GN, Menezes AH, VanGilder JC: Symptomatic Chiari malformations. An analysis of presentation, management, and long-term outcome. **J Neurosurg** 71:159-168, 1989
6. Gardner WJ: Hydrodynamic mechanism of syringomyelia: its relationship to myelocele. **J Neurol Neurosurg Psychiatry** 28:247-259, 1965
7. Heiss JD, Eidsath A, Talbot T, et al: Craniospinal decompression increases intracranial compliance and reduces subarachnoid pressure in patients with Chiari I syringomyelia. Congress of Neurological Surgeons Annual Meeting, October 1994 (Abstract)
8. Isu T, Sasaki H, Takamura H, et al: Foramen magnum decompression with removal of the outer layer of the dura as treatment for syringomyelia occurring with Chiari I malformation. **Neurosurgery** 33:845-850, 1993
9. Jack CR Jr, Kokmen E, Onofrio BM: Spontaneous decompression of syringomyelia: magnetic resonance imaging findings. Case report. **J Neurosurg** 74:283-286, 1991
10. Levy WJ, Mason L, Hahn JF: Chiari malformation presenting in adults: a surgical experience in 127 cases. **Neurosurgery** 12:377-390, 1983
11. Logue V, Edwards MR: Syringomyelia and its surgical treatment—an analysis of 75 patients. **J Neurol Neurosurg Psychiatry** 44:273-284, 1981
12. Matsumoto T, Symon L: Surgical management of syringomyelia—current results. **Surg Neurol** 32:258-265, 1989
13. Milhorat TH, Capocelli AL, Anzil AP, et al: Pathological basis of spinal cord cavitation in syringomyelia: analysis of 105 autopsy cases. **J Neurosurg** 82:802-812, 1995
14. Milhorat TH, Johnson WD, Miller JI, et al: Surgical treatment of syringomyelia based on magnetic resonance imaging criteria. **Neurosurgery** 31:231-245, 1992
15. Mullan S, Raimondi AJ: Respiratory hazards of the surgical treatment of the Arnold-Chiari malformation. **J Neurosurg** 19: 675-678, 1962
16. Oldfield EH, Muraszko K, Shawker TH, et al: Pathophysiology of syringomyelia associated with Chiari I malformation of the cerebellar tonsils. Implications for diagnosis and treatment. **J Neurosurg** 80:3-15, 1994
17. Park TS, Cail WS, Broaddus WC, et al: Lumboperitoneal shunt combined with myelotomy for treatment of syringohydromyelia. **J Neurosurg** 70: 721-727, 1989
18. Pillay PK, Awad TA, Little JR, et al: Symptomatic Chiari malformation in adults: a new classification based on magnetic resonance imaging with clinical and prognostic significance. **Neurosurgery** 28: 639-645, 1991
19. Rhoton AL Jr: Microsurgery of Arnold-Chiari malformation in adults with and without hydromyelia. **J Neurosurg** 45:473-483, 1976
20. Saez RJ, Onofrio BM, Yanagihara T: Experience with Arnold-Chiari malformation, 1960 to 1970. **J Neurosurg** 45:416-422, 1976
21. Sahuquillo J, Rubio E, Poca MA, et al: Posterior fossa reconstruction: a surgical technique for the treatment of Chiari I malformation and Chiari I/syringomyelia complex—preliminary results and magnetic resonance imaging quantitative assessment of hindbrain migration. **Neurosurgery** 35:874-885, 1994
22. Santoro A, Delfini R, Innocenzi G, et al: Spontaneous drainage of syringomyelia. Report of two cases. **J Neurosurg** 79:132-134, 1993
23. Schlesinger EB: Letter to the editor. **Surg Neurol** 38: 161-163, 1992
24. Sgouros S, Williams B: A critical appraisal of drainage in syringomyelia. **J Neurosurg** 82:1-10, 1995
25. Stevens JM, Serva WAD, Kendall BE, et al: Chiari malformation in adults: relation of morphological aspects to clinical features and operative outcome. **J Neurol Neurosurg Psychiatry** 56:1072-1077, 1993
26. Tachibana S, Iida H, Yada K: Significance of positive Queckenstet test in patients with syringomyelia associated with Arnold-Chiari malformations. **J Neurosurg** 76:67-71, 1992
27. Williams B: A critical appraisal of posterior fossa surgery for communicating syringomyelia. **Brain** 101: 223-250, 1978

CHAPTER 13

SHUNTING PROCEDURES FOR SYRINGOMYELIA IN CHIARI MALFORMATIONS

MATTHEW B. KERN, MD, AND JOHN A. ANSON, MD

Syringomyelia, named by Charles P. Ollivier d'Angers in 1827, is a clinical entity whose exact pathophysiology and ideal treatment still eludes surgeons today. Its frequent association with Chiari I malformations and presence in up to 32% of these patients raises intriguing questions about the relationship of cerebrospinal fluid (CSF) flow through the foramen magnum to the formation and progression of cavitation within the spinal cord. Surgical interventions to reduce the size of syringomyelic cavities have been reported for over 100 years.[1] Since the early myelotomy and drainage procedures performed by Abbé and Coley in the 1890s, a wide variety of surgical procedures have been attempted to treat hindbrain abnormality-related syringes. The variety of shunting procedures attempted to reverse or halt the progression of symptoms associated with syringomyelia underscores the current lack of understanding of the pathophysiology involved in formation of these cavities.

NATURAL HISTORY

Although surgical intervention is predicated on an expected worse natural outcome without treatment, this has been somewhat difficult to document in syringomyelia. Boman and Iivanainen[4] stated that the natural history of this disease is that of slow progression with intermittent stationary periods. In 1967, they reported the natural history of 55 patients from the University of Helsinki followed between 1920 and 1965.[4]

None of these patients underwent surgery and all suffered slow progression of the disease. In this group, although the disease in all patients progressed, approximately one-half had symptomatic plateaus of up to 10 years. Of the 12 patients reported by Conway[6] in 1967, six refused surgery. Five of these had stepwise progression of their neurological status. Although not uniform or consistent, it appears that in many instances the neurological deficits associated with syringomyelia show a slowly progressive coarse.

SYMPTOMATOLOGY AND INDICATIONS FOR SHUNTING

Six clinical syndromes based on presenting neurological patterns were described by Saez and associates.[22] Their classification was based on a review of 60 patients treated at the Mayo Clinic between 1960 and 1970. The six patterns include: 1) paroxysmal intracranial hypertension, 2) foramen magnum compression, 3) central cord disturbance, 4) cerebellar dysfunction,

5) spasticity, and 6) bulbar palsy.[22] Paul et al[18] later clustered these six syndromes into three, combining paroxysmal intracranial hypertension with foramen magnum compression, spasticity and bulbar palsy with the central cord syndrome, leaving cerebellar dysfunction as its own clinical syndrome. Components of cerebellar dysfunction include truncal and limb ataxia, nystagmus, and dysarthria. The central cord syndrome (dissociated sensory loss, long tract signs, and segmental weakness) is the most common of the three syndromes and may be seen in up to 65%, implying the presence of a syrinx related to the hindbrain abnormality.[18] Saez believed that with decompression alone, patients with the central cord syndrome had the poorest prognosis, whereas the prognosis was better in patients with either foramen magnum syndrome or cerebellar dysfunction. This suggests that shunting may be the best alternative for patients with the central cord syndrome due to large syringes. Due to the morbidity associated with syrinx progression and the lack of significant improvement with any one particular procedure, multiple shunting techniques have been attempted. Currently, there are many proponents of craniovertebral or foramen magnum decompression and duraplasty without shunting as the primary treatment modality of syringomyelia associated with Chiari I malformations.[1,7,16,18,21] Given the wide variety of presenting symptoms in Chiari malformations associated with syringomyelia, strict indications for shunting have not yet been established.

SHUNTING PROCEDURES

Multiple shunting procedures have been attempted with the purpose of reducing the size of syringes. The results have been mixed and included simple myelotomy with syringostomy and syringocisternostomy, as well as syringosubarachnoid, lumbo/thecoperitoneal, and syringopleural shunts. Fourth ventriculostomy associated with foramen magnum decompression was evaluated in 1982 by Cahan and Bentson,[5] who concluded that the "results of the 12 patients in whom a tube had been placed to drain the fourth ventricle were no different than in the other 13." However, in 1989 Lanford and Tulipan[12] reported four patients in whom fourth ventriculostomy combined with foramen magnum decompression resulted in good early postoperative function. Terminal ventriculostomy has also been evaluated as a direct way of decompressing the syrinx cavity. There is also a case report of syrinx resolution with ventriculoatrial shunting causing resolution of syringomyelia.[24]

Prior to modern microsurgical technique, decompression of a syrinx was often attempted by a means other than direct fenestration of the spinal cord. In 1983, Williams and Fahy[28] published a review of terminal ventriculostomy. This procedure involves excision of the filum terminale and tip of the conus in an attempt to provide an outlet for the syrinx at the end of the central canal. Of 31 patients, 29 had either deterioration or no improvement.[28] Of the clinical series in which procedures specifically aimed at syrinx decompression were evaluated, patients who underwent terminal ventriculostomy have generally met with poor results.

Syringocisternostomy, a technique in which the syrinx is shunted to the posterior fossa cisterns, has been described by Milhorat et al.[15] Milhorat's theory is that when an obstruction to CSF flow is present rostral to the level of the syrinx, then shunting to the spinal subarachnoid space is not suitable due to the inability of this space to decompress itself when a cephalad obstruction occurs. Milhorat believes that this procedure is less complicated than extraspinal shunting and may require fewer revisions than other shunting procedures. All of the four Chiari patients in his series had radiographic collapse or disappearance of the syrinx and complete resolution of symptoms. In their article published in 1992, it was stressed that more experience was needed to effectively evaluate this procedure.[15] This procedure has not gained widespread acceptance.

Lumboperitoneal shunting has been described as being effective for treatment of syringohydromyelia. It is thought to be useful in decreasing the transmural pressure gradient across the spinal cord which may contribute to syrinx formation. Park et al[17] described improvement in four of seven patients who underwent this treatment. This series included five patients with Chiari II malformation and it is not known whether or not the one patient with Chiari I improved after the procedure.[17]

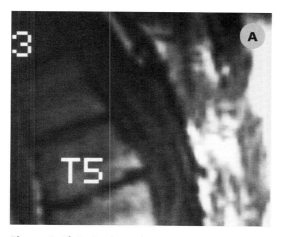
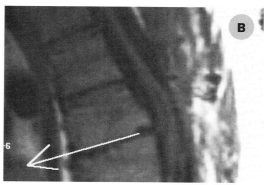

Figure 1: A) Sagittal MRI showing a thoracic syrinx in a 25-year-old man. **B)** MRI showing collapse of the syrinx following syringopleural shunting. The shunt tube can be seen to enter the dorsal aspect of the subarachnoid space at the level of the T4-5 disc space.

Thecoperitoneal shunting as described in 1991 by Vengsarkar et al[26] is analogous to a lumbar shunt in that the proximal catheter lies within the subarachnoid space, in some cases near the syringomyelic cavity. The series by Vengsarkar et al is extremely small (three patients), making critical appraisal difficult. In their series, all three patients with Chiari I malformation exhibited improvement in their myelopathies. These studies may lend some credibility to the use of theco/lumboperitoneal shunts. These procedures are clearly safer than myelotomy and may be performed percutaneously.

Phillips[19] in 1981 and Lesoin[13] in 1986 described syringoperitoneal shunting. In Lesoin's study of eight patients undergoing shunting, three had Chiari malformation. All three improved after the procedure. Phillips reported four patients, three of whom improved and one who stabilized neurologically. Barbaro et al[2] also described favorable results following syringoperitoneal shunting. Like syringoperitoneal shunting, syringopleural shunting offers placement of the distal catheter into a seemingly low-pressure extrathecal site. The selection criteria between the use of syringopleural and syringoperitoneal shunting is not clear and may depend on body habitus and prior abdominal surgeries. In both procedures, the use of an intervening low pressure valve is advocated (Figure 1).

Most recently, attention has been focused on syringosubarachnoid shunting versus the primary use of foramen magnum decompression. Once again, multiple investigators claim success using their treatments. After a critical appraisal comparing foramen magnum decompression and syringosubarachnoid shunting, in 1995, Hida et al[10] recommended syringosubarachnoid shunts as an initial procedure to treat patients with large syringes. This view is supported by Isu et al.[11] Although not associated with Chiari malformation, Tator et al[25] performed syringosubarachnoid shunting on 20 patients with isolated syringomyelia or only minimal cerebellar ectopia. Of the four patients in whom minimal cerebellar ectopia was present, two had poor results with syringosubarachnoid shunting. Although there is some support for the use of syringosubarachnoid shunting when treating isolated syringomyelia, possible poorer results are suggested when a Chiari malformation is present.[25]

Batzdorf,[3] Sgouros and Williams,[23] and Oldfield et al[16] came to the opposite conclusion. They believe that foramen magnum decompression alone is effective treatment for syringomyelia associated with Chiari malformation. Pillay et al[20] divided patients into two groups, those with and those without syringes, and performed foramen magnum decompression on all patients. Eleven of 20 patients had improvement in syrinx size and symptoms.[20] Fujii et al[7] performed foramen magnum decompression on all of their patients but combined the procedure with either a syringoperitoneal or syringopleural shunt if the syringo-cord ratio was greater than 35%. Both groups had improvement in syrinx size.[7] They found no advantage between peritoneal or pleural shunting.

SURGICAL TECHNIQUE

Effective decompression of a syrinx utilizing a shunting procedure first requires the opening of the syrinx. Multiple options exist, including: simple midline myelotomy without regard to possible eccentricity of the syrinx, myelotomy through the visibly thinnest portion of the syrinx, opening along the dorsal root entry zone, or a posterolateral myelotomy. Currently, many surgeons perform the posterolateral myelotomy as described by Rhoton[21] and emphasized by both Hida et al[10] and Isu et al.[11]

Most authors would agree that the shunt tube should consist of a nonreactive material such as silicone (Figure 2). In the past, K- or T-configured tubes have been advocated. This has given way to placement of a straight tube with multiple fenestrations.[11,25] The catheter is usually directed upward from the most-caudal aspect of the syrinx. Potential problems include septated syringes that do not allow passage of the tube. In this case, attempts should be made to place the tube in the largest syrinx cavity. Meticulous hemostasis should be obtained, especially when a subarachnoid shunt is being placed because blood in the subarachnoid space may cause meningeal irritation and arachnoiditis which will cause the shunt to fail. When the shunt is in position, it is secured to the pia with a 7-0 or 8-0 nylon suture; the arachnoid and dura are then closed with 6-0 nylon suture.

The distal end of the catheter is then passed into the body cavity of choice. Lesoin et al[13] recommended the use an intervening one-way, low-pressure valve in the case of syringoperitoneal shunts. This would seem appropriate if the cavity of drainage has the potential to be in a state of positive pressure, such as during straining. In this sense, one-way valves should be used for pleurally placed shunts as well.

If the distal end is to be placed within the subarachnoid space, it should be passed in a caudal direction. The length of the distal catheter is variable, although 3-6 cm appears to be optimal.[11,25] It is important to pass the catheter completely within the subarachnoid space. If the distal end of the catheter lies within the subdural space, the shunt will not function. If necessary, the arachnoid trabeculae can be sectioned. If possible, the arachnoid should be closed completely. This can be done either as a separate closure from the dura or as a single layer, as long as care is taken to incorporate both dura and arachnoid in each bite of the suture.

The most common complication related to shunting is malfunction of the shunt. When performed carefully, immediate neurological deterioration appears to be a rare complication. More commonly, neurological deterioration is an indication of shunt malfunction, which may occur by dislodgment of the proximal or distal ends, development of local arachnoiditis obliterating the distal catheter, incomplete penetration of syrinx septations, or of course, infection. It appears that there is a learning curve and that complications related to shunt malfunction decrease as investigators gain experience in performing their preferred method of shunting.

RESULTS

The surgical treatment of patients with Chiari malformation and associated syringomyelia has evolved over time. Both surgical correction of the Chiari malformation and specific measures to improve the syringomyelia have been attempted. Because Chiari malformation and syringomyelia are closely associated and may share a common pathophysiology, a strict separation of a discussion on treatment of Chiari malformation versus treatment of syringes is difficult. Most series evaluate the effects of various forms of treatment on the improvement or progression of the syringomyelia, including those treatments that are not specifically directed at the syrinx itself.

Until recently, surgical procedures for the treatment of syringomyelia have been predicated on two predominant theories of the pathophysiological formation and progression of syringomyelia.[8,9,27] In both Gardner's and Williams' theories, a communication between

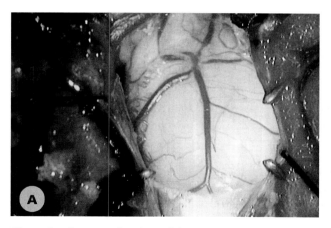

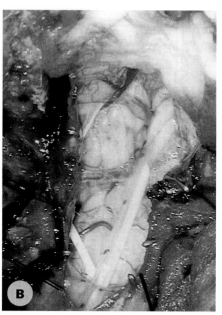

Figure 2: A) Inoperative view of the upper cervical spinal cord in a patient with a large syrinx, showing marked expansion and dilatation of the cord. **B)** Intraoperative view after placing both a fourth ventricular-to-subarachnoid shunt (seen midline between the tonsils) and a T-tube configuration syrinx-to-subarachnoid shunt (coursing laterally). The spinal cord can be seen to be markedly reduced in size.

the fourth ventricle and the central canal is necessary for progression of the syrinx to occur and, if true, then procedures to either occlude the opening of the syrinx or decrease the force of the CSF[8] through the syrinx from the intraventricular space should be efficacious. In 1958, Gardner and Angel[9] published their report of 74 patients with Chiari malformation. Of the 74 cases, 62 had an associated syrinx.[9] All of the patients in this series underwent a posterior fossa decompression and plugging of the central canal at the obex. Seventy percent of the patients showed postoperative improvement. This formed the basis of Gardner's theory of syrinx formation and the practice of plugging the obex during decompressive surgery to facilitate a decrease in the size of the syrinx cavity. Subsequently, mixed results have been reported, without elimination of the syrinx in all patients.[14] In Gardner's own series, 14% did not improve, 8% deteriorated, and five patients (6%) died in the early postoperative period.[8]

Recently, Oldfield et al[16] reviewed seven patients with progressive syringomyelia associated with Chiari I malformation. In no patient did they find evidence of communication between the fourth ventricle and the syrinx cavity, and all patients were effectively treated with decompression of the Chiari malformation alone.

These results and the use of dynamic magnetic resonance imaging (MRI) have led to a newer theory on the formation and progression of syringomyelia. The theory is based on the observation that as the brain expands during systole, the rapid movement of CSF out of the basal cisterns is accommodated in normal subjects by the spinal subarachnoid space. In patients with Chiari malformation, impaction of the cerebellar tonsils in the foramen magnum does not allow flow of CSF. This causes the tonsils to move in the manner of a piston with each systole. This, in turn, causes an abrupt pressure increase in the spinal subarachnoid space, which compresses the surface of the cord and causes the fluid in the syrinx to move longitudinally, thereby increasing the size of the syrinx. It is postulated that this pressure wave in the perivascular and interstitial spaces may be responsible for the initial formation of the syrinx as well.[16] Based on this theory and the clinical results of syrinx resolution in all seven patients treated within 6 months of surgery, Oldfield recommended that the most effective treatment is bony and dural decompression of the foramen magnum alone, without entering the arachnoid, nor placement of any type of shunt.

In 1983, Levy et al[14] published a comprehensive review of surgical experience treating 127 patients with Chiari I malformations. At that time, the majority of patients underwent decompression alone or decompression with plugging of the obex. In their series, only 16 patients had a concurrent shunting procedure. Their surgical results were similar to other small series because the percentage of patients who had improvement with decompression and shunting was similar to the results obtained when decompression alone was used. Overall, 43% of patients improved and 18% progressed. Levy concluded that syrinx shunting did not help the clinical course and that review of the literature supports this theory.

Recently in England, Sgouros and Williams[23] reviewed their experience in Chiari patients who underwent either some form of shunting procedure with or without decompression or decompression alone. Their results implied that patients who had undergone decompresion alone fared better than either of the other two groups.[23] This result is based on patient followup which showed the effectiveness of craniovertebral decompression alone to be greater than 90% at 5 years. There was less than 60% effectiveness in patients with craniovertebral decompression and drains, and all who underwent syringosubarachnoid shunting had progression at 5 years.[23] This series would imply that shunting is not an effective modality.

In 1990, Isu et al[11] published the results of 28 patients with syringomyelia who underwent syringosubarachnoid shunting without decompression. There was an average follow-up of 3 years 9 months and Isu et al claimed an 82% improvement rate, thus concluding that shunting is effective without the need for decompressive surgery. Although the authors claim that improvement was noted in both the sensory deficit and motor weakness, no patient in that series actually had objective improvement in functional grade postoperatively.[11]

Hida et al[10] reported results in 70 patients who underwent either foramen magnum decompression or syringosubarachnoid shunting, based on the symptoms of the patient. If a large syrinx (>50% syrinx-cord ratio) with symptoms predominantly of cavitation was present, then the patient underwent syringosubarachnoid shunting. If, on the other hand, the patient was experiencing symptoms of foramen mag-

num compression (nystagmus, lower cranial nerve palsy, and cerebellar signs), then the patient underwent foramen magnum decompression. In their series, neurological improvement was claimed in 82% of patients in the foramen magnum decompression group and in 97% of the syringosubarachnoid shunting group.[10] They also reported a decrease in syrinx size in 94% of the foramen magnum decompression group and in 100% of the syringosubarachnoid shunting group. Although seemingly high, the improvement rates associated with a selective approach to the surgical interventions in this study based on symptomatology and radiographic criteria would indicate that the forces maintaining syringes are multimodal and that, if reproducible, this study may provide a basis by which to provide selective criteria for initial surgery.

Based on the understanding of syrinx formation, it would appear prudent to base operative recommendations on the basis of symptomatology and not just pathological anatomy. If a patient has predominant symptoms of a spinal cord syndrome, than shunting as an initial procedure may be warranted. However, if the complaints and symptomatic complex appear to be secondary to foramen magnum compression and/or tonsillar herniation, then other treatment modalities should be entertained.

CONCLUSION

The literature is rich in theories on the formation of syringes and results of procedures used in their treatment. There is still considerable debate about the appropriate initial treatment for this disorder. Even recently, opposing recommendations have been put forth by different authors. As microsurgical techniques improve it would seem reasonable that, in patients with syringomyelia related to Chiari malformation, unless the syrinx is of very large size or syringomyelic symptoms are predominant and progressive, then foramen magnum decompression with duraplasty and no shunt may be the best initial procedure.

When foramen magnum decompression is unsuccessful, shunting is appropriate, although the best type of shunting procedure to use remains unclear. Because most investigators perform the procedure that they are most comfortable with, the results are skewed. It appears that there is probably no true advantage to any one of the common shunting procedures. For reasons of relative technical ease and significant series of patients, syringosubarachnoid shunting appears to be the best procedure. Although lumboperitoneal shunting is technically easier to perform and is less morbid, the small numbers of patients with lumboperitoneal shunts reported in the literature preclude its recommendation as a preferred treatment modality.

REFERENCES

1. Abbe R, Coley WB: Syringo-myelia, operation—exploration of cord—withdrawal of fluid—exhibition of patient. J Nerv Ment Dis 19:512-520, 1892
2. Barbaro NM, Wilson CB, Gutin PH, et al: Surgical treatment of syringomyelia. Favorable results with syringoperitoneal shunting. J Neurosurg 61:531-538, 1984
3. Batzdorf U: Chiari I malformation with syringomyelia. Evaluation of surgical therapy by magnetic resonance imaging. J Neurosurg 68:726-730, 1988
4. Boman K, Iivanainen M: Prognosis of syringomyelia. Acta Neurol Scand 43:61-68, 1967
5. Cahan LD, Bentson JR: Considerations in the diagnosis and treatment of syringomyelia and the Chiari malformation. J Neurosurg 57:24-31, 1982
6. Conway LW: Hydrodynamic studies in syringomyelia. J Neurosurg 27:501-514, 1967
7. Fujii K, Natori Y, Nakagaki H, et al: Management of syringomyelia associated with Chiari malformation: comparative study of syrinx size and symptoms by magnetic resonance imaging. Surg Neurol 36:281-285, 1991
8. Gardner WJ: Hydrodynamic mechanism of syringomyelia: its relationship to myelocele. J Neurol Neurosurg Psychiatry 28:247-259, 1965
9. Gardner WJ, Angel J: The cause of syringomyelia and its surgical treatment. Cleve Clin Q 25:4-8, 1958
10. Hida K, Iwasaki Y, Koyanagi I, et al: Surgical indication and results of foramen magnum decompression versus syringosubarachnoid shunting for syringomyelia associated with Chiari I malformation. Neurosurgery 37:673-679, 1995
11. Isu T, Iwasaki Y, Akino M, et al: Syringo-subarachnoid shunt for syringomyelia associated with Chiari malformation (Type I). Acta Neurochir 107:152-160, 1990
12. Lanford GB, Tulipan N: Fourth ventriculostomy for Chiari malformation. J Tenn Med Assoc Sept, 1989, pp 477-479
13. Lesoin F, Petit H, Thomas CE III, et al: Use of the syringoperitoneal shunt in the treatment of syringomyelia. Surg Neurol 25:131-136, 1986
14. Levy WJ, Mason L, Hahn JF: Chiari malformation presenting in adults: a surgical experience in 127 cases. Neurosurgery 12:377-390, 1983
15. Milhorat TH, Johnson WD, Miller JI: Syrinx shunt to posterior fossa cisterns (syringocisternostomy) for bypassing obstructions of upper cervical theca. J Neurosurg 77:871-874, 1992
16. Oldfield EH, Muraszko K, Shawker TH, et al: Pathophysiology of syringomyelia associated with Chiari I malformation of the cerebellar tonsils. Implications for diagnosis and treatment. J Neurosurg 80:3-15, 1994
17. Park TS, Cail WS, Broaddus WC, et al: Lumboperitoneal shunt combined with myelotomy for treatment of syringohydromyelia. J Neurosurg 70:721-727, 1989
18. Paul KS, Lye RH, Strang FA, et al: Arnold-Chiari malformation. Review of 71 cases. J Neursurg 58:183-187, 1983
19. Phillips TW, Kindt GW: Syringoperitoneal shunt for syringomyelia: a preliminary report. Surg Neurol 16:462-466, 1981
20. Pillay PK, Awad IA, Little JR, et al: Symptomatic Chiari malformation in adults: a new classification based on magnetic resonance imaging with clinical and prognostic significance. Neurosurgery 28:639-645, 1991
21. Rhoton AL: Microsurgery of Arnold-Chiari malformation in adults with and without hydromyelia. J Neurosurg 45:473-483, 1976
22. Saez RJ, Onofrio BM, Yanagihara T: Experience with Arnold-Chiari malformation, 1960-1970. J Neurosurg 45:416-422, 1976
23. Sgouros S, Williams B: A critical appraisal of drainage in syringomyelia. J Neurosurg 82:1-9, 1995
24. Sullivan LP, Stears JC, Ringel SP: Resolution of syringomyelia and Chiari I malformation by ventriculoatrial shunting in a patient with pseudotumor cerebri and a lumboperitoneal shunt. Neurosurgery 22:744-747, 1988
25. Tator CH, Meguro K, Rowed DW: Favorable results with syringosubarachnoid shunts for treatment of syringomyelia. J Neurosurg 56:517-523, 1982
26. Vengsarkar US, Panchal VG, Tripathi PD, et al: Percutaneous thecoperitoneal shunt for syringomyelia. Report of three cases. J Neurosurg 74:827-831, 1991
27. Williams B: On the pathogenisis of syringomyelia: a review. J R Soc Med 73:798-806, 1980
28. Williams B, Fahy G: A critical appraisal of "terminal ventriculostomy" for the treatment of syringomyelia. J Neurosurg 58:188-197, 1983

CHAPTER 14

COMPLICATIONS AND DETERIORATION FOLLOWING SURGERY

ULRICH BATZDORF, MD

ROUTINE COMPLICATIONS

This chapter addresses complications of the two general types of surgical procedures performed for syringomyelia and hindbrain herniation (Chiari malformation): posterior fossa decompression procedures and cyst shunting procedures. The relative merits of these two approaches have been examined elsewhere in this book.

Posterior Fossa Decompression Procedures

Posterior fossa decompression procedures may involve complications with the following: anesthesia, craniectomy, opening of the dura and arachnoid, intradural intra-arachnoid exploration, dural closure, hematoma, and infection.[4]

Anesthesia

As in patients with cervical cord or medullary compression due to other causes, acute neck hyperextension should be avoided during intubation in patients with posterior fossa decompression. Fiberoptic intubation in the awake patient is the preferable technique. When the cervical spinal cord is distended from within by a large cyst, it is particularly vulnerable to

further injury by neck hyperflexion and hyperextension; this represents a potential source of neurological worsening.

In the author's experience and at the University of California Los Angeles Medical Center, posterior fossa decompression procedures are now performed with the patient in the prone position on the operating table, thus avoiding the potential complications of operating on the patient in the sitting position. Hemostatic control is generally not a problem when the wound is opened in the midline, so that blood runoff, the sometimes cited advantage of the sitting position, is not really an issue. Problems of blood pressure maintenance and of air embolism are minimized when the patient is in the prone position. It is important to avoid hypotension, which would jeopardize perfusion of an already compromised spinal cord. The head is firmly secured in a Mayfield clamp.

Craniectomy

Patients with Chiari malformation appear to have a relatively small posterior fossa; this may play a role in the etiology of this disorder.[2] The small size may make it more likely for protrusion or ptosis of the cerebellum through the surgical craniectomy opening of patients with Chiari malformation; however, other factors may also be involved. It has been observed in several patients that an overly large suboccipital craniectomy for decompression of the cerebellar tonsils permits ptosis of the cerebellum through the newly fashioned enlarged opening, which may re-establish a subarachnoid block at the margins of the craniectomy.[6] This can result in the re-establishment of hydrodynamic conditions favoring the filling mechanism of the syrinx (i.e., recurrence of syringomyelia). The author has not found a satisfactory means for dealing with this complication other than shunting the recurrent cyst, so that avoiding the problem by limiting the size of the craniectomy is of paramount importance. The opening should be no larger than 3 cm in width and 2.5 cm from the edge of the foramen magnum. The procedure should best be regarded, and named, as an enlargement of the foramen magnum.

Opening of the Dura and Arachnoid

Currently, there is controversy regarding the opening of the dura and arachnoid.[5,9,11] Theoretically, if only the dura is opened and the arachnoid stays intact, potential complications related to cerebrospinal fluid (CSF) leakage are avoided. In practice, it is extremely difficult to avoid even a pinpoint opening in the arachnoid; sealing of a small perforation with bipolar current has been recommended, but does not always work. The arachnoid appears to leak fluid, as if it were somewhat porous, even in the absence of a recognizable perforation. Fibrin glue constituted from autologous cryoprecipitate mixed in situ with commercial thrombin and calcium[12] has been used to cover the arachnoid in situations in which an intra-arachnoid exploration is not carried out. The author's current treatment preference for patients who have a Chiari I malformation without an associated syringomyelic cavity is to cover the intact arachnoid with a dural graft.

Intradural Intra-Arachnoid Exploration

The author prefers to perform an intra-arachnoid exploration in patients with Chiari

malformation who also have syringomyelia. Fine tethering arachnoid strands are divided. Shrinkage of the cerebellar tonsils with bipolar current or subpial resection of the tonsils helps to establish free outflow of CSF from the fourth ventricle and, thereby, favors collapse of the syrinx cavity.[5] In performing this maneuver, magnification should always be used; it is important to stay well away from the posterior inferior cerebellar arteries and even to avoid heat conduction to major posterior fossa vessels. Vascular injury with serious consequences may otherwise result.

Dural Closure

If the arachnoid and dura are opened, it is important either to close the dura in watertight fashion with a graft or to achieve a watertight closure of muscle and fascia.[5,13] The aim, by either technique, is to enlarge the cisterna magna so that primary reapproximation of the dura should never be performed. Primary approximation of the dura has been encountered once as a source of failure to improve following a suboccipital decompression. The inability to achieve a watertight seal when the dural graft is sutured in place allows the CSF to leak into the soft tissue planes; while small amounts of fluid are absorbed, a persistent leak will result in pseudomeningocele formation (see below). Perioperative steroids are not necessary for the majority of patients with syringomyelia-Chiari problems and are rarely used for such patients, since they might delay healing of the suture line.

A central tack-up suture is placed through the dural graft and anchored to the deep cervical fascia. The author prefers to use defatted autologous fascia lata or pericranium, which was recently recommended by Wolfhard Caspar (personal communication, 1995). It is presumed that a tack-up suture may prevent the graft from lying against the neural tissue and that it will maximize the size of the newly created cisterna magna. For the same reason, we avoid placing deep muscle approximating sutures, which would have the effect of forcing the graft against the posterior fossa structures.

When wound closure is performed as advocated by Williams,[15] leaving the dura widely open and relying on a tight fascial closure to provide a watertight seal, there may be somewhat greater immediate risk of CSF leakage from the wound. Lumbar CSF drainage may be necessary, but should be employed judiciously; overdrainage may encourage cerebellar tonsil descent. Antibiotic therapy should be instituted until the wound is dry and the lumbar drain has been removed. Patients treated by this technique also are more likely to complain of headache and nausea, and occasionally show subtle signs of meningeal irritation.

It has been our experience that the risk of CSF leakage and pseudomeningocele formation is greatly increased in patients undergoing reoperation through the same incision. Firm scar tissue at the wound edge does not seal or heal as quickly as tissue that has not undergone prior surgical trauma. Resection of scar at the wound edge should always be performed in patients undergoing reopening of a healed wound.

As a precaution against placing excessive stress against the suture line while it is healing, patients are advised to avoid heavy lifting, straining, or bending for a period of 3 months after surgery; cough suppressant medication is recommended if necessary.

Hematoma

Meticulous hemostasis is necessary throughout the procedure, and great care must be taken to minimize bleeding into the open subarachnoid space. Bleeding from the dural sinus at the upper edge of the dural opening needs to be well controlled; this tends to be a particularly troublesome area. Bleeding may appear to be controlled when the triangular dural flap is hinged back during the exploration, only to recur when the small flap is "unhinged." It is in this area that overzealous coagulation of the dural edge may lead to suture pull-out at the necrotic dural edge.

Fibrin glue has excellent hemostatic properties;[12] in addition, for 3 days following the procedure, we maintain patients at a 30° head-elevated position whenever recumbent.

A posterior fossa hematoma was encountered in a patient early in our experience, when the posterior fossa decompression procedure was still being performed with the patient in the sitting position. It is assumed that this patient developed venous bleeding after the procedure, while in the supine position.

Infection

All patients treated by the author for Chiari malformation and syringomyelia are given prophylactic antibiotics. With the exception of patients with a known allergy, it is our practice to administer 1 gm cefazolin intravenously at the time of the skin incision; the same dose is repeated every 8 hours during the first 24 hours beginning with the hour of surgery; thereafter, antibiotics are discontinued. Wound infection has not been encountered in over 50 patients who have undergone suboccipital decompression procedures.

Cyst Shunting Procedures

The routine complications of cyst shunting procedures include wound hematoma formation and wound infection. These problems are managed as with any neurosurgical procedure, including the use of prophylactic antibiotics (see above).[3,8]

Shunt malfunction is a more specific problem (Batzdorf U: Syringomyelia shunting: a critical appraisal. 10th European Congress of Neurosurgery, Berlin, May 7-12, 1995). Most often it is diagnosed in presumptive fashion when a shunt is shown, by imaging studies, to be within the cord, yet the syringomyelic cavity persists or enlarges. When a chamber has been left in-line in the shunt system, the shunt can be tested for patency.[10] Obstruction seems to occur primarily at the proximal end, as the cyst collapses around the shunt tip, and in such instances, the shunt must be replaced. In two patients, the shunt tip was firmly anchored and needed to be excised by a myelotomy approach. Flow-restricting valves should not be used for cyst shunts. We have encountered one patient who developed meningitis and a shunt infection, necessitating removal of the system.

Shunts may also act to tether the spinal cord and thereby contribute to later neurological deterioration.

Pseudomeningoceles

Fortunately, pseudomeningoceles are rarely encountered. However, the significance of this formation after posterior fossa decompression warrants separate consideration. Depending on their size, such fluid collections may give rise to headache or neck pain, brought on particularly when the patient flexes the neck, thereby tightening the neck muscles over the fluid collection.

Of even greater importance is the fact that escape of fluid into a pseudomeningocele (from which it may be slowly absorbed into the soft tissues) weakens the pressure pulse wave transmitted against the pial surface of the spinal cord and therefore prevents optimal reduction in size of the syringomyelic cavity, leading to failure of the procedure.

Pseudomeningoceles develop when there is a relatively small opening in the dural closure suture line; when the dura is deliberately left open and tacked back, as recommended by Williams, the resulting enlarged cisterna magna, although strictly speaking a pseudomeningocele, does not behave as such. Small openings in the dural closure suture line result from: 1) sutures placed too far apart; 2) sutures that tear out of the dural edge, sometimes because the dura has been coagulated too vigorously for hemostasis; and 3) use of a synthetic membrane that cannot achieve a watertight seal for dural closure. As stated above, the use of perioperative steroids, all too often employed "routinely," is avoided so as not to jeopardize rapid dural healing. Autologous fascia lata and pericranium, recommended by Wolfhard Caspar (personal communication, 1995), seem to heal particularly well.

When a patient has a pseudomeningocele that is symptomatic or is associated with a persistent syringomyelic cavity, the wound should be reopened, the edges of the dura defined, and the suture line repaired or the graft replaced with a tissue graft. Grafts of synthetic material should always be removed and replaced with tissue grafts (Figure 1). The edges of the dural opening tend to be firm, yet not hold a suture well, and patience and ingenuity are often necessary to accomplish a dural closure in this situation. The same precautions noted above (see Dural Closure) are strictly enforced.

Neurological Deterioration After Surgery

Acute Deterioration

Fortunately, immediate or acute neurological worsening following posterior fossa decompression as employed by the author rarely occurs. In our experience, one patient developed acute respiratory failure within hours of the operation, and it is believed that there may have been a neurogenic component to this complication; this patient was treated and has recovered fully. However, it has since been our policy to maintain all patients who undergo this procedure under observation in the intensive care unit for the day and night following the operation. The author is aware of one patient who developed cerebellar ataxic symptoms, presumably due to vasospasm of a major blood vessel supplying the cerebellum; the symptoms resolved gradually in this patient.

Acute deterioration has also been seen in a patient treated with dural opening only, leaving the arachnoid intact. This patient was also treated with lumbar CSF drainage after her operation to reduce the likelihood of CSF leakage from the wound. She developed tonsillar herniation approximately 2 weeks after the operation, and it is assumed that persistent CSF leakage through multiple lumbar puncture sites may have played a role in the development of the problem. She made a full recovery after resection of the cerebellar tonsils and placement of a fascia lata dural graft.

The appearance of a new sensory deficit is not uncommonly seen in patients who undergo myelotomy for placement of a shunt to drain the syringomyelic cavity. Truncal sensory deficits may, however, be of little consequence.

Delayed Deterioration

In patients treated for syringomyelia, a distinction needs to be made between neurological deterioration seen in the presence of a distended syrinx cavity and deterioration encountered in patients in whom the syrinx cavity has

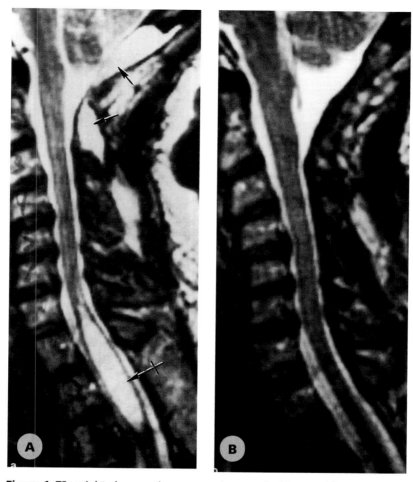

Figure 1: T2-weighted magnetic resonance images of a 50-year-old woman who had undergone surgery for a Chiari malformation 5 years previously; a synthetic dural substitute was used to expand the cisterna magna. **A)** Preoperative scan showing pseudomeningoceles *(arrows)* as well as a cervical syrinx cavity *(crossed arrow)*. **B)** Scan obtained approximately 6 months after operation revealing disappearance of the syringomyelic cavity following repair of pseudomeningocele.

been treated adequately. In the former situation, it must be assumed that the surgical procedure, of whatever type, failed. Failure of suboccipital decompression or hindbrain herniation to achieve reduction in size of the syringomyelic cavity has been encountered only twice in the author's experience: one was a patient who also had an unrecognized fungal meningitis, and the other patient had a coexisting Osler-Weber-Rendu syndrome as well as a history of a significant head injury. Both patients subsequently

required shunting of their syringomyelic cavity. It should be recognized, however, that reduction in size of the syrinx cavity may occur over the course of many weeks and even months following suboccipital decompression.

Patients who develop an enlarged syringomyelic cavity after a syrinx cavity shunting procedure must be suspected of having a mechanical failure of the shunt system. As in all shunt systems, one must consider proximal and distal obstruction as well as shunt disconnection. The author has encountered proximal shunt obstruction in two patients; this is a very troublesome complication since glial tissue from the walls of the collapsed syringomyelic cavity grows into the shunt tip perforations, necessitating sharp excision of the tip by myelotomy. In one of these patients, the shunt system had become infected and the patient developed a spinal cord abscess at the site of the embedded shunt tip.

Delayed neurological deterioration has been reported to occur in the presence of a collapsed syringomyelic cavity. The author has seen only very subtle deterioration in a small number of patients who underwent suboccipital decompression, and it is the impression that such deterioration does not follow a progressive course. It has been postulated that gliosis may proceed alongside the walls of the syringomyelic cavity, even though the cyst is no longer distended. When a patient with a cyst shunt shows delayed evidence of neurological deterioration, consideration should be given to shear stress, due to the anchored shunt itself, causing further spinal cord problems.

Persistence of dysesthetic pain after syringomyelia therapy should not be confused with neurological deterioration. This type of "central" pain is very resistant to treatment and may remain troublesome for patients who are otherwise doing well.[7]

FAILURES OF
SURGICAL THERAPY

The adage that the first surgeon to operate on a given problem has the best opportunity for effecting a cure seems to apply particularly well to the treatment of syringomyelia associated with hindbrain herniation (Chiari malformation). An inevitable consequence of all surgical procedures, scar tissue forms to different degrees in different individuals. Scarring within the subarachnoid space has the potential of reducing CSF pulsatile flow; dissociation of fluid pressures in the cranial and spinal compartments has long been considered a part of the underlying pathogenetic mechanism of syringomyelia,[13,14] and extensive subarachnoid scar formation may defeat the technically best performed procedure. It is for this reason that the author is extremely careful to minimize the spillage of blood from the wound edges into the subarachnoid space in the course of a surgical procedure for syringomyelia. Blood that does enter the subarachnoid space should be irrigated out of the wound. Postoperative meningitis would also favor the development of subarachnoid scar tissue.

Failure of suboccipital decompression may be considered as an inability to restore adequate CSF flow at the level of the foramen magnum and surrounding the spinal cord. This may result from: 1) inadequate flow of CSF from the fourth ventricle, which may be due either to a pre-existing dense arachnoid scar enveloping the cerebellar tonsils and cervical medullary junction, inadequate decompression of the cerebellar tonsils when tightly compressed tonsils retard the outflow of CSF from the fourth ventricle, or, theoretically, the presence of a ventricular shunt into the peritoneal cavity or other extracavitary location, which may diminish the CSF pressure wave and prevent full collapse of a syringomyelic cavity; 2) recurrent subarachnoid obstruction due to ptosis of the cerebellum into the craniectomy; 3) loss of CSF from the wound surface due to a pseudomeningocele or leakage around a synthetic dural graft; or 4) coexisting subarachnoid scarring distal to the craniocervical junction that could be due to coexisting inflammatory arachnoiditis (tuberculosis, fungal infection, prior meningitis) or to the prior presence of subarachnoid blood.

When a syringomyelic cavity persists or enlarges and none of the above considerations apply, one might consider re-exploration of the posterior fossa area. A cardiac-gated magnetic resonance CSF flow study[1] or even a computed tomography scan with metrizamide may be of help in assessing the problem. The risk of re-exploration is the formation of additional arachnoid scar tissue; these risks must be weighed against those of long-term results with shunting procedures, the only alternative at the present time. The results of re-exploring a well-performed suboccipital decompression procedure are generally disappointing.

Failure of shunt therapy may result from mechanical obstruction or disconnection of the shunt system, as discussed above. When shunting has failed in the treatment of syringomyelia associated with hindbrain herniation (Chiari malformation) and the patient has never undergone suboccipital decompression, such a procedure should be considered.

REFERENCES

1. Armonda RA, Citrin CM, Foley KT, et al: Quantitative cine-mode magnetic resonance imaging of Chiari I malformations: an analysis of cerebrospinal fluid dynamics. **Neurosurgery 35:**214-224, 1994
2. Badie B, Mendoza D, Batzdorf U: Posterior fossa volume and response to suboccipital decompression in patients with Chiari I malformation. **Neurosurgery 37:**214-218, 1995
3. Barbaro NM, Wilson CB, Gutin PH, et al: Surgical treatment of syringomyelia. Favorable results with syringoperitoneal shunting. **J Neurosurg 61:**531-538, 1984
4. Batzdorf U: Chiari malformation and syringomyelia, in Apuzzo MLJ (ed): **Brain Surgery: Complication Avoidance and Management**. New York, NY: Churchill Livingstone, 1993, Vol 2, pp 1985-2002
5. Batzdorf U: Syringomyelia related to abnormalities at the level of the craniovertebral junction, in Batzdorf U (ed): **Syringomyelia: Current Concepts in Diagnosis and Treatment**. Baltimore, Md: Williams & Wilkins, 1991, pp 163-182
6. Duddy MJ, Williams B: Hindbrain migration after decompression for hindbrain hernia: a quantitative assessment using MRI. **Br J Neurosurg 5:**141-152, 1991
7. Dyste GN, Menezes AH, VanGilder JC: Symptomatic Chiari malformations. An analysis of presentation, management, and long-term outcome. **J Neurosurg 71:**159-168, 1989
8. Edgar RE. Surgical management of spinal cord cysts. **Paraplegia 14:**21-27, 1976
9. Isu T, Sasaki H, Takamura H, et al: Foramen magnum decompression with removal of the outer layer of the dura as treatment for syringomyelia occurring with Chiari I malformation. **Neurosurgery 33:**845-850, 1993
10. La Haye PA, Batzdorf U: Posttraumatic syringomyelia. **West J Med 148:**657-663, 1988
11. Oldfield EH, Muraszko K, Shawker TH, et al: Pathophysiology of syringomyelia associated with Chiari I malformation of the cerebellar tonsils. Implications for diagnosis and treatment. **J Neurosurg 80:**3-15, 1994
12. Shaffrey CI, Spotnitz WD, Shaffrey ME, et al: Neurosurgical applications of fibrin glue: augmentation of dural closure in 134 patients. **Neurosurgery 26:**207-210, 1990
13. Williams B: Cerebrospinal fluid pressure-gradients in spina bifida cystica, with special reference to the Arnold-Chiari malformation and aqueductal stenosis. **Dev Med Child Neurol Suppl 35:**138-150, 1975
14. Williams B: Simultaneous cerebral and spinal fluid pressure recording. 2. Cerebrospinal dissociation with lesions at the foramen magnum. **Acta Neurochir 59:**123-142, 1981
15. Williams B: Surgery for hindbrain related syringomyelia. **Adv Tech Stand Neurosurg 20:**107-164, 1993

CHAPTER 15

CONCLUSION: THOUGHTS ON SYRINGOMYELIA AND THE CHIARI MALFORMATIONS

EDWARD C. BENZEL, MD, JOHN A. ANSON, MD, AND
ISSAM A. AWAD, MD, MSC, FACS

The chapters throughout this volume present sometimes disparate views on the pathogenetic theories of syringomyelia and the Chiari malformations. Although recent research has perhaps brought us closer to an accurate understanding of these disorders, many questions remain about their pathophysiology and optimal treatment. In fact, the terms "syringomyelia" and "syringohydromyelia" themselves engender as much confusion as they accomplish description. They encompass a wide variety of neural elements, anatomical and geometrical alterations, etiopathogeneses, and histomorphological findings. Although syringomyelia is often considered a single syndrome, it clearly is not (perhaps explaining the confusion). This latter point is illustrated in part by its inconsistent pattern of development and response to therapeutic interventions. There are dramatic differences from patient to patient. Finally, congenital anomalies, tumor, and trauma play a role in the development and maintenance of a syrinx cavity in many cases. Similar problems cloud our crisp understanding and management approach to the Chiari malformations.

The thrust of this book has been, in many respects, traditional. This is particularly true with respect to theories regarding etiologies and management options. Therefore, it may be appropriate to focus this final chapter on some "nontraditional" aspects of these disorders. Four such aspects include "nontraditional" theories, "atypical" clinical and imaging presentations, "nontraditional" schemes of management, and concluding thoughts on the Chiari malformations. These are discussed separately.

NONTRADITIONAL THEORIES OF SYRINGOMYELIA

The etiology of spinal cord dilatation from cystic cavitation is associated and synonymous with syringomyelia (syringohydromyelia). It is clearly multifactorial. Ependymal-lined cavities versus gliotic tissue-lined cavities reflect somewhat on the histomorphology and pathology. By no means, however, does it strongly correlate with the hydrodynamics of the pathological process.

A variety of theories regarding the cystic enlargement of the spinal cord have been championed. The inability of each theory to achieve enthusiastic acceptance further underscores the importance of the multifactorial nature of the pathological process. The underlying difference in processes is most likely related to the anatomical and geometrical differences between the individuals afflicted with similar clinical and pathological syndromes. This implies that the central process producing cystic spinal cord enlargement is hydrodynamic in nature. However, if this is so, why are the successful management schemes so varied? That they are is clearly the basis for the multiple proposed underlying mechanisms for the syndrome.

Many questions still are deserving of answers. Why does lumbar thecal drainage (lumboperitoneal shunting) provide relief for central medullary enlargement, when the pressure within the spinal cord is theoretically greater than that of the extramedullary thecal space? Why is shunting of the cystic space (syrinx) inconsistently associated with anatomical or clinical improvement? Is the pathological process associated with increased parenchymal compliance, rather than increased intramedullary pressure? If so, can treatment by pressure alteration (e.g., by pressure reduction via shunting) be effective? Finally, is syringomyelia induced by a pressure phenomenon? Does it progress from a pressure-related problem to a compliance-related problem in some cases? If so, this may explain the long-term ineffectiveness of individual treatment regimens in the majority of clinical and imaging situations, particularly posttraumatic and idiopathic syringomyelia. The latter scenario is deserving of explanation in greater detail.

Spinal Cord Compliance: A Comparison With Normal Pressure Hydrocephalus

It is probable that normal pressure hydrocephalus is a syndrome that is manifested neurologically by the sequelae associated with ventricular enlargement, not increased intraventricular pressure. If increased intraventricular (intracranial) pressure were the underlying nidus for the neurological manifestations, the clinical picture would be more consistent with diffuse intracranial pressure elevation. Stupor and coma, rather than a decline of intellectual function, would be observed. A uniform, rather than focal (lower extremity), loss of motor control function would be similarly observed. The diminution of lower extremity function, at least theoretically, is the result of the course of affected neurons (around the ventricles) and their distortion as a result of lateral ventricle enlargement. The latter is not related to pressure, but rather to a distortion effect.

If normal pressure hydrocephalus is a com-

pliance- rather than a pressure-related pathological process, how did it become established? An increase in ventricular fluid pressure results in an increase in intraventricular pressure and volume.

An interesting observation regarding normal pressure hydrocephalus may be pertinent here. Hypertension-related vasculopathy can result in subcortical white matter injuries. This increases the probability of long-term parenchymal tissue injury. Injured tissues lose their elastance, thus increasing their compliance (allowing ventricular dilatation at "normal pressures").

The tension on the wall of the sphere is described by the law of Laplace ($P = 2T/R$; where P = pressure within the sphere, T = wall tension of the sphere, and R = radius of the sphere). Therefore, the increasing radius of a sphere increases the tension on its wall proportionally. In the case of the hydrocephalic ventricle this, in turn, further increases the propensity for ventricular enlargement by an obligatory increase in wall tension. Thus, the cycle continues (assuming that the pressure remains constant). Of importance, this decreases the pressure requirement for cavity (e.g., ventricle) enlargement; thus, the observation of a normal pressure in the majority of cases of normal pressure hydrocephalus.

A pressure-related phenomenon may be the nidus for hydrocephalus development (etiology). At some point, however, a transformation from a pressure-related (or, analogously, a hypertensive vasculopathy-related) process to a compliance-related process may ensue.

Since shunting procedures decrease pressure and do not alter compliance, their efficacy is theoretically greatest during the initial phases of the disease (i.e., during the period of time when compliance is minimally elevated). This theory is supported clinically by reports that demonstrate a decrease in the efficacy of shunting procedures during the later stages of the normal pressure hydrocephalus syndrome. Although decreasing the pressure can overcome, to one degree or another, a compliance-related problem, as the compliance effect becomes more and more significant, it becomes increasingly difficult to reverse this effect by altering or lowering the pressure within the sphere (e.g., ventricle or syrinx). Neuronal loss (dropout) is assumed.

These aforementioned factors may, indeed, play a role in the evolution of syringomyelia and syringohydromyelia. They also may explain, in part, the variation of responses to treatment schemes.

Shunting Procedures

Lowering the pressure within the fluid-filled cavity often helps improve the clinical status of the patient. However, if the compliance is high (and the cavity wall tension even greater), a significant reduction of pressure may be required to effect a clinically significant volume reduction and clinical improvement. This "overcompensation" of a compliance problem by a pressure reduction management scheme invariably will meet a point of diminishing returns.

Lumbar Thecal Drainage Procedures

Does lumbar thecal drainage occasionally decrease syrinx size and result in clinical improvement? If so, why? Several reports have demonstrated a clinical and imaging improvement associated with lumbar thecal drainage (lumboperitoneal shunt) for the management of syringomyelia. On the one hand, spinal subarachnoid space pressure reduction may lead to a further decrease in spinal cord parenchymal pressure. This should increase, not decrease, the chances of developing and propagating a syrinx by increasing the transparenchymal pressure gradient. On the other hand, in the face of a subarachnoid block (e.g., from an impacted foramen magnum or from traumatic injuries), a one-way valve effect may exist. In these cases, spinal fluid may enter the intracranial subarachnoid space (or the space above the lesion) during episodes of Valsalva, as a result of the effect of the dilated veins and arteries. This effect can cause a "sloshing" of the spinal canal contents (as described by Williams) and cause an egress of spinal subarachnoid fluid into the intracranial compartment as a result of the intracranial-spinal pressure gradient reversal that is brought about by the underlying cranial-spinal pressure dissociation (caused by the one-way valve effect)

and the transient water-hammer effect related to the Valsalva maneuver. Although a lumboperitoneal shunt increases the pressure gradient between the cranial and spinal compartments, it may lessen the reversal of spinal fluid flow from the spinal subarachnoid space into the cranial subarachnoid space. The effect of the aforementioned water-hammer effect is, thus, diminished.

The natural history of syringomyelia of a traumatic origin is that of a "ratcheting" downhill course that is usually only temporarily affected by surgical intervention. Many explanations for ultimate management failure exist; however, a likely explanation for failure following an initial positive response is that of shunt failure or obstruction. Often, narrow shunt tubing is employed for syrinx or subarachnoid shunting procedures. Both flow and resistance to flow are related to shunt failure. Therefore, a narrower shunt tube, as well as a long tube, will respectively impact upon flow by increasing resistance to flow (Poiseuille's law). This is complicated, in turn, by thick or proteinaceous fluid where viscosity may be beyond the tolerance of the combination of flow and resistance to flow by the shunt system. The narrower the diameter of the tube, the greater the resistance to flow. The longer the tube, the greater the resistance to flow. The lesser the flow, the greater the chance for stagnation and obstruction, particularly if the fluid may congeal because of consistency alteration (primarily as a result of increased protein content).

The latter observations regarding shunt patency and shunt failure underscore the importance of syrinx management by addressing the underlying etiology, if possible. These include decompression of areas of impaction by decompressing the brain and foramen magnum (including dural band constriction in cases of Chiari malformation) and the employment of ventricular shunting techniques when hydrocephalus is present. The latter usually involves the employment of larger tubing and is less frequently associated with shunting fluid that contains a high protein content.

No single mechanism is yet understood that explains the function and progression of all syringomyelia. The various factors involved, however, are increasingly understood and will allow therapies to be directed at causative pathophysiology as well as at reversing anatomical changes.

Concluding Thoughts About the Chiari Malformations

The most consistent concept in recent reports about the entity described by Chiari more than a century ago is the idea of *different disease processes*, hence the plural "malformations," in reference to congenital crowding of posterior fossa structures and hindbrain herniation. For decades, clinicians recognized "types" of hindbrain herniation associated with a spectrum of symptomatology. Pathologists documented a myriad of associated neuraxis abnormalities, including giant diencephalic massa intermedia, beaking of the mesencephalic tectal plate, low-lying torcular and flattening of the tentorium, herniation of the medulla along with the cerebellar tonsils, a variety of spinal dysraphic anomalies, spinal cord cavitation (syringomyelia), and hydrocephalus. Clinical presentation earlier in life and more severe clinical manifestations seemed to reflect the severity of associated dysmorphism. Treatment was primarily guided toward such associated dysmorphism (i.e., the repair of myelomeningocele and shunting of hydrocephalus).

More recently, clinicians have recognized that adults with Chiari malformation may develop progressive symptoms later in life, an apparent paradox in light of the concept of congenital dysmorphism. Why do these patients appear to "decompensate" later in life? In one subgroup, imaging studies clearly revealed associated syringomyelia, a likely cause of progressive symptomatology. These cases may respond favorably to posterior fossa decompression (treatment of the presumed primary problem), often with demonstrated collapse of the syrinx on magnetic resonance imaging. This can occur regardless of whether or not the syrinx itself is shunted, and with or without plugging of the obex. There seems to be a consensus that the craniocervical decompression procedure should include dural opening (achieving lysis of any compressive dural bands) and intradural lysis of arachnoid

adhesions which are frequently quite dense at the foramen of Magendie (accomplishing opening of the fourth ventricular outlet). The symptomatic benefit is not always long-lasting, and many patients do not achieve relief of subjective dysesthetic pain and other disabling sensory complaints. The disappointing outlook in many of these cases calls for innovative therapeutic strategies and perhaps earlier treatment before recalcitrant myelopathic symptoms.

In other cases without associated cord cavitation, the cause of symptom progression remains a mystery. These cases exhibit primarily cerebellar symptoms, including gait disturbance, dysequilibrium, and oscillopsia. These symptoms very frequently resolve with posterior fossa decompression, and such relief is usually more dramatic and more lasting than in cases with associated syringomyelia. Yet, many patients with radiological evidence of Chiari malformation are diagnosed incidentally in the course of evaluation of unrelated or nonspecific complaints. The natural history of these cases is poorly understood. For example, could the Chiari malformation account for nonspecific but often severe occipital pain and cephalgia, and should these cases undergo surgical decompression even in the absence of focal neurological symptoms and signs? Are there thresholds of posterior fossa volume or extent of tonsillar herniation which invariably predict symptomatic progression, and what may be other factors contributing to clinical worsening? Of practical and medicolegal concern is what role (if any) does trauma potentially play in clinical symptomatology? Should patients with incidentally discovered Chiari malformation be restricted from vigorous physical activities such as contact sports? The elucidation of mechanisms leading to symptomatic transformation and progression would allow us to predict and not just explain clinical events, and to apply management decisions more rationally.

The *de novo* development of radiological hindbrain herniation and its occasional symptomatic transformation have recently been recognized after lumbar cerebrospinal fluid (CSF) diversion procedures. Controlled risk factor studies have not been reported to date, nor has there been any analysis of underlying posterior fossa volume in these cases. Does this apparently acquired form of Chiari malformation occur exclusively in predisposed individuals? Should lumbar CSF diversion procedures be avoided in such cases in particular? What does this phenomenon of *de novo* Chiari malformation tell us about the presumably more common congenital form? Do some cases with adult onset clinical presentation of Chiari malformation represent unrecognized acquired disease from idiopathic or as yet unknown etiology?

Lastly has come the recognition that the Chiari malformation may occur as a genetically determined and inherited trait rather than a presumed sporadic developmental anomaly. Care-

ful phenotype-genotype correlations have not been performed to date. It is expected that the elucidation of specific molecular mechanisms associated with such apparently rare genetic disease might shed unexpected light on the pathophysiology of the more common sporadic cases.

Answers to many of these questions will undoubtedly be clarified during this second century after Hans Chiari's description of the congenital hindbrain herniation. A better understanding of this fascinating and complex disease will evolve, and optimal clinical management may in the future aim as much at prevention as at treatment of its clinical sequelae.

PATIENT INFORMATION AND PEER SUPPORT INFORMATION

For a fact sheet on syringomyelia:

Syringomyelia (No. 94-3780)
NIH Neurological Institute
Office of Scientific and Health Reports
P.O. Box 5801
Bethesda, MD 20824
(800-352-9424 or 301-496-5751)

For peer support and patient information:

American Syringomyelia Alliance Project, Inc. (ASAP)
P.O. Box 1586
Longview, TX 75606-1586
(800-ASAP-282 or 903-236-7079)
(e-mail: 102563.3507@compuserve.com)

Spina Bifida Association of America
4590 MacArthur Boulevard, NW
Suite 250
Washington, DC 20007
(800-621-3141 or 202-944-3285)

Ann's Neurological Trust Society (ANTS)
Self Help Group for Syringomyelia Sufferers
c/o Mrs. Sue Adshead
1 Abbey Drive
Little Haywood
Stafford, England
ST18 0QQ

Irish Ann's Neurological Trust Society
c/o Gena Scott
Castleblayney, Ireland

Recently established to promote teaching and research:

Bernard Williams Syringomyelia Research Fund
80 Farquhar Road
Edgbaston
Birmingham, England
B15 2QJ

QUESTIONS FOR

Syringomyelia and the Chiari Malformations

The following questions have been provided to give physicians the option of testing their comprehension of the material provided in *Syringomyelia and the Chiari Malformations*. The test is to be self-scored. Answers may be found in the back of this book. A Continuing Medical Education (CME) certificate will be mailed upon the return of the enclosed test evaluation/feedback card along with a $25 administrative fee. Telephone 847-692-9500 to order additional evaluation/feedback cards or for more information about other CME products from the American Association of Neurological Surgeons.

After reading this book, a physician should be able to:
- understand the pathophysiological mechanisms thought to cause syringomyelia
- apply appropriate surgical techniques to the treatment of syringomyelia
- understand the classification schemas and complications of Chiari malformation
- apply appropriate surgical techniques to the treatment of Chiari malformation.

CHAPTER 1

HISTORICAL CONSIDERATIONS

1. The first person to describe cavities within the spinal cord was:
   (A) Ollivier d'Angers.
   (B) Vesalius.
   (C) Estienne.
   (D) Morgagni.

2. Ollivier restricted the definition of "syringomyelia" to:
   (A) all cavities within the spinal cord.
   (B) pathological dilatation of the central canal.
   (C) the clinical syndrome only.
   (D) dilatation of the central canal in association with hindbrain deformities.

3. The first person to coin the term "hydromyelia" was:
   (A) Stilling.
   (B) Simon.
   (C) Charcot.
   (D) Schlesinger.

4. The first description of the classic clinical syndrome was given by:
   (A) Portal.
   (B) Rullier.
   (C) Schultze.
   (D) Simon.

5. Evidence brought forth to support the early theories of a congenital origin of syringomyelia included:
   (A) the association between spina bifida and syringomyelia.
   (B) the presence of ependymal cells lining the cavities.
   (C) the frequent coexistence of hydromyelia and hydrocephalus.
   (D) all of the above

6. The first person to recognize the association between hindbrain anomalies and cystic cavitations within the spinal cord was:
   (A) Chiari.
   (B) Cleland.
   (C) Arnold.
   (D) Schwalb.

7. The first person to coin the term "gliosis" to describe the degeneration of an abnormal proliferation of ependymal cells was:
   (A) Simon.
   (B) Schultze.
   (C) Schlesinger.
   (D) Oppenheim.

8. The infectious theory of the origin of syringomyelia was initially elaborated by:
   (A) Charcot and Joffroy.
   (B) Joffroy and Achard.
   (C) Camus and Roussy.

9. The reason why post-traumatic syringomyelia was not recognized until relatively recently can be attributed to:
   (A) the lack of autopsy material.
   (B) the short life span of paraplegic and quadriplegic patients.
   (C) the inability to image the spinal cord with magnetic resonance imaging.

10. Which of the following was *not* offered as supporting evidence for the hydrodynamic theory of Gardner?
    (A) Die injected into the lateral ventricles could be recovered from syringes.
    (B) The fluid aspirated from the syrinx at the time of surgery was found to be identical in composition to cerebrospinal fluid (CSF).
    (C) Venous distention in the face of defective intracranial drainage resulted in CSF being forced into the central canal.
    (D) Chronic adhesive arachnoiditis in the experimental animal led to both communicating hydrocephalus and cavitation within the spinal cord.

11. The reason that radiation therapy was utilized in preference to surgery in the early part of the century can be largely attributed to:
    (A) the excessively high mortality of operations involving the spinal cord.
    (B) the theory that syringomyelia resulted from an excessive proliferation of neuroglia.
    (C) the widespread availability of radiation therapy equipment.
    (D) all of the above

12. Contrast myelography was initially utilized
    to outline syringomyelic cavities by:
    (A) Abbe and Coley.
    (B) Frazier and Rowe.
    (C) Sicard, Haguenau, and Mayer.
    (D) Westberg and Ellertson.

13. Plugging of the obex has been gradually
    abandoned, largely because:
    (A) the hydrodynamic theory of
        syringomyelia has lost favor.
    (B) the procedure was associated with a
        significant morbidity.
    (C) simple decompression often produced
        as good results.
    (D) all of the above

CHAPTER 2

CLASSIFICATION OF CHIARI
MALFORMATIONS AND
SYRINGOMYELIA

1. Classification of disease most typically
   reflects which of the following?
   (A) a rigid scheme dictating treatment
   (B) a firm biological understanding of the
       disease
   (C) a permanent framework for disease
       management
   (D) an evolving understanding of the dis-
       ease with practical implications

2. Which of the following is *true* about the
   initial description of the Chiari malforma-
   tions?
   (A) described by Arnold more than three
       centuries before Chiari
   (B) described by Hans Chiari in 1891
   (C) included no mention of hindbrain
       herniation
   (D) proposed by James Gardner before
       Arnold or Chiari

3. Recent magnetic resonance imaging
   (MRI) studies have shown all of the fol-
   lowing about the Chiari malformation
   except:
   (A) consistent evidence of cerebrospinal
       fluid flow disturbance.
   (B) frequent associated syringomyelia.
   (C) small posterior fossa volume.
   (D) frequent associated dysmorphism
       along the neuraxis.

4. Which of the following is *true* about
   Chiari malformation when associated
   with syringomyelia?
   (A) It is rarely symptomatic.
   (B) There is consistent symptomatic
       relief with shunting.
   (C) There is consistent symptomatic
       relief with craniocervical decompres-
       sion.
   (D) It has worse clinical prognosis than
       Chiari malformation without
       syringomyelia.

5. Which of the following is *not true* about
   the definition of syringomyelia?
   (A) Syringomyelia includes the entity
       "hydromyelia."
   (B) Syringomyelia includes cases which
       are idiopathic.
   (C) Syringomyelia refers to white matter
       cavitation exclusively.
   (D) Syringomyelia can be caused by
       spinal trauma.

6. Careful analysis of MRI in syringomyelia
   has revealed all of the following *except*:
   (A) an established etiology in every case.
   (B) central and paracentral cavitations.
   (C) an occasional occult neoplasia.
   (D) an occasional association with Chiari
       malformation.

7. Which of the following is *not true* about
   "acquired Chiari malformations"?
   (A) They are frequently documented
       after lumboperitoneal shunting.
   (B) They have been reported after multi-
       ple lumbar punctures.
   (C) They have been reported to develop
       de novo without apparent cause.
   (D) They are always symptomatic.

8. Which of the following is *not true* about posttraumatic syringomyelia?
   (A) It may be related to adhesive arachnoiditis.
   (B) It may result from traumatic hemorrhage.
   (C) It frequently represents an occult neoplasm.
   (D) It typically is eccentric rather than central syrinx.

9. Vascular causes of syringomyelia may include which of the following?
   (A) intramedullary vascular malformation
   (B) previous spinal infarction
   (C) dural arteriovenous malformation
   (D) all of the above

10. Which of the following is *true* about the current classification of syringomyelia?
   (A) It strictly includes acquired and congenital categories.
   (B) It excludes neoplastic causes.
   (C) It excludes vascular causes.
   (D) It will likely evolve with better understanding of the disease.

CHAPTER 3

PATHOGENESIS AND DEVELOPMENT THEORIES

1. Current optimal primary treatment for Chiari malformations with syringomyelia consist of:
   (A) plugging of the obex.
   (B) posterior fossa decompression and enlargement of cisterna magna.
   (C) syringoperitoneal shunting.
   (D) all of the above

2. Obex plugging as a treatment for Chiari malformation with syringomyelia:
   (A) is based on the fact that there always is communication between the fourth ventricle and the syrinx cavity.
   (B) stops cerebrospinal fluid (CSF) from entering the syrinx cavity.
   (C) is a benign procedure that can be added to all other forms of treatment.
   (D) none of the above

3. Subarachnoid fluid is believed to be chemically identical with syringomyelic cavity fluid in patients with hindbrain herniation and posttraumatic syringomyelia. The fluid is thought to communicate:
   (A) as a tissue transudate.
   (B) by a to-and-fro flow.
   (C) along Virchow-Robin spaces or dorsal roots.
   (D) through vascular filtration.
   (E) by a mechanism analogous to entry of metrizamide.
   (F) A and C
   (G) C and E

4. The principle underlying current treatment for syringomyelia is based on:
   (A) draining the cyst fluid.
   (B) lowering cyst fluid pressure.
   (C) eliminating pressure dissociation.
   (D) diverting fluid flow.
   (E) enhancing fluid resorption.

5. Cranial-spinal pressure dissociation as proposed by Williams:
   (A) envisions a complete subarachnoid block at the foramen magnum.
   (B) results in hydrocephalus in most patients.
   (C) is relieved by shunting the syrinx cavity.
   (D) is relieved by posterior fossa decompression.

6. Hindbrain descent may be seen in conjunction with lumboperitoneal shunts in children:
   - (A) because there is a common association between hydrocephalus and Chiari malformation.
   - (B) children are generally more likely to develop hindbrain descent.
   - (C) but is never associated with syringomyelia.
   - (D) is reversible if the shunt is removed.

7. The ependyma of the central canal:
   - (A) could theoretically play a role in the development of syringomyelia if the central canal were partly blocked.
   - (B) produces CSF which normally drains into the fourth ventricle.
   - (C) has been demonstrated to produce CSF in adults.
   - (D) remains in continuity throughout adult life in humans.

8. Bony abnormalities seen in association with hindbrain descent or Chiari malformation include:
   - (A) basilar invagination.
   - (B) platybasia.
   - (C) assimilation of the atlas.
   - (D) small posterior fossa.
   - (E) all of the above

9. Spinal-spinal pressure dissociation and syringomyelia may be seen after:
   - (A) spine trauma.
   - (B) tuberculous meningitis.
   - (C) postoperative spinal cord tumor surgery.
   - (D) all of the above

10. Effective treatment options for hindbrain descent (Chiari malformation) include:
    - (A) a large posterior fossa bone decompression.
    - (B) removing the rim of the foramen magnum and leaving the dura intact.
    - (C) opening the dura but leaving the arachnoid intact.
    - (D) shunting the lateral ventricles.

CHAPTER 4

IMAGING OF SYRINGOMYELIA AND THE CHIARI MALFORMATIONS

1. The most common plain film finding in syringomyelia is:
   - (A) widening of the spinal canal.
   - (B) fused vertebrae.
   - (C) a neuropathic shoulder joint.
   - (D) scoliosis.

2. Dynamic magnetic resonance imaging (MRI) demonstrates flow in:
   - (A) the posttraumatic syrinx.
   - (B) myelomalacia.
   - (C) intratumoral cysts.
   - (D) none of the above

3. Which of the following is *true* regarding tonsillar position in Chiari I malformation?
   - (A) Position is best determined on T1-weighted coronal images.
   - (B) Tonsillar descent occurs with increasing patient age.
   - (C) Herniation greater than 10 mm is always symptomatic.
   - (D) When tonsils descend more than 5 mm, clinical symptoms are more likely to develop.

4. Which of the following is *not true* concerning Chiari malformations?
   - (A) Syringomyelia occurs more frequently in Chiari I malformations.
   - (B) Hydrocephalus occurs more frequently in Chiari II malformations.
   - (C) Tectal beaking suggests the presence of Chiari II malformations.
   - (D) Myelomeningocele signifies the presence of Chiari II malformations.

5. Which of the following MRI artifacts can mimic syringomyelia?
   (A) partial volume averaging
   (B) beam hardening artifact
   (C) truncation artifact

6. In syringomyelia:
   (A) high signal intensity on T2-weighted images adjacent to the syrinx signifies tumor.
   (B) enhanced scans help differentiate a neoplastic from a non-neoplastic syrinx.
   (C) the presence of fibroglial septations suggests a neoplastic syrinx.
   (D) the optimal time for delayed computed tomography scanning is 1 hour postintrathecal injection of water-soluble contrast medium.

7. Which of the following is associated with Chiari II malformation?
   (A) small massa intermedia
   (B) dilatation of the lateral and third ventricles
   (C) enlarged cisterna magna
   (D) polymicrogyria
   (E) absence or fenestration of the septum pellucidum

8. Concerning dynamic imaging:
   (A) T2-weighted MRI without flow compensation is more sensitive to flow than cine-phase contrast images.
   (B) caudal flow in the cervical arachnoid space occurs during diastole.
   (C) stationary tissue is black on cine-phase contrast images.
   (D) downward motion of the tonsils and brain stem occurs during cardiac systole.

9. Concerning Chiari II malformation:
   (A) lacunar skull disappears following ventricular shunting.
   (B) the fourth ventricle is normal in size.
   (C) dysgenesis of the corpus callosum is common.
   (D) the vermian peg typically extends caudad to the medullary kink.

10. Regarding MRI of syringomyelia:
    (A) on T1-weighted images, syrinx fluid may be slightly higher in signal intensity than cerebrospinal fluid.
    (B) optimal scan parameters include a large field of view and 5-mm sagittal cuts.
    (C) performing both sagittal and axial images of the cervical and thoracic spine results in a significant cumulative radiation dose.
    (D) none of the above are true

CHAPTER 5

THE CHIARI I MALFORMATION

1. Chiari I malformations typically present with clinical symptoms at which of the following ages?
   (A) birth
   (B) early childhood
   (C) early adult life
   (D) geriatric ages

2. The most common presenting symptom of type I malformations is:
   (A) cranial nerve dysfunction.
   (B) neck pain/headache.
   (C) spasticity.
   (D) hand weakness.
   (E) hydrocephalus.

3. What percentage of patients with Chiari I malformations present with cranial nerve abnormalities?
   (A) 75% to 90%
   (B) 50% to 60%
   (C) 35% to 50%
   (D) 10% to 25%

4. Using magnetic resonance imaging criteria, the neuroradiographic diagnosis of a Chiari I malformation could be made appropriately in all of the following cases *except*:
   (A) herniation of the medulla into the spinal canal with the cerebellar tonsils located at the level of C2, not associated with myelodysplasia.
   (B) normal position of the brain stem with the cerebellar tonsils located 3 mm below the level of the foramen magnum.
   (C) normal position of the brain stem with the cerebellar tonsils located 5 mm below the level of the foramen magnum.
   (D) normal position of the brain stem with the cerebellar tonsils 4 mm below the level of the foramen magnum and a 14-mm elongated cyst appearing in the center of the cervical spinal cord.

5. Anterior decompression of a Chiari malformation is indicated in which of the following?
   (A) Klippel-Feil syndrome
   (B) hydrocephalus caused by foramen magnum obstruction
   (C) ventral compression of the brain stem or cervicomedullary junction
   (D) cervical stenosis

6. What percentage of patients undergoing anterior transoral decompression in combination with posterior decompression will have instability at the craniocervical segment?
   (A) 20%
   (B) 40%
   (C) 50%
   (D) 75%
   (E) 100%

7. For the characteristic patient with an unoperated Type I malformation, the recommended first surgical procedure in the absence of complicating associated conditions would be:
   (A) suboccipital craniectomy, upper cervical laminectomy, plugging of the obex with muscle, and duraplasty.
   (B) suboccipital craniectomy, upper cervical laminectomy, syringopleural shunting, and standard dural closure.
   (C) suboccipital craniectomy, upper cervical laminectomy, and duraplasty.
   (D) suboccipital craniectomy, upper cervical laminectomy, syringo-subarachnoid shunt, and duraplasty.
   (E) any of the above

8. In counseling patients preoperatively, which of the following deficits have the least likelihood for postoperative improvement?
   (A) ataxia
   (B) muscle atrophy
   (C) cranial neuropathy
   (D) hydrocephalus
   (E) spasticity

9. Acquired Chiari malformations may be seen in patients with which of the following?
   (A) tethered spinal cord
   (B) spinal cord injury
   (C) following lumboperitoneal shunting procedures
   (D) following ventricular shunting procedures

10. The goals of the first surgical procedure for Chiari I malformation should include which of the following?
    (A) decompression of the foramen magnum
    (B) restoration of cerebrospinal fluid (CSF) flow with an enlarged subarachnoid space
    (C) restoration of CSF egress from the fourth ventricle
    (D) all of the above

CHAPTER 6

THE CHIARI II MALFORMATION OF THE HINDBRAIN AND THE ASSOCIATED HYDROMYELIA

1. The Chiari II malformation is caused by:
   (A) fetal hydrocephalus.
   (B) traction on the hindbrain by the tethered spinal cord.
   (C) lückenschädel of the skull.
   (D) decompression of the embryonic vesicles.

2. The Chiari II malformation is almost invariably associated with:
   (A) lipomas of the spinal cord.
   (B) sacral agenesis.
   (C) myelomeningocele.
   (D) diastematomyelia.

3. Hydrocephalus in children with a myelomeningocele:
   (A) is caused by the Chiari II malformation.
   (B) causes the Chiari II malformation.
   (C) is always present in early fetal life.
   (D) invariably produces a large head at birth.

4. Which is not part of the Chiari II malformation?
   (A) beaked collicular plate
   (B) large massa intermedia
   (C) upward herniation of the cerebellum
   (D) absence of the cerebellar vermis

5. The signs and symptoms of hindbrain problems in children with the Chiari II malformation include:
   (A) stridor.
   (B) apnea.
   (C) tracheal-esophageal reflux.
   (D) all of the above

6. Deterioration in neurological function in a child with a Chiari II malformation must first establish:
   (A) the severity of the Chiari II by magnetic resonance imaging.
   (B) the optimal function of the shunt.
   (C) the presence of hydromyelia.
   (D) if the spinal cord is tethered.

7. Presence of an open central canal of the spinal cord in a child with the Chiari II malformation:
   (A) requires intervention.
   (B) may be due to atrophy or dysplasia.
   (C) may equal shunt malfunction.

8. Holocord hydromyelia in the Chiari II malformation may respond to
   (A) posterior decompression.
   (B) shunt revision.
   (C) placement of hydromyelia-to-pleural shunt.
   (D) all of the above

9. Segmental hydromyelia in the child with Chiari II malformation and a worsening neurological deficit is most likely to respond to:
   (A) tethered cord release.
   (B) fenestration of the hydromyelia.
   (C) ventriculoperitoneal shunt revision.
   (D) posterior decompression.

10. Hydromyelia in the presence of the Chiari II malformation:
    (A) is rare.
    (B) is invariably holocord.
    (C) communicates with the fourth ventricle.
    (D) none of the above

CHAPTER 7

THE CHIARI III AND IV MALFORMATIONS

1. Which of the following statements is *true*?
    (A) The Chiari III malformation is more common than the type II malformation.
    (B) The Chiari III malformation is less common than the type IV malformation.
    (C) The Chiari II malformation is more common than the type IV malformation.
    (D) The Chiari I malformation is more common than the type III malformation.

2. The one feature not usually associated with the Chiari III malformation is:
    (A) myelomeningocele.
    (B) displacement of the cerebellum below the foramen magnum into a cervical encephalocele.
    (C) displacement of the medulla into the cervical canal.
    (D) variable degrees of cerebellar and tectal dysplasia.

3. The Chiari III malformation can be:
    (A) a cervical encephalocele.
    (B) an occipital encephalocele.
    (C) an occipitocervical encephalocele.
    (D) any of the above

4. The encephalocele in patients with Chiari III malformations may contain any of the following *except*:
    (A) cerebellum.
    (B) occipital lobes.
    (C) temporal lobes.
    (D) brain stem.

5. Diagnosis of the Chiari III malformation is best established with the aid of:
    (A) computed tomography.
    (B) magnetic resonance (MR) imaging.
    (C) MR angiography.
    (D) angiography.

6. Which of the following vessels does *not* supply the encephalocele in Chiari III malformations?
    (A) the posterior inferior cerebellar artery
    (B) the anterior inferior cerebellar artery
    (C) the external carotid artery
    (D) the middle cerebral artery

7. Hydrocephalus is associated with the Chiari III malformation in what percent of patients?
    (A) 25%
    (B) 50%
    (C) 75%
    (D) 100%

8. Which of the following management principles for Chiari III malformation patients is *not* correct?
    (A) Early closure of the defect is required if cerebrospinal fluid leakage occurs or if neural tissue is exposed.
    (B) Resection of nonviable neural tissue is required to allow for adequate closure of most encephaloceles.
    (C) Anatomical layers are closed over the defect (e.g., dura and skin).
    (D) Shunting of hydrocephalus prior to treatment of the encephalocele will usually allow for easier reduction of the posterior fossa encephalocele contents.

9. The morphological features described for Chiari IV malformations include all of the following *except*:
    (A) aplasia or severe hypoplasia of the cerebellar hemispheres.
    (B) funnel-shaped posterior fossa without displacement of cerebellar tissue out of the posterior fossa.
    (C) normal-shaped brain stem.
    (D) marked dilatation of the fourth ventricle and cisterna magna without enlargement of the third and lateral ventricles.

10. The Chiari IV malformation is most similar to the:
    (A) Chiari I malformation.
    (B) Chiari II malformation.
    (C) Chiari III malformation.
    (D) Dandy-Walker malformation.

CHAPTER 8

THE RELATIONSHIP BETWEEN SYRINGOMYELIA AND THE CHIARI MALFORMATIONS

1. Which one of the following is *not* a typical finding in Chiari I malformations?
   (A) medullary kinking
   (B) tonsillar impaction at the foramen magnum
   (C) dense arachnoid scar at foramen of Magendie
   (D) gliosis of the tonsils
   (E) loss of folia pattern on the tonsils

2. Which of the following is associated with Chiari II malformations?
   (A) descent of medulla and pons
   (B) tonsillar and vermion herniation
   (C) enlarged massa intermedia
   (D) A and C
   (E) all of the above

3. Which of the following are indications for placement of a fourth ventricle to subarachnoid shunt?
   (A) hydrocephalus
   (B) ventral brain stem compression
   (C) syringohydromyelia
   (D) concomitant myelodysplasia

4. Which of the following are common bony abnormalities associated with the Chiari malformations?
   (A) scoliosis
   (B) shallow posterior fossa with flattening of the squamous-occipital bones
   (C) platybasia or basilar invagination
   (D) Klippel-Feil syndrome
   (E) all of the above

5. Which of the following correctly describes the histological findings on section spinal cords?
   (A) age-dependent stenosis of the central canal

(B) squamous epithelial lining
(C) pseudostratified ciliated epithelial lining of the central canal
(D) A and C
(E) all of the above

6. Holochord syringes are more common in:
   (A) elderly patients.
   (B) women.
   (C) younger patients.
   (D) men.
   (E) all of the above

7. Which of the following is *not* a key feature of posterior fossa decompression?
   (A) duraplasty
   (B) plugging of the obex
   (C) lysis of adhesions
   (D) fourth ventricle to subarachnoid shunt in select patients

8. Which theory regarding the pathogenesis of syringohydromyelia is the best explanation?
   (A) Williams
   (B) Gardner
   (C) Aboulker
   (D) Oldfield
   (E) No single theory explains all findings of Chiari malformations

9. Syringosubarachnoid shunts should be:
   (A) routinely used in patients with syringohydromyelia.
   (B) placed in all Chiari decompression procedures.
   (C) only required in Chiari II malformations.
   (D) reserved for rare cases of persistent syringohydromyelia following all other attempts at treatment or for syringes without associated Chiari malformation.

10. The proper initial treatment for hydrocephalus associated with a Chiari malformation is:
    (A) early Chiari decompression.
    (B) ventriculoperitoneal shunt.
    (C) fourth ventricle to subarachnoid shunt.
    (D) A and C
    (E) all of the above

CHAPTER 9

POSTTRAUMATIC SYRINGOMYELIA

1. Communicating syringomyelia is defined as a communication between:
   (A) the central canal of the spinal cord and the syrinx.
   (B) the posterior fossa and the syrinx.
   (C) the fourth ventricle and the syrinx.
   (D) the cyst cavity and the subarachnoid space.

2. The reported incidence of posttraumatic syrinx is:
   (A) less than 1%.
   (B) 1% to 4.5%.
   (C) 20%.
   (D) 51%.

3. Possible etiological factors for posttraumatic syrinx include:
   (A) resolving hematomyelia.
   (B) production of free radicals.
   (C) spinal cord necrosis.
   (D) vascular spinal cord injury.
   (E) all of the above

4. Which of the following statements is *true* concerning posttraumatic syrinx and arachnoiditis?
   (A) Arachnoid adhesions may form one-way passages causing accumulation of spinal fluid in the spinal cord parenchyma.
   (B) In experimental studies, arachnoiditis does not increase the incidence of posttraumatic syrinx.
   (C) Posttraumatic syrinx is more commonly associated with arachnoiditis in the cervical spine than in the thoracic spine.
   (D) Arachnoiditis may cause enlargement of the Virchow-Robin spaces, providing a pathway for spinal fluid into the spinal cord.
   (E) A and D

5. Common symptoms of posttraumatic syrinx include:
   (A) a capelike distribution of diminished pain and temperature sensation.
   (B) atrophy of the hands.
   (C) neck, arm, or hand pain.
   (D) loss of proprioception and vibratory sense.
   (E) A, B, and C

6. Unusual symptoms of posttraumatic syrinx include:
   (A) segmental hyperhidrosis.
   (B) hiccups.
   (C) tinnitus.
   (D) episodic unconsciousness.
   (E) all of the above

7. Scoliosis may be the first presenting symptom of syrinx.
   (A) true
   (B) false

8. Single minor trauma is the most common cause of posttraumatic syrinx.
   (A) true
   (B) false

9. Ascending neurological loss in a spinal cord-injured patient may indicate syrinx.
   (A) true
   (B) false

10. Magnetic resonance imaging is the diagnostic study of choice for evaluating syrinx.
    (A) true
    (B) false

CHAPTER 10

SYRINGOMYELIA ASSOCIATED WITH INTRASPINAL NEOPLASMS

1. Postulated mechanisms for formation or sustainment of syringomyelic cavities in association with spinal cord tumors include:
   (A) edema.
   (B) blockage of the perivascular spaces with resultant tissue fluid stasis.
   (C) cavitation secondary to disordered spinal cord circulation.
   (D) spontaneous intratumoral hemorrhage or autolysis.
   (E) all of the above

2. Clinical presentations which should alert the examiner to the possibility of tumor-associated syringomyelia include which of the following:
   (A) torticollis
   (B) scoliosis
   (C) back pain in a child
   (D) bowel and bladder dysfunction
   (E) all of the above

3. In patients with hemangioblastoma, resection of the tumor nidus will result in obliteration of the syrinx without the necessity for additional shunting procedures.
   (A) always
   (B) often
   (C) rarely
   (D) never

4. Cauda equina tumors produce syringomyelia.
   (A) always
   (B) often
   (C) rarely
   (D) never

5. Discovery of a syrinx in the absence of a hindbrain malformation should prompt:
   (A) aggressive search for an underlying neoplasm.
   (B) shunting of the syrinx without further investigation.
   (C) trial of cervical traction.
   (D) percutaneous puncture in the office.
   (E) shunting of the patient to a neurologist.

CHAPTER 12

SUBOCCIPITAL AND CERVICAL DECOMPRESSION

1. Both Gardner's and Williams' theories of syrinx formation associated with the Chiari malformation assume:
   (A) a direct communication between the fourth ventricle and the syrinx.
   (B) abnormal flow of cerebrospinal fluid (CSF).
   (C) a pressure dissociation between the intracranial and spinal CSF.
   (D) A and B
   (E) B and C

2. The difference between Gardner's and Williams' theories of syrinx formation associated with the Chiari malformation is:
   (A) Gardner's theory assumes a direct communication between the fourth ventricle and the syrinx but Williams' does not.
   (B) obstruction of CSF flow occurs at the foramen magnum by Williams' theory and at the outlet of the fourth ventricle by Gardner's theory.
   (C) both of the above
   (D) neither of the above

3. The syringomyelia associated with the Chiari malformation based on magnetic resonance imaging of CSF flow is caused by obstruction of CSF at the:
   (A) foramen magnum
   (B) obex
   (C) upper cervical spinal cord
   (D) none of the above

4. According to Oldfield's theory of syrinx formation, CSF enters the syrinx:
   (A) via a direct communication with the fourth ventricle.
   (B) from the subarachnoid space via perivascular and interstitial spaces.
   (C) via a direct communication with the central canal.

5. The presence of a direct communication between the fourth ventricle and syrinx has been disputed by:
   (A) cadaver studies.
   (B) ultrasound.
   (C) MRI.
   (D) all of the above
   (E) A and C

6. The indication for operating on a Chiari malformation is:
   (A) diagnosis by MRI even when asymptomatic.
   (B) only if symptomatic with or without a history of progression of symptoms.
   (C) when the patient is severely neurologically compromised so that the benefits outweigh the risks.

7. To adequately decompress the foramen magnum in patients with the Chiari malformation, current surgical philosophy leans toward:
   (A) opening the outer layer of dura only.
   (B) opening the dura but leaving the arachnoid intact.
   (C) dissecting the arachnoid off the tonsils.
   (D) mobilizing the tonsils.

8. According to current thinking, treatment of syringomyelia associated with the Chiari malformation requires:
   (A) suboccipital and cervical decompression only as a first step.
   (B) plugging of the obex and opening of the fourth ventricular outlet.
   (C) posterolateral myelotomy and placement of a drainage catheter.
   (D) A, B, and C

9. The symptoms that are most likely to improve after suboccipital and cervical decompression for Chiari malformation and associated syringomyelia are:
   (A) symptoms of intracranial hypertension and cerebellar dysfunction.
   (B) dysesthetic pain and dissociated sensory loss.
   (C) motor weakness and atrophy requiring the use of a wheelchair.
   (D) A and B

10. Preoperative features associated with a poor outcome for suboccipital and cervical decompression for Chiari malformation and associated syringomyelia are:
    (A) symptoms for longer than 2 years.
    (B) bulbar symptoms.
    (C) nystagmus.
    (D) muscle atrophy.
    (E) all of the above

CHAPTER 13

SHUNTING PROCEDURES FOR SYRINGOMYELIA IN CHIARI MALFORMATIONS

1. Syringomyelia was named by:
   (A) A. Earl Walker
   (B) Harvey Cushing
   (C) Charles P. Ollivier d'Angers
   (D) Walter Dandy

2. The most common course of syrinx progression associated with Chiari I malformation is:
   (A) rapid progression and quadriplegia.
   (B) fixed deficit that rarely progresses.
   (C) no symptoms associated with lesion.
   (D) slowly progressive or stepwise progression of neurological deficit.

3. Of the following patterns of neurological involvement, which one is *not* described?
   (A) paroxysmal intracranial hypertension
   (B) eye movement abnormalities with ocular bobbing
   (C) cerebellar dysfunction
   (D) bulbar palsy

4. The most recently proposed theory on syrinx formation is which of the following?
   (A) The constant heartbeats cause consistent, transient rises in intracranial pressure which causes increased cerebrospinal fluid (CSF) pressure. This in turn forces CSF into the central canal thereby expanding the syrinx.
   (B) A decreased ability to reabsorb fluid within the central canal and syrinx causes expansion of the syrinx.
   (C) Every time a person strains, fluid is forced into the central canal and enlarges the syrinx.
   (D) Impaction of the cerebellar tonsils causes an increase in spinal subarachnoid pressure, causing longitudinal flow of CSF into the syrinx.

5. Which of the following has not been used as a treatment for syringes?
   (A) syringosubarachnoid shunt
   (B) syringopleural shunt
   (C) syringoatrial shunt
   (D) fourth ventriculostomy

6. The theory behind terminal ventriculostomy is which of the following?
   (A) By separating the filum terminale, the spinal cord is more mobile and the syrinx is less likely to grow.
   (B) Opening allows drainage of the syrinx.
   (C) Opening allows better equilibrium of pressure within the central canal and spinal subarachnoid space, inhibiting growth of syrinx.
   (D) all of the above

7. When placing a syringopleural or syringoperitoneal shunt, it is important to:
   (A) place an antisiphon device.
   (B) place at least 30 cm of tubing in distal cavity.
   (C) suture tubing to either the chest or the abdominal wall.
   (D) place a low-pressure valve.

8. The most recently advocated site of myelotomy is:
   (A) directly in midline.
   (B) visibly through the thinnest portion of syrinx.
   (C) a point 0.5 cm lateral to midline.
   (D) posterolaterally.

9. The best material for shunts is:
   (A) galvanized rubber.
   (B) silicone.
   (C) multipolymer plastic.
   (D) polyvinyl chloride.

10. The most appropriate placement of the shunt tube into the syrinx is:
    (A) caudad.
    (B) straight into the syrinx.
    (C) cephalad.
    (D) both caudad and cephalad with a T-configured tube.

CHAPTER 14

COMPLICATIONS AND DETERIORATION FOLLOWING SURGERY

1. The optimal treatment for syringomyelia associated with Chiari malformation is:
   (A) marsupialization of the syrinx.
   (B) enlarging the foramen magnum.
   (C) plugging of the obex with muscle.
   (D) large decompression of the posterior fossa.
   (E) none of the above

2. Decompression of a Chiari malformation may consist of:
   (A) removing bone at the posterior margin of the foramen magnum.
   (B) performing a laminectomy of C1.
   (C) opening of the dura over the craniocervical junction.
   (D) opening the dura at the craniocervical junction but leaving the arachnoid intact.
   (E) all of the above

3. Advantages of decompression of the foramen magnum over shunting a syringomyelic cyst, include all but which one of the following?
   (A) Decompression brings about an immediate collapse of the syrinx cavity.
   (B) Decompression relieves craniospinal pressure dissociation.
   (C) Decompression does not involve placement of synthetic material.
   (D) Decompression is more likely to be followed by long-term syrinx decrease.
   (E) Decompression is less likely to become obstructed again.

4. In the usually placed syrinx shunting procedure, one may anticipate:
   (A) immediate collapse of the entire syrinx cavity, since these cavities are rarely septated.
   (B) relief of hand atrophy and weakness.
   (C) relief of dysesthetic pain.
   (D) further downward herniation of the hindbrain.
   (E) none of the above

5. The least desirable material to use for grafting the posterior fossa dura in patients with hindbrain herniation is:
   (A) autologous fascia lata.
   (B) Vicryl mesh.
   (C) lyophilized dura.
   (D) pericranium.
   (E) bovine pericardium.

6. Shunting a syringomyelic cavity requires:
   (A) an on-off valve system.
   (B) a horizontal-vertical valve system.
   (C) a high-pressure reed valve.
   (D) periodic shunt irrigation.
   (E) none of the above

7. Suboccipital decompression may fail to reduce the size of a syringomyelic cavity associated with a hindbrain herniation for all but which of the following?
   (A) The cisterna magna is not adequately enlarged.
   (B) The cerebellar tonsils are encased in scar tissue.
   (C) The syringomyelic cavity has not been opened.
   (D) The patient has a functioning lumboperitoneal shunt.
   (E) The suboccipital craniectomy was too large.

8. Malfunction of a syringomyelic cyst shunt is easily diagnosed because:
   (A) magnetic resonance imaging shows the site of shunt obstruction.
   (B) the usual cause is shunt disconnection.
   (C) a Valsalva maneuver fails to increase cyst fluid outflow.
   (D) meningitis can be detected by clinical evaluation.
   (E) none of the above

9. Coughing or straining may produce headache in patients with Chiari malformation because:
   (A) the tonsils are momentarily more impacted.
   (B) dural stretch is increased.
   (C) there is transient increase in intracranial pressure.
   (D) venous outflow from the cranial cavity is transiently diminished.
   (E) all of the above

10. Hindbrain herniation with syringomyelia is:
   (A) always due to a congenital abnormality at the foramen magnum.
   (B) may be caused by high-speed motor-vehicle accidents.
   (C) can be treated conservatively since the syrinx cavity, once established, is unlikely to enlarge.
   (D) is an indication for emergency surgery.
   (E) none of the above

INDEX

Page numbers for figures and tables are followed by *f* and *t*, respectively.

Syringomyelia and the Chiari Malformations
ANSWERS TO CME QUESTIONS

Chapter 1

1. C	2. B	3. B	4. C	5. D
6. B	7. B	8. B	9. B	10. C
11. B	12. C	13. D		

Chapter 2

1. D	2. B	3. A	4. D	5. C
6. A	7. D	8. C	9. D	10. D

Chapter 3

1. B	2. D	3. G	4. C	5. D
6. D	7. A	8. E	9. D	10. C

Chapter 4

1. D	2. A	3. D	4. A	5. C
6. B	7. E	8. D	9. C	10. A

Chapter 5

1. C	2. B	3. D	4. B	5. C
6. D	7. C	8. B	9. C	10. D

Chapter 6

1. D	2. C	3. A	4. D	5. D
6. B	7. B	8. D	9. A	10. D

Chapter 7

1. C	2. A	3. D	4. C	5. B
6. D	7. C	8. D	9. C	10. D

Chapter 8

1. A	2. E	3. C	4. E	5. D
6. C	7. B	8. E	9. D	10. B

Chapter 9

1. C	2. B	3. E	4. E	5. E
6. E	7. A	8. B	9. A	10. A

Chapter 10

1. E	2. E	3. B	4. C	5. A

Chapter 12

1. D	2. B	3. A	4. B	5. C
6. B	7. B	8. A	9. A	10. E

Chapter 13

1. C	2. D	3. B	4. D	5. C
6. B	7. C	8. D	9. B	10. C

Chapter 14

1. B	2. E	3. A	4. E	5. B
6. E	7. C	8. E	9. E	10. E

Previously Published Books in the
Neurosurgical Topics Series

Neurosurgical Aspects of Pregnancy
Edited by Christopher M. Loftus, MD

Endovascular Neurological Intervention
Edited by Robert J. Maciunas, MD

Benign Cerebral Glioma, Volume II
Edited by Michael L. J. Apuzzo, MD

Benign Cerebral Glioma, Volume I
Edited by Michael L. J. Apuzzo, MD

*Contemporary Management of
Spinal Cord Injury*
Edited by Edward C. Benzel, MD, and
Charles H. Tator, MD

Philosophy of Neurosurgery
Edited by Issam A. Awad, MD

Neurosurgical Emergencies, Volume II
Edited by Christopher M. Loftus, MD

Neurosurgical Emergencies, Volume I
Edited by Christopher M. Loftus, MD

Interactive Image-Guided Neurosurgery
Edited by Robert J. Maciunas, MD

Spinal Instrumentation
Edited by Edward C. Benzel, MD

*Current Management of
Cerebral Aneurysms*
Edited by Issam A. Awad, MD

*Spinal Trauma: Current
Evaluation and Management*
Edited by Gary L. Rea, MD, and
Carole A. Miller, MD

*Surgery of the Cranial Nerves of the
Posterior Fossa*
Edited by Daniel L. Barrow, MD

Degenerative Disease of the Cervical Spine
Edited by Paul R. Cooper, MD

Neurosurgery for the Third Millennium
Edited by Michael L.J. Apuzzo, MD

*Cerebrovascular Occlusive Disease and Brain
Ischemia*
Edited by Issam A. Awad, MD

*Practical Approaches to Peripheral Nerve
Surgery*
Edited by Edward C. Benzel, MD

Complications and Sequelae of Head Injury
Edited by Daniel L. Barrow, MD

Neurosurgical Aspects of Epilepsy
Edited by Michael L.J. Apuzzo, MD

Complications of Spinal Surgery
Edited by Edward C. Tarlov, MD

*Contemporary Diagnosis and Management
of Pituitary Adenomas*
Edited by Paul R. Cooper, MD

*Neurosurgical Treatment of
Disorders of the Thoracic Spine*
Edited by Edward C. Tarlov, MD

Intracranial Vascular Malformations
Edited by Daniel L. Barrow, MD

Malignant Cerebral Glioma
Edited by Michael L.J. Apuzzo, MD

*Management of Posttraumatic
Spinal Instability*
Edited by Paul R. Cooper, MD

For order information call (847) 692-9500.